Workbook to Accompany

CLINICAL MEDICAL ASSISTING:

A Professional, Field Smart Approach to the Workplace

Workbook to Accompany

CLINICAL MEDICAL ASSISTING:
A Professional, Field Smart Approach to the Workplace

Second Edition

Prepared by:
Virginia Busey Ferrari, MHA, BA, CEHRS
Michelle E. Heller, CMA (AAMA)

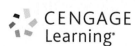

Australia • Brazil • Mexico • Singapore • United Kingdom • United States

CENGAGE
Learning·

Workbook to Accompany Clinical Medical Assisting: A Professional, Field Smart Approach to the Workplace, Second Edition
Virginia Ferrari, Michelle Heller

SVP, GM Skills & Global Product Management:
Dawn Gerrain

Product Director: Matthew Seeley

Product Team Manager: Stephen Smith

Senior Director, Development:
Marah Bellegarde

Product Development Manager: Juliet Steiner

Senior Content Developer: Lauren Whalen

Product Assistant: Mark Turner

Vice President, Marketing Services:
Jennifer Ann Baker

Marketing Manager: Jessica Cipperly

Senior Production Director: Wendy Troeger

Production Director: Andrew Crouth

Senior Content Project Manager:
Thomas Heffernan

Senior Art Director: Jack Pendleton

Manager, Digital Production: Jamilynne Myers

Media Producer: Virginia Harrison

Cover image(s): ©stevecoleimages/Getty
Images

For product information and technology assistance, contact us at
Cengage Learning Customer & Sales Support, 1-800-354-9706

For permission to use material from this text or product,
submit all requests online at **www.cengage.com/permissions.**
Further permissions questions can be e-mailed to
permissionrequest@cengage.com

Library of Congress Control Number: 2007940733

ISBN: 978-1-305-11138-7

Cengage Learning
20 Channel Center Street
Boston, MA 02210
USA

Cengage Learning is a leading provider of customized learning solutions with employees residing in nearly 40 different countries and sales in more than 125 countries around the world. Find your local representative at **www.cengage.com**

Cengage Learning products are represented in Canada by Nelson Education, Ltd.

To learn more about Cengage Learning, visit **www.cengage.com**

Purchase any of our products at your local college store or at our preferred online store **www.cengagebrain.com**

Notice to the Reader

Publisher does not warrant or guarantee any of the products described herein or perform any independent analysis in connection with any of the product information contained herein. Publisher does not assume, and expressly disclaims, any obligation to obtain and include information other than that provided to it by the manufacturer. The reader is expressly warned to consider and adopt all safety precautions that might be indicated by the activities described herein and to avoid all potential hazards. By following the instructions contained herein, the reader willingly assumes all risks in connection with such instructions. The publisher makes no representations or warranties of any kind, including but not limited to, the warranties of fitness for particular purpose or merchantability, nor are any such representations implied with respect to the material set forth herein, and the publisher takes no responsibility with respect to such material. The publisher shall not be liable for any special, consequential, or exemplary damages resulting, in whole or part, from the readers' use of, or reliance upon, this material.

Printed in the United States of America
Print Number: 01   Print Year: 2016

C O N T E N T S

PART 1 **Chapter Assignment Sheets**   **1**

Chapter 1   Journey to Professionalism   3
Chapter 2   Clinical Trends in Health Care   11
Chapter 3   The Complete Medical Record and Electronic Charting   19
Chapter 4   Fundamentals of Documentation   29
Chapter 5   Conducting a Patient Screening   45
Chapter 6   Assisting Patients with Special Needs   55
Chapter 7   Health Coaching and Patient Navigation   63
Chapter 8   Principles of Infection Control   69
Chapter 9   Sterilization Procedures, Instrument Identification,
            and Surgical Supplies   77
Chapter 10 Assisting with Minor Office Surgeries and Wound
            Care Procedures   89
Chapter 11 Vital Signs and Measurements   97
Chapter 12 The Physical Exam   107
Chapter 13 Eye and Ear Exams and Procedures   115
Chapter 14 Cardiovascular Exams and Procedures   123
Chapter 15 Pulmonary Examinations and Procedures   133
Chapter 16 Gastrointestinal Exams and Procedures   141
Chapter 17 Women's Health Issues: Obstetrics and Gynecology   149
Chapter 18 Urology and Male Reproductive Exams and Procedures   157
Chapter 19 Other Specialty Procedures   165
Chapter 20 Diet and Nutrition   173
Chapter 21 Evaluation and Care of the Pediatric Patient   181
Chapter 22 Orthopedics, Rehabilitation, and Physical Therapy   189
Chapter 23 Fundamentals of the Medical Laboratory   197
Chapter 24 Blood Collection Techniques   207
Chapter 25 Urinalysis   217
Chapter 26 Hematology and Coagulation Studies   231
Chapter 27 Microbiology   243
Chapter 28 Clinical Chemistry and CLIA-Waived Testing   257
Chapter 29 Diagnostic Imaging   271
Chapter 30 Fundamentals of Pharmacology   281
Chapter 31 Dosage Calculations   295
Chapter 32 Administration of Parenteral Medications   307
Chapter 33 Responding to Medical Office Emergencies   321

PART 2   **Competency Checklists**   **331**

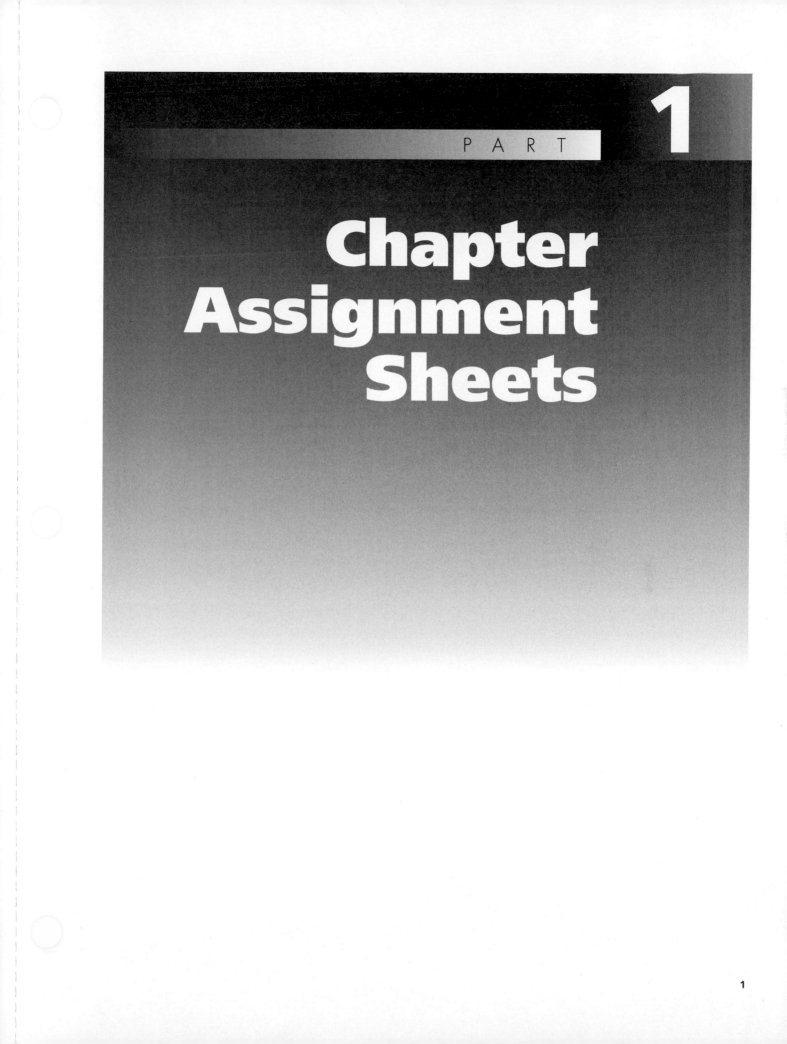

PART 1

Chapter Assignment Sheets

C H A P T E R **1**

Journey to Professionalism

VOCABULARY REVIEW

Assignment 1-1: Matching

Match the term with its definition and place the corresponding letter in the blank.

____ 1. Empathy

____ 2. Initiative

____ 3. Compassion

____ 4. Attitude

____ 5. Tact

____ 6. Professionalism

____ 7. Dependability

____ 8. Appearance

____ 9. Service

____ 10. Integrity

A. To be reliable or trustworthy; starts with an internal mind-set and works its way outward in the form of an action

B. Conducting oneself with responsibility (a duty or obligation), integrity, accountability, and excellence; communicating effectively and appropriately and always finding a way to be productive

C. Having the ability to put yourself in another person's shoes

D. To possess sound character

E. To show concern and empathy

F. To extend help to others

G. A character trait; sensitive to what is appropriate and suitable when dealing with other individuals (sometimes referred to as diplomacy)

H. To take the lead or to work independently

I. The way you feel about someone or something

J. The patient's initial impression about you as a trustworthy professional

Assignment 1-2: Vocabulary Builder

Find the words below that are misspelled; circle them and then correctly spell them in the spaces provided. Then fill in the blanks in the following sentences with the correct vocabulary terms from the list.

Appearance	Certification	Credantialing
Attitude	Compassion	Service
Dependebility	Integrity	Tact
Collaboration	Licencing	Communication
Impathy	Profesionalism	Curtesy
Initiative	Registration	Assertive
Aggressive	Adaptibility	Engajement
Diplomasy	Dinamics	Respect
Mindfullness	Passive	
Accountability	Confidantiality	

_____   _____   _____

_____   _____   _____

_____   _____   _____

_____   _____   _____

In the development of professionalism, there are important traits or characteristics the medical assistant must evaluate in order to succeed in the profession. (1) Your _____ helps mold your personality and is the way you feel about someone or something. (2) _____ is one of the most important keys to possess as a professional; it means that you are reliable and trustworthy. (3) _____ is a character trait that you exhibit when you are sensitive to what is appropriate and suitable when dealing with other individuals. (4) _____ is what the patient bases his or her initial impression about you as a professional.

In the medical office, it is important to ensure patient (5) _____ at all times in order to protect the patient's private information. Truthfulness, honesty, and honor are all qualities of a person who possesses (6) _____.

As you become more seasoned in the field of medical assisting, you will demonstrate more (7) _____, the emotional commitment you have to the organization and its goals, performing to the best of your ability with enthusiasm, excellence, work ethic, and initiative. Extending help to others is an example of providing (8) _____. The AAMA offers the (9) _____ credential. (10) _____ demonstrates to your patients and supervisors that you are worthy to be working in the capacity in which you have been entrusted. Types of credentialing include: (11) _____, which is a *legal document* that permits or authorizes you to perform specific tasks; (12) _____, which signifies that you have fulfilled the necessary requirements of a specific organization to perform specific tasks, usually through formal testing; and (13) _____, which means to enroll your name in a register, based on successful completion of a specific program and/or passing an examination designed specifically for that particular specialty.

CHAPTER REVIEW

Assignment 1-3: Abbreviation Review

Write what each of the following abbreviations stands for.

1. ABHES: _____

2. AAMA: _____

3. AMT: _____

4. ARMA: _____

5. CMA (AAMA): _____

6. CAAHEP: _____

7. NCCT: _____

8. NHA: _____

9. RMA (AMT): _____

Assignment 1-4: Short Answer

1. List five factors that may contribute to some patients holding clinical personnel to a higher degree of professionalism than those working in administrative settings.

    A. _____

    _____

    B. _____

    _____

    C. _____

    _____

    D. _____

    _____

    E. _____

    _____

    _____

    _____

2. List at least four organizations that credential medical assistants.

    _____

    _____

3. List the *professionalism keys* and components of professional behavior that are essential for a medical assistant to have.

A. _____

B. _____

C. _____

D. _____

E. _____

F. _____

G. _____

H. _____

4. List two different types of communications.

A. _____

B. _____

5. How does empathy play a role in patient relations?

_____

_____

6. In order to share patient information with other individuals, you must first obtain _____ from the patient.

CERTIFICATION PRACTICE

Assignment 1-5

Choose the best answer and place the corresponding letter in the blank.

____ 1. Medical assistants may take the AAMA examination to obtain which credential?

A. AMT

B. RMA

C. CPC

D. CMA (AAMA)

____ 2. A person with integrity:

A. is reliable.

B. maintains high standards.

C. is honest and dependable.

D. All of the above

____ 3. Which of the following traits or characteristics would not be considered desirable in a medical assistant?

A. Initiative

B. A self-serving attitude

C. Dependability

D. Empathy

____ 4. Which of the following would convey a professional appearance to the patient?

A. A clean uniform that is free of wrinkles

B. Duty or athletic shoes that follow institutional guidelines

C. A name tag worn on the uniform that identifies the medical assistant's name and credential.

D. All of the above

___ 5. The term that means to be reliable or trustworthy is:

   A. initiative.

   B. dependability.

   C. tactful.

   D. All of the above

___ 6. Identify which of the following descriptions best describes empathy.

   A. Showing concern for a patient

   B. Conveying compassion toward a patient

   C. The ability to put yourself in another person's shoes

   D. All of the above

___ 7. Ethics can be defined as:

   A. the innate knowledge of right and wrong.

   B. cultural and religious-based distinctions of right and wrong.

   C. maintaining personal integrity regardless of the legal aspect of the situation.

   D. All of the above

___ 8. The diagnostic and treatment process that is reasonable and prudent that a clinician should follow for a certain type of patient, illness, or clinical circumstance is known as:

   A. scope of practice.

   B. standard of care.

   C. Patient's Bill of Rights.

   D. All of the above

___ 9. A way to communicate a patient's legal rights while under the care of a provider or facility is known as:

   A. The Patient Protection and Affordable Care Act.

   B. HIPAA Privacy Act.

   C. Americans with Disabilities Act Amendments Act.

   D. The Patients' Bill of Rights.

___ 10. Being able to articulate and express your ideas, needs, and feelings in a way that is honest and direct is known as which type of communication?

   A. Aggressive

   B. Assertive

   C. Passive

   D. All of the above

SKILL APPLICATION CHALLENGES

Assignment 1-6: Research Activity

1. Research employment opportunities for medical assistants using the Internet, newspapers, and/or other sources. Find at least three openings for medical assistant positions. Find at least one opening outside your state. Take note of the titles of the positions advertised. On each of the listings, highlight the information that identifies educational requirements, credentialing requirements, personal qualities, and other useful information. Consider what you have learned regarding professionalism and how you would use that knowledge when applying for a position.

2. Chapter 1 lists examples of professional and unprofessional appearance for a medical assistant. Using magazines, newspapers, the Internet, or any other sources available, find three pictures of medical assistants dressed in professional attire. Cut out each picture and secure it to a standard piece of 8½ ×11 paper. Describe in detail how each person looks professional. Is there anything in the photograph that looks substandard in regard to professional appearance?

FIELD APPLICATION CHALLENGE
Assignment 1-7

Read the following Field Application Challenges and respond to the questions following each scenario.

1. A medical assistant getting ready to perform an ECG notices that the disposable electrodes are missing from the stand that holds the ECG unit. The patient is in a hurry and needs to get back to work. The medical assistant remembers that there was an entire box of electrodes on the stand that morning when he ran an ECG on his first patient. The practice usually only goes through one pack of leads per month and the leads are only good for a certain amount of time after opening. He quickly searches areas in which the leads may be located but to no avail. Sarah is another medical assistant who just performed an ECG before him; she is now with a new patient and will not be out of the patient's room for several minutes. From the choices below, what would be the *best* solution for obtaining the leads?

   A. Confront the other medical assistant about the leads in front of the new patient.

   B. Open a new box of leads.

   C. Wait until the medical assistant comes out of the patient's room to inquire about the leads.

   D. _____

   _____

   _____

   _____

   _____

   _____

2. Your provider finishes up with patients early today. You notice that Megan, the medical assistant who works for Dr. Thompson, is running severely behind schedule. The other medical assistants refuse to help her because they have other commitments and frankly they are not very fond of her. Megan mentioned to you that she was supposed to attend a birthday dinner for her mother tonight but that she is now going to be very late for the dinner. You have plans of your own and worked very hard to get done early so that you can leave early today as well. Are you committed to staying later to help Megan after you worked very hard to finish early so that you could leave on time? Reflect on which of the professionalism keys you would use to handle this situation, and apply them to your answer.

   _____

   _____

   _____

   _____

JOURNALING EXERCISE
Assignment 1-8

What content within this chapter was most meaningful to you? Why? List some of the professionalism keys that you feel are your strongest. Why do you feel that way? List some of the professionalism keys that you feel you need to work on. Why do you feel that way? What steps can you take to improve those skills? List some examples of how you might apply information contained in this chapter, both during your training and after you enter the health care field.

C H A P T E R **2**

Clinical Trends in Health Care

VOCABULARY REVIEW

Assignment 2-1: Matching

Match the term with its definition and place the corresponding letter in the blank.

____ 1. Health information technology

____ 2. Fee for service

____ 3. Accountable care organization

____ 4. Triple Aim Initiative

____ 5. Pay for performance organization

____ 6. Pay for coordination

____ 7. Patient-centered

____ 8. National Committee for Quality Assurance

A. Groups of doctors, hospitals, and other health care providers who come together voluntarily to give coordinated high-quality care to Medicare patients (sometimes referred to as medical communities)

B. Health care model designed to facilitate partnerships between patients and their health care team; ensures that patients receive continuity of care, and care provided is patient-centric

C. The most common health care delivery model where the provider is reimbursed according to the type and amount of services provided with no emphasis on patient outcomes

D. The exchange of health information between providers, payers, and consumers in a secure electronic environment

E. A type of health care delivery model that is often used in medical home environments and involves payment for specified care coordination services; the provider leads a team of professionals to oversee and coordinate the patient's overall health

F. A non-profit organization which strives to improve the quality of health care through accreditation

G. A movement by the Institute for Healthcare Improvement developed to address three dimensions: patient experience of care, improving health populations, and to reduce the per capita cost of health care

H. A model of care that emphasizes care coordination; places the needs and preferences of the patient at the core of health care

___ 9. Patient-centered medical home

I. Health care model using a team approach where providers are rewarded and reimbursed by way of care processes and measurable goals related to outcomes and patient satisfaction

Assignment 2-2: Grammar Challenge

Select/underline the correct word.

1. How will the change in health care delivery models (affect, effect) patients?

2. The provider will (advice, advise) you if a patient needs to be scheduled for a consultation.

3. Be sure to properly (sight, site, cite) the consultation report in the description.

4. By involving patients in the decision-making process, the manager was satisfied with the reduction in the (amount, number) of missed appointments.

5. The issue of the morning huddle will be (further, farther) discussed at the next staff meeting.

6. Using (two, too, to) models of health care delivery allow the practice (to, too, two) see better patient outcomes, without generating (two, to, too) many duplicate orders.

CHAPTER REVIEW

Assignment 2-3: Abbreviation Review

Write what each of the following abbreviations stands for.

1. ACO: _____

2. AHRQ: _____

3. CMS: _____

4. HIT: _____

5. IBHC: _____

6. IHI: _____

7. IOM: _____

8. NCQA: _____

9. PCMH: _____

10. PPACA: _____

Assignment 2-4: Short Answer

1. List the six NCQA PCMH 2014 Standards and provide a summary of the requirements.

   A. _____
   _____

   B. _____
   _____

   C. _____
   _____
   _____

   D. _____
   _____

E. _____

_____

F. _____

_____

_____

2. (A) Define PCMH and (B) describe the relationship between an ACO and a PCMH.

A. _____

_____

_____

_____

B. _____

_____

_____

_____

3. Describe the differences between fee for service health care delivery systems and pay for performance organizations.

_____

_____

_____

_____

_____

_____

_____

_____

_____

_____

_____

_____

4. Describe the medical assistant's role in the newer health care models, and describe how the role impacts the patient, employer, and nation.

_____

_____

_____

_____

_____

_____

_____

_____

_____

CERTIFICATION PRACTICE

Assignment 2-5

Choose the best answer and place the corresponding letter in the blank.

____ 1. The implementation of electronic health records (EHR) is an essential component of:

    A. ANHQ.

    B. PCMH.

    C. HIT.

    D. the Triple Aim Initiative.

____ 2. The most common health care delivery model used for reimbursing providers in the Unites States is the _____ model.

    A. pay for coordination

    B. patient-centered

    C. fee for service

    D. pay for performance

____ 3. Which model of health care emphasizes quantity of services rather than quality of services?

    A. Pay for coordination

    B. Fee for service

    C. Pay for performance

    D. PCMH

____ 4. The two major provisions of the PPACA that directly impact health care providers are _____ *and* _____.

    A. Obamacare; quality affordable health care for all Americans

    B. quality affordable health care for all Americans; prevention of chronic disease and improving health

    C. improving quality and efficacy of health care; prevention of chronic disease and improving health

    D. pay for performance; improving quality and efficacy of health care

____ 5. _____ health care models, which are sometimes referred to as medical communities, are groups of doctors, hospitals, and other health care providers who come together voluntarily to give coordinated high-quality care to their Medicare patients.

    A. PCMH

    B. ACO

    C. HMO

    D. All of the above

____ 6. The health care team working collaboratively with patients is referred to as:

    A. a patient-centered approach to health care.

    B. HIPAA compliant.

    C. a pay for coordination approach.

    D. None of the above

____ 7. There is(are) _____ level(s) of NCQA PCMH Recognition.

    A. three

    B. six

    C. one

    D. None of the above

___ 8. The medical assistant can help implement care plans in the new health care delivery models by:

    A. entering orders into the electronic health record.

    B. carefully screening patients and sharing findings with the provider.

    C. tracking the patient to make certain he or she follows through with outside testing.

    D. All of the above

___ 9. The Institute for Healthcare Improvement (IHI) has initiated a movement referred to as the *Triple Aim Initiative*. The initiative hopes to do the following:

    A. Improve the patient experience of care, improve the health populations, and reduce the per capita cost of health care

    B. Improve the HIPAA Privacy Act, improve the patient experience of care, and reduce the per capita cost of health care

    C. Incorporate the HIPAA Privacy Rule, the HIPAA Security Rule, and the Americans with Disabilities Act Amendments Act

    D. Improve the Patient Bill of Rights, improve the health populations, and reduce the per capita cost of health care

___ 10. Health care reform is necessary due to:

    a. surging health care debt and poor outcomes.

    b. violations of HIPAA Privacy and HIPAA Security Rules.

    c. more and more providers entering the health care field.

    d. All of the above

SKILL APPLICATION CHALLENGES

Assignment 2-6: Research Activity

1. Research the various types of health care models (PCMH, ACO, Pay for performance, etc.). Which type of health care model do you consider the most effective? How did you reach your conclusion?

2. Based on each type of health care model, how can you apply your skills to maintain or lower costs while at the same time increasing patient outcomes and satisfaction levels? Consider how to apply the *professionalism keys* you possess to develop and integrate a plan to improve patient outcomes and satisfaction. Support your conclusion with facts.

Assignment 2-7: Role Play

1. Pair up with a classmate and practice your patient interviewing skills.

2. Pair up with a classmate and practice your medication reconciliation skills.

3. Reverse order (or change classmate) and repeat #1 and #2.

FIELD APPLICATION CHALLENGE

Assignment 2-8

Read the following Field Application Challenges and respond to the questions following each scenario.

1. As the medical assistant for Dr. Endo, you are getting ready to reconcile patient Jane Morgan's medication. The practice recently converted to electronic health records (EHR) and no medications, supplements, or allergies have been entered. You have the patient's paper chart but this is her first visit since the practice converted from paper to electronic charts. From the choices below, what would be the *best* solution for obtaining and reconciling the patient's medications?

   A. Scan a copy of the medication history page from the paper chart.

   B. Ask the patient if she has a copy of her medication list, and scan into the electronic health record.

   C. _____

   _____

   _____

   D. Ask the medical records department to update the list.

2. Having completed the medication reconciliation, you will document the chief complaint (reason for the visit by Ms. Morgan today). You note that in the electronic scheduling module, the reason for visit was noted as "Follow-up". Your provider and the practice are following a PCMH model, and your responsibilities include performing the patient interview to record an accurate chief complaint. Everyone is running behind since it is taking more time to update and enter information in the electronic health record than it was using the paper chart. Dr. Endo likes to run on time and you are responsible for keeping him on schedule. How would you be sure to obtain the accurate information from Ms. Morgan? Reflect on which of the professionalism keys you would use to handle this situation, and apply them to your answer.

   _____

   _____

   _____

   _____

   _____

   _____

   _____

JOURNALING EXERCISE

Assignment 2-9

With the rapidly and ever-changing health care field, what content within this chapter was most meaningful to you? Why? Do you think the PPACA and the new health care models can improve patient's health, outcomes, and satisfaction? Do you see any pitfalls of all the new regulations? If so, what are your concerns? How can the professionalism keys help you be a better medical assistant in today's health care delivery models? List some examples of how you might apply information contained in this chapter, both during your training and after you enter the health care field.

C H A P T E R **3**

The Complete Medical Record and Electronic Charting

VOCABULARY REVIEW

Assignment 3-1: Matching

Match the term with its definition and place the corresponding letter in the blank.

____ 1. Shingling

____ 2. Assessment

____ 3. Electronic health record

____ 4. Business associate agreement

____ 5. Notice of privacy practices

____ 6. Subjective impressions

____ 7. Problem list

____ 8. Reverse chronological order

____ 9. Progress notes

____ 10. Objective impressions

____ 11. Flow sheet

____ 12. Plan

____ 13. Electronic medical record

A. A patient's medical record in digital format

B. Describes exactly how protected information is to be handled between business partners

C. Provider's plans to perform diagnostic and lab testing to assist in confirming a diagnosis and plans for treating the patient

D. The heart of the patient record; a chronological listing of the patient's overall health status

E. The way information is stored within the patient's chart; the most recent notes, reports, and forms are always on top

F. The method for filing lab reports when reports are not the size of a standard piece of paper

G. An interpretation of the subjective and objective findings

H. Logs found in the patient's chart that assist the provider in monitoring specific repetitive information, at one glance

I. A record of specific problems that are identified from the patient history form; it should list new problems as they arise; each problem is numbered and should include the name of the problem or diagnosis

J. Patients should receive a notice for how their personal medical information may be used

K. A generic term for all electronic patient care systems

L. Requires that you de-identify information: PHI with all HIPAA identifiers removed

M. Patient's vital signs, height and weight, laboratory results, or other diagnostic data

___ 14. Personal health record

N. A copy of the patient's own personal health information that can be shared with all providers

___ 15. Minimum necessary

O. The patient's chief complaint or an explanation of why the patient is here

Assignment 3-2: Vocabulary Builder

Find the words below that are misspelled; circle them and then correctly spell them in the spaces provided. Then complete the following sentences with the correct vocabulary terms from the list.

advance direcktive

Computer Practice Order Entry (CPOE)

scrub

meaningful use

practice management

minimum neccessary

_____   _____   _____

The portion of the electronic health record that performs the administrative functions is known as (1) _____ _____ software. The administrative function known as (2) _____ verifies that the procedure codes selected are supported with appropriate diagnosis codes. One of the advantages of an EHR is that it contains (3) _____, an application for medication and orders that will allow results to be automatically checked for potential errors or problems. Medical assistants will document whether or not the patient has (4) a(n) _____, a term for the legal document that allows people to convey their wishes should they become unable to do so. HIPAA's (5) _____ rule requires that you only provide PHI in the amount to accomplish the purpose for which the disclosure is sought. (6) _____ is the set of standards defined by CMS incentive programs that governs the use of EHRs and allows eligible providers and hospitals to earn incentive payments by meeting specific criteria.

CHAPTER REVIEW

Assignment 3-3: Abbreviation Review

Write what each of the following abbreviations stands for.

1. CCHIT: _____

2. HIT: _____

3. HITECH: _____

4. HIPAA: _____

5. PHI: _____

6. POMR: _____

7. SOAP: _____

8. SOMR: _____

Assignment 3-4: Short Answer

1. List the commission that was the oldest and best known of the six EHR-certifying agencies recognized by the ONC as responsible for certifying electronic medical records.

   _____

2. Why are flow sheets used in the medical record?

   _____

   _____

   _____

3. List the two major types of formats that are used for documenting in the patient's paper medical record.

   a. _____

   b. _____

4. List what each of the letters stand for in the SOAP acronym and describe information that would be included in each section.

   S: _____

   O: _____

   _____

   A: _____

   P: _____

   _____

5. List four advantages of the POMR.

   _____

   _____

   _____

6. Describe how long medical records need to be retained and how to properly dispose of paper medical records.

   _____

   _____

   _____

7. EHRs have many positives, but what may be some pitfalls associated with an EHR?

   _____

   _____

   _____

   _____

   _____

8. Provide at least three examples of phone reports that may need to be documented either on a progress note or onto a special phone form and placed within a special section of the paper chart. (*Note—messages and reports will be electronically recorded in an EHR.*)

   _____

   _____

9. List at least six functions of EHRs.

_____

_____

_____

_____

_____

_____

_____

_____

_____

_____

_____

10. Explain the shingling method for filing in a paper chart and list examples of some reports that may be shingled.

_____

_____

_____

_____

11. Why would an office manager conduct a comprehensive audit trail?

_____

_____

_____

_____

_____

_____

_____

_____

_____

Assignment 3-5: Matching I

Information found in a SOAP note is listed below. Identify the part of the note in which the information would be found. Match the information with the answers listed. Record the answer in the blank provided. Each answer may be used more than once.

S—Subjective   A—Assessment

O—Objective   P—Plan

____ a. Temperature 99.9°F

____ b. Patient c/o sore throat

____ c. Lymph nodes enlarged upon palpation

____ d. Strep throat

____ e. Abdomen and groin area shows rash

____ f. Lungs are clear

____ g. Patient states slight headache above right eye

____ h. Will perform an ECG and run a metabolic panel

____ i. Results of rapid strep test

Assignment 3-6: Matching II

Match the section of the chart in which you would find the following information. (Sections may be used more than once or not at all.)

Information	Sections of the chart
____ 1. Patient's chief complaint	A. Demographic information
____ 2. CBC or complete blood count	B. Insurance section
____ 3. Referral form (this may vary from office to office)	C. Correspondence
____ 4. Registration form	D. Diagnostic/X-ray reports
____ 5. MRI report	E. Lab reports
____ 6. Letter from the cardiologist	F. Medication information
____ 7. Social history	G. Progress note
____ 8. Copy of the patient's insurance card	H. Medical history
____ 9. Copy of the patient's privacy statement, living will, and advance directive	I. Consultation report
____ 10. Prescription information	J. Legal

CERTIFICATION PRACTICE

Assignment 3-7

Choose the best answer and place the corresponding letter in the blank.

_____ 1. This is an analysis of the patient's health status.

    A. Patient's record

    B. Medical record

    C. Flow sheets

    D. Objective impressions

_____ 2. This is the person who developed the POMR system.

    A. Larry Word

    B. Larry Reed

    C. Lawrence Weed

    D. Robert Weed

_____ 3. This is the section of the medical record that contains letters written about the patient from an assessment made by a specialist.

    A. Progress notes

    B. Discharge summary

    C. Correspondence

    D. Consultation reports

_____ 4. This is the section of the chart in which you would find a biopsy study.

    A. Laboratory section (pathology report)

    B. Correspondence

    C. Insurance section

    D. Progress notes

_____ 5. A Lipid Panel and Basic metabolic panel (BMP) would be filed in which of the following sections of the chart?

    A. Diagnostic section

    B. Laboratory section

    C. Progress notes

    D. Medication section

_____ 6. Which of the following does not belong with the others?

    A. Assessment

    B. Impression

    C. Diagnosis

    D. Examination

_____ 7. Which of the following is not a use of the medical record?

    A. Medical research and education

    B. Legal documentation

    C. Tracking patient's progress

    D. To check the patient's financial balance

____ 8. All of the following are found in the administrative section of the record *except:*

    A. demographics.

    B. patient insurance.

    C. correspondence.

    D. prescription information.

____ 9. The physical outer part of the paper medical record belongs to the practice; however, information stored within the chart is property of the:

    A. patient.

    B. practice.

    C. Both A and B

    D. None of the above

____ 10. The information in a POMR includes:

    A. problem list.

    B. plan.

    C. progress notes.

    D. All of the above

SKILL APPLICATION CHALLENGE

Assignment 3-8: Documentation Exercise

From the following dictation, put the information into a SOAP note format on the paper progress note provided.

Rx: Accutane. Allergies: Latex and SULFA. Vital Signs: T 99.2°F. BP: 110/76, R: 20, P: 78.
"I have pain when I go to the bathroom. I go all the time, especially at night." + abdominal pain(6), –back pain, + fever (99.6° to 101°F), LMP 05-06-2010. OTC; Urostat (no relief). Abdominal tenderness and guarding in the mid-hypogastric region of the abdomen. Urinalysis: Urine bright orange due to the Urostat: Unable to read urine dipstick. Microscopic examination of urine revealed a large amount of white blood cells and bacteria. Few red blood cells. Diagnosis: Urinary tract infection. Will send urine out for a C&S and start the patient on Bactrim DS, sig 1 tab/day × 7 days. Pt. to return to office in 10 days for a recheck on urine.

S: _____

_____

_____

_____

O: _____

_____

_____

_____

A: _____

_____

_____

_____

P: _____

_____

_____

_____

FIELD APPLICATION CHALLENGE
Assignment 3-9

Read the following Field Application Challenge and respond to the questions following the scenario.
Mr. Snodgrass calls to request his wife's lab results. Mrs. Snodgrass is traveling today and will not have access to a phone until after the office is closed. Mr. Snodgrass states that his wife is most anxious about the results and does not want to wait until tomorrow for the results. Mr. Snodgrass is listed on the privacy sheet as being able to accept lab results for the patient. You just placed the chart on the provider's desk because the results just came back. The results are normal but the provider is out of the office and will not return until the next day. The policy of the office is that no test results are given to a patient until they have been signed off by the provider.

1. What makes it all right for this particular patient's spouse to receive his wife's lab results?

   _____

   _____

2. Would it be okay to share the results with the spouse since the results are normal?

   _____

   _____

3. Are there any other options for giving the spouse the information?

   _____

   _____

   _____

JOURNALING EXERCISE
Assignment 3-10

Incomplete documentation in the patient medical record is like having a book with missing pages. Every office visit is a new chapter and the physician depends on the MA to maintain accurate records of each patient experience. How will you apply the professionalism keys to demonstrate your commitment to excellence in completing documentation in the patient health record?

C H A P T E R **4**

Fundamentals of Documentation

VOCABULARY REVIEW

Assignment 4-1: Matching

Match the term with its definition and place the corresponding letter in the blank.

____ 1. Joint Commission

____ 2. Participating provider

____ 3. Addendum

____ 4. Institute for Safe Medication Practices (ISMP)

____ 5. "Do Not Use" Abbreviation List

____ 6. Directed exchange

____ 7. Consumer-mediated exchange

A. An addition or supplement to a previous chart note

B. A list of abbreviations that are commonly misinterpreted and may no longer be used when documenting orders within the patient's medical record, or when writing orders that are to be sent to other health care facilities

C. Separate organization that specifically seeks ways to promote medication safety; has also compiled a list which is referred to as "List of Error-Prone Abbreviations, Symbols, and Dose Designations"

D. A facility that contracts with the insurance company to provide laboratory or diagnostic services

E. A national organization that focuses on improving the quality and safety of care provided by health care organizations; published a "Do Not Use List" of medication abbreviations as part of its 2006 National Patient and Safety Goals

F. A means that is often used to communicate with patients. Example: Patients' health portal.

G. Used by providers to easily and securely send patient information such as laboratory orders and results, patient referrals, or discharge summaries directly to another health care professional.

Assignment 4-2: Sentence Completion

Fill in the blanks below with essential terms from this chapter.

Lisa works for Dr. Beachler who is not seeing patients this afternoon. Lisa is catching up on some paper work. She pulls the charts for tomorrow's patients, completes the callbacks, and prepares the lab specimens for the courier. One of Dr. Beachler's patients, Mark Stevens, had some chest pain last week so Dr. Beachler ordered a heart ultrasound on the patient. The test came back abnormal so Dr. Beachler now wants Lisa to send the patient to Dr. Wong, a well-respected cardiologist. The cardiology group asks Lisa to send over the most recent, relevant (1) _____ (follow-up information from previous visits) in advance along with the patient's (2) _____ (reason the patient is being seen). Dr. Wong's office also asks Lisa to call the patient and have him get some blood work performed before his first visit. Lisa looks in the UHC directory to see which lab is a(n) (3) _____. Lisa calls the lab, sets up the testing for the patient, and calls the patient back with the information. She then records the information in the patient's chart. In addition, Lisa will include as part of the new patient paperwork for Mr. Stevens to complete, the (4) _____ (a legal document advising patients prior to a procedure the nature of the treatment, possible benefits, risks, and alternative treatments available). After completing her tasks, Lisa discovers after signing off the entry that she forgot to list the time of the testing. She makes a(n) (5) _____ to the entry to include the time of the test.

CHAPTER REVIEW

Assignment 4-3: Abbreviation Review

Write what the following abbreviations stand for.

ISMP: _____

JC: _____

Assignment 4-4: Short Answer

1. Fill in the chart below with 11 "Documentation Dos" and 5 "Documentation Don'ts" when documenting in the medical record.

Dos	
1.	7.
2.	8.
3.	9.
4.	10.
5.	11.
6.	

Don'ts	
1.	4.
2.	5.
3.	

2. List the steps that should be taken when making a correction or an addendum to both a paper-based and a paperless record.

Paper-based: _____

_____

_____

_____

Paperless: _____

_____

_____

3. Describe proper etiquette guidelines that should be adhered to when sending electronic exchanges or entering information into the patient portal. .

_____

- _____

_____

- _____

_____

- _____

- _____

- _____

- _____

- _____

- _____

- _____

- _____

- _____

4. The following chart entry contains nine errors. Many of the errors are the result of using "Do Not Use" abbreviations (see Appendix B). Highlight the errors using a highlighter in the chart entry and transfer the errors to the lines listed below the entry. Describe why each error is incorrect and write in what may be used in place of the error.

05/31/20xx 9:30 a.m. Allergy serum, 0.5 cc, sub-q, R. arm per Dr. Armstrong. Small

wheal formed > than the size of a ▇ (CORR Lisa Brown, RMA 05/31/20xx) at the injection

^(dime)

site follwing the injections. +erythema and edema, pt. states the site is sore and tender to

the touch. −Resp sx. Appleid ice to area. Informed doctor of reaction. Dr. would like dose to be

reduced from 0.5 cc to 0.3 ml next visit. LB, RMA (AMT) ————————————

---

1. _____

2. _____

3. _____

4. _____

5. _____

6. _____

7. _____

8. _____

9. _____

CERTIFICATION PRACTICE

Assignment 4-5

Choose the best answer and place the corresponding letter in the blank.

____ 1. When documenting in the medical record, the entry should be:

   A. accurate and thorough.

   B. typed or written in black ink.

   C. neat and legible.

   D. All of the above

____ 2. The chief complaint is the reason that the patient is being seen. The complaint should be all of the following *except*:

   A. Accurate

   B. Concise

   C. Flow well

   D. Judgmental

___ 3. The medical office in which you work uses EHR. The provider sends a message to your electronic task box with a high priority symbol asking you to contact Rebecca Harting instructing her to change the way that she is taking her Dilantin. You notify the patient and document the phone call within the electronic message template. You reopen the message template and discover that you made an error. What is the correct method for correcting an error or making an addendum in the EHR?

    A. Open a new note and type in the correction.

    B. Click on the addendum or change button and follow the directions.

    C. There is no way to correct an error once the message has been created.

    D. Notify your clinical supervisor and she will fix the error.

___ 4. The way that a provider discovers the reason for the patient's office visit is by reading:

    A. the patient's H&P.

    B. the patient's lab reports.

    C. the patient's social history.

    D. the patient's chief complaint.

___ 5. One pitfall that should be avoided in regard to documentation is:

    A. procrastination.

    B. initiative.

    C. completeness.

    D. accuracy.

___ 6. Which of the following would be regarded as a "Documentation Don't"?

    A. Use standard abbreviations

    B. Use illegible handwriting

    C. Use correct spelling

    D. Document accurately

___ 7. A follow-up note from a previous visit is a:

    A. chief complaint.

    B. lab report.

    C. patient education.

    D. progress note.

___ 8. Items that should be included when documenting an in-office procedure includes all of the following *except*:

    A. the name of the procedure.

    B. the name of the provider ordering the procedure.

    C. any complications during or following the procedure.

    D. the name and address of the facility.

___ 9. Information that should be included in a medication entry includes all of the following *except*:

    A. the lot number of any syringes that are used to administer the medication.

    B. the name of the medication.

    C. the strength of the medication.

    D. the route of the medication.

___ 10. Information that should be included when documenting an educational session includes all but which of the following?

    A. The date and time of the session

    B. The topic of the session

    C. The patient's highest level of education

    D. Who was present for the session

SKILL APPLICATION CHALLENGES

Assignment 4-6: Flash Card Connection

1. Refer to Appendix A in the back of the textbook. Make up a set of flash cards for each abbreviation. (Helpful hint: Using different colors of flash cards for the different groups of abbreviations may assist in quicker memorization of the abbreviations.)

2. Refer to Appendix B in the back of the textbook. Make up a set of flash cards for the "Do Not Use" abbreviations. These abbreviations should be placed on bright neon-colored flash cards as a reminder not to use them.

Assignment 4-7: Documentation Exercise

Rewrite the following chart note in long hand.

03-15-20XX 10:15 am: Pt. C/O R. sided abd pain (7) x 3 days. + N/V, Last BM 4 days ago. Fever X 2 days (99-102°F) ↓appetite. LMP: 02-14-2010, OTC Med: Tums (-relief) -RX, NKDA. Colleen Frye, CMA (AAMA) ——————————————

Assignment 4-8: Completing Special Forms

The following assignments are to assist you in completing special forms and in learning how to document information onto a progress note. Each assignment will list which forms are necessary to complete the assignment.

Assignment 4-8A: Documenting a Progress Note

Work Form Necessary: FORM 4-1

Directions: Transfer the following information in proper documentation format onto the progress note, Work Form 4-1.

February 08, 20XX 10:00 a.m.: Jillian Longfellow, born 03/11/1969, is here for a follow-up appointment from her last visit regarding her UTI. Jillian finished the Macrobid as directed, but still feels the urge to urinate. Pain upon urination; urinating 3 times per hour. Has visible blood in the urine (shows up on tissue paper when she wipes). Patient is complaining of moderate lower back pain (around an 8 on the pain scale). Taking OTC: Aleve 220 mg every four hours (very little relief). Erika Simmons, RMA

Assignment 4-8B: Documenting Lab Results onto a Reporting Form and onto a Progress Note

Work Forms Necessary: FORM 4-1, FORM 4-2, and FORM 4-3

Directions: Transfer the following information to Work Forms 4-1, 4-2, and 4-3. (*Note:* You will continue to use Work Form 4-1, which you started in Assignment 4-8A. To learn how to document the full procedure onto a progress note, refer to Table 4-1, Items Listed When Documenting Lab Procedures, in the textbook.

After examining Jillian Longfellow, Dr. Brown asks the medical assistant, Erika Simmons, to perform a physical and chemical urinalysis on the patient's urine. Results to the physical and chemical urinalysis are below. Please transfer the results of the physical and chemical urinalysis to the urine reporting form (Work Form 4-2) and the urinalysis log (Work Form 4-3), and make a note on the progress note. Since the lab result information is already on the lab form you will just need to state that the tests were performed and where to find the results on the progress note, for example, 02/08/20XX 10:30 a.m. Physical & Chemical UA per Dr. Brown. Results can be found on the urinalysis reporting form in the lab section of the chart.

02/08/20XX 10:30 a.m. Location (Long Street Office)

Lab results were as follows: Physical & Chemical UA: Color: Amber, Appearance: Cloudy, Odor: Strong Ammonia: Leukocyte (Moderate), Nitrite (Positive), Urobilinogen (Normal), pH (7.5), Protein (30+), Blood (Moderate), Specific Gravity (1.030), Ketones (Negative), Bilirubin (Negative), Glucose (250)

Tested by Erika Simmons, RMA (AMT)

Assignment 4-8C: Documenting an Outside Appointment onto a Progress Note

Work Form Necessary: FORM 4-1

Directions: Document the information from the phone call onto Work Form 4-1. (*Note:* Again, continue using Work Form 4-1.) Table 4-7 in the textbook lists steps for recording outside procedures, which is very similar for recording outside appointments.

After reviewing the results, Dr. Brown decides to refer Jillian to an urologist. He is concerned that the patient is not responding to treatment. Since Jillian belongs to an HMO plan, Erika (Dr. Brown's medical assistant) needs to set up a referral for the patient. Erika first calls the urologist to make certain that she can get an appointment for the patient.

Erika contacts Dr. Michael Hale's office, a urologist listed on Jillian's HMO plan and speaks with Terri Kissler (a scheduler for Dr. Hale). The time the call takes place is 10:45 a.m. Terri expresses to Erika that the first appointment available is on Tuesday, February 12, 20XX at 10:00 a.m. Erika pauses for a moment to ask Jillian, who is standing next to the phone, if the date and time works with her schedule. She states that it does. Erika accepts the appointment for the patient and tells Terri that she will send the referral just as soon as she completes it. Erika hangs up the phone and shares all of the information with Jillian who appears to have a clear understanding of the instructions.

Assignment 4-8D: Documenting a Medication

Work Form Necessary: FORM 4-4

Directions: Using the information below, document a medication on Work Form 4-4. Refer to Table 4-3 in the textbook for steps for documenting a medication.

Patient's name: Timothy Heller

DOB: 12-10-1968

Doctor's order: Dr. Henderson orders the patient to have a flu immunization.

Today's date: 06/15/XX

Time of administration: 0900

The standard adult dose is 0.5 mL.

Name of manufacturer: Prevention Inc

Lot number: 27A119

Exp. date: 06/20XX

Route: IM

Location: R. Deltoid

Medical assistant's name and title: Brad Green, RMA

No complications during or following the injection.

Assignment 4-8E: Documenting a Procedure

Work Form Necessary: FORM 4-4

Directions: Using the information given below, document the procedure on Work Form 4-4. Refer to Table 4-2 in the textbook for steps for documenting a procedure.

Patient's name: Timothy Heller

Doctor's order: Dr. Henderson ordered a 12-Lead ECG

Today's date: 06/15/XX

Time of ECG: 0915

No complications. Gave a copy of the ECG to Dr. Henderson.

Medical assistant's name and title: Brad Green, RMA (AMT)

Assignment 4-8F: Documenting a Prescription

Work Form Necessary: FORM 4-5

Directions: Using the information given below, document the prescription on Work Form 4-5. Refer to Table 4-4 in textbook for steps for documenting prescriptions.

Patient's name: Holly Hatfield

Patient's DOB: 02/15/1989

Provider's name: Chelsie Wong

Date: 03/18/XX

Time prescription prepared: 11:15 a.m.

Name of Rx: Paxil CR 12.5 mg Tablets Number Dispensed 30

Instructions: Take 1 daily

0 Refills

Name of medical assistant: Sasha Disorov, CMA (AAMA)

Assignment 4-8G: Documenting a Patient Education Session

Work Form Necessary: FORM 4-5

Directions: Using the information given below, document the patient education session, using Work Form 4-5. Refer to Table 4-5 in the textbook for steps for documenting a patient education session.

Patient's name: Holly Hatfield

Provider's name: Chelsie Wong

Date: 03/18/XX

Time of session: 11:30 a.m.

Name of session: Living with Anxiety

Mother present for session: Both Holly and mother appeared to comprehend all of the information. The medical assistant explained how to reduce anxiety and provided tips for what to do when anxiety is present. The patient was given several brochures on anxiety and instructed to call the office if symptoms worsen. Both the mother and patient appeared to comprehend the information.

Name of medical assistant: Sasha Disorov, CMA (AAMA)

FIELD APPLICATION CHALLENGE

Assignment 4-9

Read the following Field Application Challenges and respond to the questions following each scenario.

1. You received a fax from Dr. O'Malley's office concerning Dorothy J. Fuller. She is not a patient at your office nor is she on the referral list. What would you do?

   _____

   _____

2. Leslie Gunther is scheduled for surgery today at 1 p.m. The hospital calls this morning to state the PAT information is not in her chart. You pull up Leslie's electronic chart and see documentation that states the information was sent electronically to the hospital three days ago. What would you do?

   _____

   _____

   _____

   _____

   _____

   _____

JOURNALING EXERCISE

Assignment 4-10

What content within this chapter was most meaningful to you? Why? List some examples of how you might apply information contained in this chapter, both during your training and after you enter the health care industry. Considering the comments from Davene (your Professionalism Mentor) how would you rate your ability to accurately and timely document in a patient's medical record? Apply the professionalism keys to your responses.

Work Form 4-1

PROGRESS NOTE		
Patient Name:		DOB:

DATE/TIME	PROGRESS NOTES	ALLERGIES

Work Form 4-2

URINALYSIS REPORTING FORM

Patient Name: _____

Tested by: _____   Time: _____

Doctor: _____ Location: _____ Date: _____

Leukocytes	Negative ☐		Trace ☐	Small+ ☐	Moderate++ ☐	Large+++ ☐	
Nitrite	Negative ☐		Positive ☐	(Any degree of pink color is Positive)			
Urobilinogen	Normal ☐	Normal 1 ☐	2 ☐	4 ☐	8 ☐		
Protein	Negative ☐	Trace ☐	30+ ☐	100++ ☐	300+++ ☐	2000 or more ++++ ☐	
pH	5.0 ☐	6.0 ☐	6.5 ☐	7.0 ☐	7.5 ☐	8.0 ☐	8.5 ☐
Blood	Negative ☐	Non-Hemolyzed Trace ☐	Non-Hemolyzed Moderate ☐	Hemolyzed Large ☐	Small + ☐	Moderate ++ ☐	Large +++ ☐
Specific Gravity	1.000 ☐	1.005 ☐	1.010 ☐ Trace	1.015 ☐ Small	1.020 ☐ Moderate	1.025 ☐ Large	1.030 ☐ Large
Ketone	Negative ☐	mg/dL	5 ☐ Small	15 ☐ Moderate	40 ☐ Large	50 ☐	150 ☐
Bilirubin	Negative ☐		+ ☐ 1/10 (tr.)	++ ☐ 1/4	+++ ☐ 1/2	☐ 1	☐ 2 or more
Glucose	Negative ☐	g/dL (%) mg/dL	100 ☐	250 ☐	500 ☐	1000 ☐	2000 ☐ or more

Microscopic

WBC _____ /HPF	EPITHELIAL CELLS _____/HPF	APPEARANCE_____
RBC _____ /HPF	TYPE _____	ODOR _____
CASTS _____ /LPF	TRICHOMONAS _____	COMMENTS: _____
TYPE _____	BACTERIA _____	_____
CRYSTALS _____	OTHER _____	_____
YEAST _____	Color _____	_____

Work Form 4-3

Urinalysis Log

Patient Name	Date	Dr	Glu	Bili	Ket	Blo	SG	pH	Pro	Uro	Nit	WBC	MA

Work Form 4-4

PROGRESS NOTE		
Patient Name:		DOB:

DATE/TIME	PROGRESS NOTES	ALLERGIES

Work Form 4-5

PROGRESS NOTE		
Patient Name:		DOB:

DATE/TIME	PROGRESS NOTES	ALLERGIES

C H A P T E R **5**

Conducting a Patient Screening

VOCABULARY REVIEW

Assignment 5-1: Spelling Review

Find the words below that are misspelled; circle them, and then correctly spell them in the spaces provided.

Active Listning	Cheif complaint	Body language
Comprehensive medical history	Family medical history	Genagram
Gesture	History of presant illness	Past history
Persunal medical history	Social history	Subgective information
Theraputic communication	Usual childhood diseases	

_____   _____   _____

_____   _____   _____

_____

Assignment 5-2: Sentence Completion

Fill in the blanks below with essential terms from this chapter. (*Hint:* Not all the words will be used.)

1. _____ may be best described as an exchange of information between the health care worker and patient that leads to the advancement of the patient's physical and emotional well-being.

2. Employing _____ along with verbal communication helps to enhance the message that is being sent and is often incorporated during the questioning phase of the patient interview.

3. Defined as a complete health history that covers the patient's personal, social, and family history is a(n) _____ .

4. A(n) _____ resembles a family tree and is incorporated as part of the family medical history.

5. _____ is defined as gestures, postures, and facial expressions by which a person manifests various physical, mental, or emotional states and communicates nonverbally with others.

6. The _____ is the reason the patient is being seen.

7. A(n) _____ includes the patient's previous health concerns, current health concerns, and current medication list.

8. Along with the chief complaint the medical assistant may also be responsible for conducting a *brief* _____, which is a series of questions that are related to the patient's complaint.

9. The _____ refers to lifestyle questions.

10. _____ involves more than just your sense of hearing; it encompasses other senses as well. Observe the patient's facial expressions and body language as they respond to certain questions. Does the patient's body language match what is being stated verbally?

CHAPTER REVIEW

Assignment 5-3: Abbreviation Review

Write what each of the following abbreviations stands for.

1. UCD: _____

2. UCHD: _____

3. PH: _____

4. PHH: _____

5. ROS: _____

6. CC: _____

7. HPI: _____

8. BMI: _____

9. OTC: _____

10. FH: _____

11. SH: _____

Assignment 5-4: Short Answer

1. List three components of body language.

   A. _____

   B. _____

   C. _____

2. Describe two types of tools that are used to collect data for the patient history.

   A. _____

   B. _____

3. What are the three parts/sections of the comprehensive medical history? Describe what information would be found in each section.

   A. _____

   _____

   _____

   _____

   _____

   _____

   B. _____

   _____

   _____

   _____

   _____

   C. _____

   _____

   _____

   _____

   _____

4. If possible, how many feet apart should the interviewer be from the patient during the patient interview?

   _____

5. What is a genogram and how is it used?

   _____

   _____

   _____

   _____

6. To be a successful communicator you must understand how the communication cycle works. In every communication encounter there is a *sender* or source. The sender is the person that conveys the message. Describe the segment of the patient interview in which you can assess the patient's comprehension of the questions at hand and an opportunity to make adjustments if necessary.

   _____

   _____

7. List and describe characteristics the medical assistant must possess to communicate in a therapeutic manner.

_____

_____

_____

_____

_____

_____

_____

_____

_____

CERTIFICATION PRACTICE

Assignment 5-5

Choose the best answer and place the corresponding letter in the blank.

____ 1. A farmer comes into the office today to be seen about a persistent sore on his face that will not go away. What part of his medical history may be especially helpful to the provider in making a diagnosis on this patient?

    A. Episodic medical history

    B. Personal medical history

    C. Family medical history

    D. Social medical history

____ 2. A 37-year-old white female is scheduled for her annual exam today. She states that her sister who is 32 years old was recently diagnosed with melanoma and her Grandma Helga was diagnosed with breast cancer at the age of 72. This information would be listed within what part of the comprehensive medical history?

    A. Episodic medical history

    B. Personal medical history

    C. Family medical history

    D. Social medical history

____ 3. Repeating or rephrasing the main idea of the sentence is called:

    A. clarification.

    B. restatement.

    C. reflection.

    D. summarizing.

____ 4. This technique is usually incorporated at the conclusion of the interview.

    A. Clarification

    B. Restatement

    C. Reflection

    D. Summarizing

____ 5. "So your mommy says that your tummy hurts. Can you point to the part of your tummy that hurts the most?" What listening technique would this example describe?

    A. Clarification

    B. Restatement

    C. Reflection

    D. Summarizing

___ 6. Which family members would *not* be included in the family medical history?

    A. Siblings

    B. Parents

    C. Cousins

    D. Grandparents (maternal and paternal)

___ 7. You have a patient coming in today who has limited English proficiency. Whose responsibility is it to arrange for an interpreter?

    A. The patient

    B. The patient's family

    C. The medical staff

    D. The provider

___ 8. Questions regarding each of the major body systems and parts are known as:

    A. ROS.

    B. CC.

    C. FH.

    D. SH.

___ 9. "How long has the pain been going on?" is an example of:

    A. an open-ended question.

    B. a closed-ended question.

    C. using a leading question.

    D. demanding an explanation.

___ 10. All of the following are good examples of "asking close-ended questions" *except*:

    A. On a scale of 0 to 10, how would you rate your pain?

    B. How many episodes of diarrhea have you experienced over the last three days?

    C. How many Extra Strength Tylenol did you take?

    D. What is the reason for your visit today?

SKILL APPLICATION CHALLENGE

Assignment 5-6: Documentation Exercise

Complete a genogram for your family. Either use the example in your textbook (Figure 5-9) to guide you in getting started or go to this website: *https://familyhistory.hhs.gov*.

    The family history should go back at least two generations.

COMPLETING SPECIAL FORMS

Assignment 5-7: Completing a Medical History

Work Form Necessary: FORM 5-1

Directions: Interview a friend, neighbor, or family member who has multiple health problems. Complete Work Form 5-1, a medical history form. On a separate sheet of notebook paper, expand on all "Yes" questions by asking the following: Duration of Condition, Course of Treatment, Current Status of Condition, and Date of Resolve (if applicable).

FIELD APPLICATION CHALLENGE
Assignment 5-8

Read the following Field Application Challenge and respond to the question following the scenario.

Bailey Tanner, a 16-year-old female, is here today for a physical examination. Bailey's mom is also present for the exam. You notice that Bailey's mom answers all of your questions before Bailey has an opportunity to respond. The last part of the history involves sensitive subject matter regarding the patient's sexual history. Should the mother be allowed to stay during this part of the questioning? List the reasons for your response. If your response is that you would ask the mother to leave, what would be an appropriate way to do so?

_____

_____

_____

_____

_____

_____

_____

_____

JOURNALING EXERCISE
Assignment 5-9

What content within this chapter was most meaningful to you? Why? Do you consider yourself a good listener? Reflect on the scenario Davene put forward in the "Professionalism Mentor" feature. How will you incorporate listening and interviewing skills, while not becoming "trapped" behind the computer? How will you demonstrate professionalism? Which of the professionalism keys would you apply in this situation?

Work Form 5-1

CONFIDENTIAL HEALTH HISTORY

Name: _____   Date: _____

Birthdate: _____   Age: _____   Date of last physical examination: _____

Occupation: _____

Reason for visit today: _____

MEDICATIONS List all medications you are currently taking	**ALLERGIES** List all allergies

SYMPTOMS   Check (✓) symptoms you currently have or have had in the past year.

GENERAL	GASTROINTESTINAL	EYE, EAR, NOSE, THROAT	MEN only
☐ Chills	☐ Appetite poor	☐ Bleeding gums	☐ Breast lump
☐ Depression	☐ Bloating	☐ Blurred vision	☐ Erection difficulties
☐ Dizziness	☐ Bowel changes	☐ Crossed eyes	☐ Lump in testicles
☐ Fainting	☐ Constipation	☐ Difficulty swallowing	☐ Penis discharge
☐ Fever	☐ Diarrhea	☐ Double vision	☐ Sore on penis
☐ Forgetfulness	☐ Excessive hunger	☐ Earache	☐ Other
☐ Headache	☐ Excessive thirst	☐ Ear discharge	
☐ Loss of sleep	☐ Gas	☐ Hay fever	**WOMEN only**
☐ Loss of weight	☐ Hemorrhoids	☐ Hoarseness	☐ Abnormal Pap Smear
☐ Nervousness	☐ Indigestion	☐ Loss of hearing	☐ Bleeding between periods
☐ Numbness	☐ Nausea	☐ Nosebleeds	☐ Breast lump
☐ Sweats	☐ Rectal bleeding	☐ Persistent cough	☐ Extreme menstrual pain
	☐ Stomach pain	☐ Ringing in ears	☐ Hot flashes
MUSCLE/JOINT/BONE	☐ Vomiting	☐ Sinus problems	☐ Nipple discharge
Pain, weakness, numbness in:	☐ Vomiting blood	☐ Vision - Flashes	☐ Painful intercourse
☐ Arms ☐ Hips		☐ Vision - Halos	☐ Vaginal discharge
☐ Back ☐ Legs	**CARDIOVASCULAR**		☐ Other
☐ Feet ☐ Neck	☐ Chest pain	**SKIN**	Date of last
☐ Hands ☐ Shoulders	☐ High blood pressure	☐ Bruise easily	menstrual period _____
	☐ Irregular heart beat	☐ Hives	Date of last
GENITO-URINARY	☐ Low blood pressure	☐ Itching	Pap Smear _____
☐ Blood in urine	☐ Poor circulation	☐ Change in moles	Have you had
☐ Frequent urination	☐ Rapid heart beat	☐ Rash	a mammogram? _____
☐ Lack of bladder control	☐ Swelling of ankles	☐ Scars	Are you pregnant? _____
☐ Painful urination	☐ Varicose veins	☐ Sores that won't heal	Number of children _____

MEDICAL HISTORY   Check (✓) the medical conditions you have or have had in the past.

☐ AIDS	☐ Chemical Dependency	☐ Herpes	☐ Polio
☐ Alcoholism	☐ Chicken Pox	☐ High Cholesterol	☐ Prostate Problem
☐ Anemia	☐ Diabetes	☐ HIV Positive	☐ Psychiatric Care
☐ Anorexia	☐ Emphysema	☐ Kidney Disease	☐ Rheumatic Fever
☐ Appendicitis	☐ Epilepsy	☐ Liver Disease	☐ Scarlet Fever
☐ Arthritis	☐ Gall Bladder Disease	☐ Measles	☐ Stroke
☐ Asthma	☐ Glaucoma	☐ Migraine Headaches	☐ Suicide Attempt
☐ Bleeding Disorders	☐ Goiter	☐ Miscarriage	☐ Thyroid Problems
☐ Breast Lump	☐ Gonorrhea	☐ Mononucleosis	☐ Tonsillitis
☐ Bronchitis	☐ Gout	☐ Multiple Sclerosis	☐ Tuberculosis
☐ Bulimia	☐ Heart Disease	☐ Mumps	☐ Typhoid Fever
☐ Cancer	☐ Hepatitis	☐ Pacemaker	☐ Ulcers
☐ Cataracts	☐ Hernia	☐ Pneumonia	☐ Vaginal Infections
			☐ Venereal Disease

CONFIDENTIAL HEALTH HISTORY

(continues)

Work Form 5-1   (continued)

HOSPITALIZATIONS

Year	Hospital	Reason for Hospitalization and Outcome

Have you ever had a blood transfusion? ☐ Yes ☐ No
if yes, please give approximate dates: _____

OCCUPATIONAL CONCERNS Check (✓) if your work exposes you to the following:	**HEALTH HABITS** Check (✓) which substances you use and indicate how much you use per day/week.	**PREGNANCY HISTORY**		
		Year of Birth	Sex of Birth	**Complications if any**
☐ Stress	☐ Caffeine			
☐ Hazardous Substances	☐ Tobacco			
☐ Heavy Lifting	☐ Drugs			
☐ Other	☐ Alcohal			

SERIOUS ILLNESS/INJURIES	**DATE**	**OUTCOME**

FAMILY HISTORY Fill in health information about your family.

Relation	Age	State of Health	Age of Death	Cause of Death	Check (✓) if your blood relatives had any of the following Disease	Relationship to you
Father					☐ Arthritis, Gout	
Mother					☐ Asthma, Hay Fever	
Brothers					☐ Cancer	
					☐ Chemical Dependency	
					☐ Diabetes	
					☐ Heart Disease, Strokes	
Sisters					☐ High Blood Pressure	
					☐ Kidney Disease	
					☐ Tuberculosis	
					☐ Other	

I certify that the above information is correct to the best of my knowledge. I will not hold my doctor or any members of his/her staff responsible for any errors or ommisions that I may have made in the completion of this form.

_____   _____
Signature   Date

_____   _____
Reviewed By   Date

C H A P T E R **6**

Assisting Patients with Special Needs

VOCABULARY REVIEW

Assignment 6-1: Matching

Match the term with its definition and place the corresponding letter in the blank.

_____ 1. ADA Standards for Accessible Design

_____ 2. Auxiliary services

_____ 3. Civil Rights Act

_____ 4. Guide dogs

_____ 5. Limited English proficiency (LEP)

_____ 6. Mental health

_____ 7. Mental illness

_____ 8. Mental impairment

_____ 9. Mentally challenged

_____ 10. Postlingual

_____ 11. Prelingual

_____ 12. Sighted guide assistance

A. English is not the primary language and the individual has a difficult time reading, speaking, or comprehending English

B. Patient who became deaf after she started talking

C. How people look at themselves, their lives, and the other people in their lives; evaluate their challenges and problems; and explore choices

D. Sighted individual who gives a blind individual assistance in walking

E. Brain functions at a subnormal intellectual level

F. Disorder that disrupts a person's ability to think, feel, and relate to others

G. Aids that will help to ensure effective communication when working with deaf patients

H. Prohibits discrimination against someone because of race, color, sex, national origin, or religion

I. Patient who became deaf before she started talking

J. Dogs specially trained to guide their visually impaired or blind owners

K. Condition or illness which impairs the mind's ability to process information in a "normal" fashion

L. Mandates construction companies to design buildings that are accessible to all persons, including those who have dexterity and limited mobility problems

Assignment 6-2: Misspelled Words

Underline the correctly spelled term.

1. demenita	dementia	dimentia
2. frale senior	frail seneor	frail senior
3. fiscal disablity	fysical disbility	physical disability
4. diversity	diverisity	divercity
5. culuture	culture	calture
6. singed English	signed Enlish	signed English
7. tellatyperighter	teleatypewriter	teletypewriter
8. activities of daily living	activitys of daily living	daily living activities
9. Alzheimer's Disease	Alltimer's Disease	Oldtimer's Disease
10. explotation	exploitation	explortation
11. oldsters abuse	elder abuse	elders abuse
12. neglect	naglect	neglact

CHAPTER REVIEW

Assignment 6-3: Abbreviation Review

Write what each of the following abbreviations stands for.

1. ADA: _____

2. ADAAA: _____

3. ADL: _____

4. ASL: _____

5. CASE: _____

6. SEE: _____

7. LEP: _____

8. TTY: _____

9. TRS: _____

10. TDD: _____

Assignment 6-4: Short Answer

1. What is the most common sign language used in the United States and parts of Canada?

   _____

2. List three tips that can be used when performing invasive procedures on a pediatric patient.

   _____

   _____

   _____

   _____

   _____

3. What are the proper steps for providing sighted guide assistance to a blind patient?

_____

_____

_____

_____

_____

_____

_____

_____

_____

_____

4. Why might a senior adult make a statement like, "You are so rough"?

_____

_____

5. What is the purpose of the Americans with Disabilities Act (ADA) and Americans with Disabilities Act Amendments Act (ADAAA)?

_____

_____

_____

_____

_____

_____

_____

_____

_____

_____

_____

6. New building codes require Braille plates for identification purposes. Name at least three locations where the plates should be placed.

_____

7. Why is it better to use a professional interpreter as opposed to a family member or friend during a patient office visit?

_____

_____

_____

_____

_____

_____

8. List four examples of auxiliary aids and services that can be used to assist hearing-impaired and deaf patients.

_____

_____

_____

_____

_____

_____

_____

9. How should a medical assistant navigate a vision impaired patient up the stairs?

_____

_____

_____

_____

_____

_____

10. List three examples of *accessible design* features that can accommodate patients with disabilities.

_____

_____

_____

_____

_____

CERTIFICATION PRACTICE

Assignment 6-5

Choose the best answer and place the corresponding letter in the blank.

____ 1. The average life expectancy in 2015 is what age?

    A. 69 years

    B. 79 years

    C. 80 years

    D. 85 years

____ 2. What is the name that most seniors prefer to be addressed as?

    A. First name

    B. Honey, Sweetie

    C. Last name

    D. Mr. or Mrs.

___ 3. What color leash would a signal dog be wearing?

    A. Orange

    B. Yellow

    C. Blue

    D. Red

___ 4. All gestures do not mean the same thing to all cultures. What gesture would be considered acceptable by most people?

    A. Direct eye contact

    B. Proxemics

    C. Warm smile

    D. Pointing a finger

___ 5. Who would be responsible for arranging for an interpreter during an office visit for an LEP patient?

    A. The provider's office

    B. The patient

    C. The family of the patient

    D. The government

___ 6. When assisting blind patients, all would be correct procedures *except*:

    A. Introduce *new* people as they enter the area and let the patient know where people are positioned in reference to the patient.

    B. Use sighted words.

    C. Use verbal cues.

    D. Move the patient's personal belongings without their knowledge.

___ 7. When working with an interpreter, the correct room arrangement would be:

    A. Place the chairs in a row.

    B. Set the room up in a circular pattern.

    C. Set the room up in a triangular pattern.

    D. Set the room up so the medical assistant is beside the patient.

___ 8. Speech reading is also known as which of the following?

    A. Tongue movement

    B. Facial gestures

    C. Reading lips

    D. Listening

___ 9. What is paramount in the eyes of most seniors?

    A. Professional behavior

    B. Work ethic

    C. Articulation of medical terminology

    D. Compliments and the nice gestures

___ 10. Impairment that restricts or prevents normal functioning of a particular limb or group of limbs would be termed:

    A. mental illness.

    B. dementia.

    C. mental impairment.

    D. physical disability.

SKILL APPLICATION CHALLENGE
Assignment 6-6: Research Activity

1. Select your own culture group or one in which you are interested (Japanese, Greek, Irish, etc.) and do an Internet search for issues related to aging in that group using "elderly". Write a half-page summary on your findings.

2. Contact an interpreting company and find out how much it would cost to have an interpreter come out to your location and provide interpreting services for one hour for the following: an Arabic interpreter, a blind interpreter, and a Spanish interpreter.

3. Go to the Department of Labor website (www.dol.gov). Research information on this website and list four federal agencies that enforce the ADA and ADAAA rules besides the Department of Labor.

4. To learn more about the ADAAA, log on to the EEOC website (www.eeoc.gov) and search for the topic ADAAA.

5. Enter the phrase "National Technical Institute for the Deaf" into an Internet browser. Bring up the home page of the website and read one of the articles under *Articles and Resources*. Write a half-page report on your findings.

6. Type the words "Alzheimer Association" into an Internet browser. Bring up the home page. Click on *Resources* and click on *Fact Sheets*. Print a fact sheet on Alzheimer's disease. Share the information with your classmates.

FIELD APPLICATION CHALLENGE
Assignment 6-7

Read the following Field Application Challenge and respond to the question following the scenario.
You work for a family practice. Joshua, an 11-year-old developmentally disabled patient, is here with his mother. He needs to have his blood drawn and have his MMR vaccination today. For the most part, Joshua does a good job of sitting still, but has a history of moving during invasive procedures. How will you approach Joshua?

_____

_____

_____

_____

JOURNALING EXERCISE
Assignment 6-8

What content within this chapter was most meaningful to you? Why? List some examples of how you might apply information contained in this chapter, both during your training and after you enter the health care industry. Reflect on Davene's "Professionalism Mentor" tips for assisting patients with special needs. How would you develop a better understanding of patient needs and apply the professionalism keys to your work as a medical assistant? If you know of a special needs patient, consider how you will apply what you have learned in this chapter.

CHAPTER **7**

Health Coaching and Patient Navigation

VOCABULARY REVIEW

Assignment 7-1: Sentence Completion

Fill in the blanks below with essential terms from this chapter.

1. A(n) _____ is usually a registered nurse (RN) who can manage and consolidate the information acquired through multiple modalities.

2. _____ involves focusing on the information at hand, not allowing your mind to wander, and observing the patient for additional cues other than what they are stating verbally.

3. A(n) _____ is a person who provides individualized evaluation and subsequent management and encouragement to achieve superior patient health outcomes.

4. _____ is a way to identify the patient's feelings and respond with understanding.

5. A(n) _____ is the way to reverse the effect of a drug.

6. A(n) _____ is an impartial party who listens to patients' concerns and provides them access to the systems in place that would resolve their conflicts.

7. A(n) _____ is the person who is able to assist a patient navigating the health system.

8. _____ means identifying and monitoring groups of patients with similar diagnoses.

Assignment 7-2: Grammar Challenge

Select/underline the correct word.

1. Policies relating to patients are developed and derived from both the legal and ethical responsibilities of the practice to (it's, its) patients.

2. Any blood pressure under 140/90 is considered controlled for most adult patients, but a goal of (fewer, less) than 150/90 is used for patients over 60 years old.

3. Patients should take their anticoagulants exactly as directed and at the same time each day and should receive education regarding foods, medications, and herbal supplements that (affect, effect) blood clotting.

4. There are times when the patient needs more (then, than) just coaching to improve their health and overall well-being.

5. As a well-informed health coach and patient navigator, you will explain the office policies and patient responsibilities, (which, that) include understanding and complying with the financial policy.

6. Medical assistants (may, might) also be called upon to develop instructional handouts and brochures for common topics within the practice where they are employed.

7. Verbal communication skills are even more important when speaking over the phone (since, because) facial expressions and body language cannot be seen.

CHAPTER REVIEW

Assignment 7-3: Short Answer

1. Describe at least two common health coaching topics presented over the phone.

   _____

   _____

   _____

2. List five barriers that can impede the educational process.

   _____

Assignment 7-4: Abbreviation Review

Write what each of the following abbreviations stands for.

1. ACO: _____

2. PCMH: _____

3. Afib: _____

4. NPP: _____

5. PPE: _____

6. HDL: _____

7. LDL: _____

8. PT: _____

9. INR: _____

10. DEXA: _____

11. FEMA: _____

Assignment 7-5: Matching

Match the term with its definition and place the corresponding letter in the blank.

_____ 1. Denial

_____ 2. Anger

_____ 3. Empathy

_____ 4. Bargaining

_____ 5. Depression

_____ 6. Acceptance

A. Way to identify the patient's feelings and respond with understanding. Used to strengthen rapport with the patient.

B. The grief stage where the person is trying to shut out the reality and magnitude of their situation, often creating a false reality.

C. The grief stage when the patient is now overcome with the reality that they are going to die but become despondent over their fate, often feeling that there is no point in going on or doing anything.

D. In this stage of grief, patients become difficult to care for because of the misplaced feelings of anger for what has happened to them.

E. The grief stage when the patient believes that somehow they can undo what has happened by changing their lifestyle or negotiating a compromise to live a little longer.

F. At this point in the stages of grief the patient has come to terms with the inevitable future and plans accordingly in preparation for their impending death.

CERTIFICATION PRACTICE

Assignment 7-6

Choose the best answer and place the corresponding letter in the blank.

_____ 1. Ways to stimulate patient compliance include:

   A. Including family members in the session.

   B. Calling the patient, one to two days after the session.

   C. Being a good role model.

   D. All of the above

_____ 2. All are common topics for health coaching *except*:

   A. smoking cessation.

   B. Medicare and Medicaid's new reimbursement procedures.

   C. diabetes management.

   D. heart health.

_____ 3. All are examples of community resources for patient health care needs *except*:

   A. social service organizations.

   B. interpreting services.

   C. Chamber of Commerce.

   D. public health and human services.

_____ 4. Barriers that may prohibit patient compliance include:

   A. transportation.

   B. interest.

   C. time.

   D. All of the above

_____ 5. Examples of educational sessions over the telephone would include all of the following *except*:

   A. self-exams.

   B. introduction of new medication.

   C. special dietary changes.

   D. instructions for the patient to see a specialist.

___ 6. Which of the following would not reflect a cholesterol number that patients should strive to achieve?

   A. Total cholesterol score less than 200

   B. LDL less than 99

   C. HDL that is less than 40

   D. All of the above

___ 7. Patients on anti-coagulation therapy should:

   A. avoid liver.

   B. take the medication exactly as directed.

   C. take the medication at the same time each day.

   D. All of the above

___ 8. Instructing patients on how to take their medications is one of the most frequent topics for health coaching. The medical assistant:

   A. need not be familiar with the medication as the pharmacy will provide an information sheet.

   B. should follow only the provider instruction with no need to know the reason the medication was prescribed.

   C. should know the economic resources of the patient as it will help in determining if compliance is even an option.

   D. All of the above

___ 9. Which of the following statements is true regarding blood pressure monitoring?

   A. Any blood pressure under 140/90 is considered controlled for most adult patients.

   B. A goal of less than 150/90 diastolic is used for patients over 60 years old.

   C. Patients should be encouraged to check their blood pressures one to two times per day and to check it at the same time each day.

   D. All of the above

___ 10. As a medical assistant, health coach, and patient navigator, you will need to know how to recognize the signs of substance abuse. Which of following is not a sign of substance abuse?

   A. Never missing school or work, a sudden interest in school activities or work, or an improvement in grades or work performance

   B. Lack of energy, motivation, or lack of interest in clothing, grooming, or looks

   C. Your discovery that money is missing or has been stolen or that items have disappeared from your home

   D. A drastic change in behavior and relationships with family and friends

SKILL APPLICATION CHALLENGE

Assignment 7-7: Research Activities

1. Select a disease or disorder about which to act as health coach to other students in your class. You can deliver a presentation using PowerPoint, you may give a speech in regards to your topic, or create a YouTube presentation. You should use a variety of visual aids. Key points should include the following: the name of the disease or condition, symptoms of the disease, risk factors for the disease, diagnostic tools used to diagnose the disease, treatment options, and tips for living with the disease. Consider the members of your audience. How would they learn best? What methods would you use to be an effective health coach? Do you have access to audiovisual equipment or the Internet? Who can provide you with additional information?

2. As a medical assistant in a pediatric office, you are given the task of updating the patient education materials. The file contains handouts on immunizations, nutrition, and healthy/exercise lifestyles. Many of the handouts are old. Do an Internet search and review the top diseases that are plaguing pediatric patients today. List five new educational topics you would include and provide materials for each one.

3. Make up a list of support groups (community resources) along with their contact information that are available in your local area. Look in the phone book, on websites, in local hospital directories, or in local newspapers. Be prepared to share this information with class members. Once all of the class has shared their findings, merge the lists so that one new list contains everyone's information. Display the list somewhere in the classroom so that it can be used as a reference when conducting health coaching and patient navigator sessions.

FIELD APPLICATION CHALLENGE

Assignment 7-8

Read the following Field Application Challenges and respond to the questions following each scenario. Utilize the Internet to help you answer the questions.

1. You work for a dermatology office. What advice might you give to an 11-year-old fair-skinned girl who is planning to visit her grandparents in Florida for the summer?

   _____

   _____

   _____

2. You work for an orthopedic office. One of your patients is a child who just had a cast put on his arm. What would be helpful information for this patient and his parents?

   _____

   _____

   _____

   _____

   _____

   _____

   _____

JOURNALING EXERCISE

Assignment 7-9

In the new health care models, how would you incorporate the professionalism keys to demonstrate your ability to be an effective health coach and patient navigator? What difference do you see in the health coach and patient navigator roles? Which of the professionalism keys do you think will be most helpful in these roles?

C H A P T E R **8**

Principles of Infection Control

VOCABULARY REVIEW

Assignment 8-1: Matching

Match the term with its definition and place the corresponding letter in the blank.

____ 1. Antigen

____ 2. Antibody

____ 3. Biohazard

____ 4. Vector

____ 5. Fomite

____ 6. Normal flora

____ 7. Opportunistic infection

____ 8. Sharps

____ 9. Bloodborne pathogens

____ 10. Epidemiology

____ 11. Medical asepsis

____ 12. Pathogen

A. Contaminated nonliving objects such as water glasses, computer keyboards, telephones, doorknobs, dressings, catheter tubing, needles, and IV tubing

B. Microorganisms present everywhere in our environment that are helpful and necessary for normal life processes of plants, animals, and humans

C. Referred to as AIDS-defining illnesses because they are typical illnesses that are seen only in patients with progressed HIV or those patients who have progressed to the end stage called AIDS

D. Protein particles produced by the lymphocytes to promote immunity and provide resistance to specific pathogens

E. The invading antagonistic organism

F. Devices such as needles, sharp instruments, scalpels, glass slides, glass tubes, and pipettes that could cause puncture wounds or other injuries to the skin

G. Any substance contaminated with blood, body fluids, or OPIM that could transmit disease

H. Carriers of microorganisms such as insects or rodents

I. Microorganisms that cause disease

J. Destruction of microorganisms after they leave the body

K. A pathogen that can be transmitted through blood or OPIM

L. The study of infectious disease

Assignment 8-2: Misspelled Words
Underline the correctly spelled term.

1. <u>disinfection</u>   dysinfection   disunfection

2. immunosupresed   imunosupresed   <u>immunosuppressed</u>

3. resistence   <u>resistance</u>   resistince

4. immunoglobulen   <u>immunoglobulin</u>   imunoglobulin

5. <u>sanitization</u>   sanitazation   sanatization

CHAPTER REVIEW

Assignment 8-3: Abbreviation Review
Write what each of the following abbreviations stands for.

1. AIDS: _____

2. OPIM: _____

3. OSHA: _____

4. PPE: _____

5. SDS: _____

6. BSI: _____

Assignment 8-4: Short Answer

1. List the five classifications of pathogenic organisms.

_____

2. List and describe the six stages of infection.

_____

_____

_____

_____

_____

3. Describe the purpose of the inflammatory response.

_____

_____

4. List both local and systemic signs of inflammation.

Local signs: _____   Systemic signs: _____

_____

5. Place the appropriate letter (B = biohazard container, S = sharps container, R = regular trash) beside each type of medical waste that corresponds with proper disposal of biohazardous wastes when following OSHA guidelines.

   A. Microbiology specimens ___

   B. Dressing that contains blood or OPIM ___

   C. Cover slips ___

   D. Empty urine container ___

   E. Surgical pathology specimens ___

   F. Used gloves with no visible blood or OPIM ___

   G. Used needles ___

   H. Stool specimen container ___

   I. Drapes with vaginal secretions ___

   J. Empty containers that held semen samples ___

6. Under what circumstances might a health care facility dispose of items contaminated with all types of body fluids—including urine, saliva, and stool—into the biohazardous trash?

   _____

   _____

7. List and describe the environmental factors or conditions that must be present in order for a microorganism to grow and prosper.

   _____

   _____

   _____

   _____

   _____

   _____

   _____

   _____

   _____

   _____

8. OSHA provides standards, guidelines, and precautions for protecting the worker/employee based on "Exposure Determination". Give examples of the types of employees (job duties) that may fit into these categories.

   _____

   _____

   _____

   _____

CERTIFICATION PRACTICE
Assignment 8-5
Choose the best answer and place the corresponding letter in the blank.

____ 1. Choose the final step in the infection cycle.

    A. Portal of exit

    B. Reservoir

    C. Susceptible host

    D. Means of transmission

____ 2. Yeasts and molds would fall under the classification of:

    A. bacteria.

    B. fungi.

    C. rickettsiae.

    D. None of the above

____ 3. In which of the following ways can a pathogen enter a susceptible host?

    A. Inhalation

    B. Ingestion

    C. Sexual transmission

    D. All of the above

____ 4. In which stage of infection would a patient be if presenting with a general complaint of malaise?

    A. Incubation

    B. Acute

    C. Prodromal

    D. Invasion and multiplication

____ 5. Which of the following would be considered a systemic sign of inflammation?

    A. Fever

    B. Pain

    C. Redness

    D. Heat

____ 6. Which of the following are components that participate in the immune response?

    A. T-cells

    B. B-cells

    C. Antibodies

    D. All of the above

____ 7. During which type of immunity are T-cells present?

    A. Humoral

    B. Cell-mediated

    C. Passive

    D. Natural

____ 8. When following standard precautions, which of the following should be considered as potentially infectious?

    A. All body fluids

    B. Non-intact skin

    C. Mucous membranes

    D. All of the above

___ 9. Which of the following would be an example of an engineering control?

    A. The method by which a task is performed

    B. Device used to separate employees from hazards

    C. Puncture-resistant sharps container

    D. Only B and C

___ 10. Which of the following must be available to all employees regarding the use of hazardous chemicals used in the facility?

    A. SDS forms

    B. Biohazard trash cans

    C. Ventilation hoods

    D. None of the above

SKILL APPLICATION CHALLENGE

Assignment 8-6: Case Study

Today's date is October 10, 20XX. Kelly L. Leonard, CMA (AAMA), is working in Dr. Pendleton's general practice and began work at 8:00 a.m this morning. At 9:40 a.m., Kelly is preparing to perform an erythrocyte sedimentation rate (ESR) on a patient sample from Grace Beavers. This requires Kelly to transfer blood using a disposable pipette from the specimen tube to a kit tube. She is wearing gloves and her lab coat. While opening the lavender top tube of blood, some of the blood splashes in Kelly's L. eye. Kelly immediately flushes her left eye, using the eyewash station for 20 minutes and reports the incident to her supervisor, Janet Vick, RN. What PPE or other precautions should Kelly have taken to prevent this exposure from occurring in the first place?

_____

_____

COMPLETING SPECIAL FORMS

Assignment 8-7: Exposure Incident Report Exercise

Work Form Necessary: FORM 8-1

Directions: Using the Case Study in Assignment 8-7 and the information below, fill out Work Form 8-1 (Employee Bloodborne Pathogen Exposure Incident Report).

Kelly's home address is 1234 Carter Lane, Toddler, OH, 14458. Date of birth is 5/19/1987, and her hiring date is 10/1/2014. The source individual gave permission for her blood to be tested for HIV and HBV and Kelly also gave permission to have her blood tested. The source individual tested positive for HBV and negative for HIV. Kelly tested negative for both. Gamma globulin was administered to Kelly on 10-10-20XX by Dr. Connor James with recommended follow-up testing in six months. The incident was logged by Kelly's supervisor, Janet Vick, RN, and assigned a case number of LEO-XX.

FIELD APPLICATION CHALLENGE

Assignment 8-8

Read the following Field Application Challenge and respond to the questions following the scenario.

The OSHA inspector drops by the medical facility for an unannounced inspection. While observing in the phlebotomy area, he notices that the medical assistant is not wearing a lab coat and is wearing only one glove on the hand used for drawing the sample. The medical assistant has also removed the index finger of the glove for better palpation of the vein. After cleansing the site, the medical assistant palpates the site again and then performs the venipuncture.

1. List the errors made by the medical assistant in the above scenario.

_____

_____

_____

_____

JOURNALING EXERCISE

Assignment 8-9

Protecting the health and safety of patients and health care workers is vital. In order to do this everyone must understand the principles of infection control. What content within this chapter was most meaningful to you? Why? List some examples of how you might apply information contained in this chapter, both during your training and after you enter the health care industry. How will you apply the professionalism keys to demonstrate your awareness and competency to apply the principles of infection control as a medical assistant?

Work Form 8-1

OSHA's Form 301
Injury and Illness
Incident Report

This *Injury and Illness Incident Report* is one of the first forms you must fill out when a recordable work-related injury or illness has occurred. Together with the *Log of Work-Related Injuries and Illnesses* and the accompanying *Summary*, these forms help the employer and OSHA develop a picture of the extent and severity of work-related incidents.

Within 7 calendar days after you receive information that a recordable work-related injury or illness has occurred, you must fill out this form or an equivalent. Some state workers' compensation, insurance, or other reports may be acceptable substitutes. To be considered an equivalent form, any substitute must contain all the information asked for on this form.

According to Public Law 91-596 and 29 CFR 1904, OSHA's recordkeeping rule, you must keep this form on file for 5 years following the year to which it pertains.

If you need additional copies of this form, you may photocopy the printout or insert additional form pages in the PDF, and then use as many as you need.

Completed by _____

Title _____

Phone (____) ____ - _____   **Date** ____ - ____ - ____
                                    Month   Day   Year

Note: *You can type input into this form and save it.*
Because the forms in this recordkeeping package are "fillable/writable" PDF documents, you can type into the input form fields and then save your inputs using the _____ . In addition, the forms are programmed to auto-calculate as appropriate.

Information about the employee

1) Full name _____

2) Street _____

3) City _____ State _____ ZIP _____

4) Date of birth ____ ____ ____
                 Month Day Year

5) Date hired ____ ____ ____
              Month Day Year
   ○ Male
   ○ Female

Information about the physician or other health care professional

6) Name of physician or other health care professional _____

7) If treatment was given away from the worksite, where was it given?

   Facility _____

   Street _____

   City _____ State _____ ZIP _____

8) Was employee treated in an emergency room?
   ○ Yes
   ○ No

9) Was employee hospitalized overnight as an in-patient?
   ○ Yes
   ○ No

Page ___ 1 ___ of ___ 1 ___

Attention: This form contains information relating to employee health and must be used in a manner that protects the confidentiality of employees to the extent possible while the information is being used for occupational safety and health purposes.

U.S. Department of Labor
Occupational Safety and Health Administration

Form approved OMB no. 1218-0176

Information about the case

10) Case number from the *Log* _____
    (Transfer the case number from the Log after you record the case.)

11) Date of injury or illness ____ ____ ____
                              Month Day Year

12) Time employee began work ____ ○ AM ○ PM

13) Time of event ____ ○ AM ○ PM   ○ Check if time cannot be determined

14) What was the employee doing just before the incident occurred? Describe the activity, as well as the tools, equipment, or material the employee was using. Be specific. *Examples:* "climbing a ladder while carrying roofing materials"; "spraying chlorine from hand sprayer"; "daily computer key-entry."

    _____

15) What Happened? Tell us how the injury occurred. *Examples:* "When ladder slipped on wet floor, worker fell 20 feet"; "Worker was sprayed with chlorine when gasket broke during replacement"; "Worker developed soreness in wrist over time."

    _____

16) What was the injury or illness? Tell us the part of the body that was affected and how it was affected; be more specific than "hurt," "pain," or "sore." *Examples:* "strained back"; "chemical burn, hand"; "carpal tunnel syndrome."

    _____

17) What object or substance directly harmed the employee? *Examples:* "concrete floor"; "chlorine"; "radial arm saw." *If this question does not apply to the incident, leave it blank.*

    _____

18) If the employee died, when did death occur? Date of death ____ ____ ____
                                                              Month Day Year

[Save Input]   [Add a Form Page]   [Reset]

Public reporting burden for this collection of information is estimated to average 22 minutes per response, including time for reviewing instructions, searching existing data sources, gathering and maintaining the data needed, and completing and reviewing the collection of information. Persons are not required to respond to the collection of information unless it displays a current valid OMB control number. If you have any comments about this estimate or any other aspects of this data collection, including suggestions for reducing this burden, contact: US Department of Labor, OSHA Office of Statistical Analysis, Room N-3644, 200 Constitution Avenue, NW, Washington, DC 20210. Do not send the completed forms to this office.

C H A P T E R **9**

Sterilization Procedures, Instrument Identification, and Surgical Supplies

VOCABULARY REVIEW

Assignment 9-1: Fill in the Blank

Fill in the blanks below with Essential Terms from this chapter.

1. _____   To cut open or cut apart

2. _____   Material used to tie off tubular structures such as the fallopian tubes or vas deferens

3. _____   Sealants in these products provide the incision site with instant strength usually within a matter of minutes of application

4. _____   Part of the instrument that the surgeon uses to hold the instrument

5. _____   Special hinge found on ring-handled instruments

6. _____   Device used to remove small foreign bodies from the eye, ear, or wound

7. _____   A type of medication that is used to produce a lack of feeling in patients during a surgical procedure

8. _____   Type of strand or fiber that is used to sew

9. _____   The amount of time the disinfecting solution may be used once the bottle has been opened

10. _____   To make sanitary or clean

11. _____   Device that cleans instruments by transmitting sound waves through a cleaning fluid

Assignment 9-2: Matching I

Match the term with its definition and place the corresponding letter in the blank.

___ 1. Atraumatic needle

___ 2. Autoclave

___ 3. Endoscopes

___ 4. Medical asepsis

___ 5. Minimum effective concentration (MEC)

___ 6. Shelf life

___ 7. Fenestrated

___ 8. Jaws

___ 9. Ratchet

___ 10. Shank

___ 11. Serrations

___ 12. Traumatic needle

A. These are found on the inside tips of some instruments; their purpose is to help improve gripping power when working with tissue that is slippery

B. The destruction of organisms after leaving the body

C. The tips of certain instruments that are used to grasp or clamp items

D. The locking mechanism that tightens or locks the tips of an instrument at varying degrees

E. Swaged needles

F. The long straight portion of the instrument that connects the handle with the tip of the instrument

G. The concentration of a high-level disinfectant that is necessary to kill bacterial spores

H. Eyed needles

I. Illuminated flexible or sometimes rigid tubes used to view body structures or organs

J. Compared to that of a pressure cooker; it displaces all the air with steam, which allows for greater pressure (15 pounds of pressure per square inch [psi]) to reach a heat of 250°F to 254°F [121°C to 123°C])

K. The amount of time the solution may be stored unopened before losing its potency (the expiration date on the container)

L. Having one or more openings

CHAPTER REVIEW

Assignment 9-3: Abbreviation Review

Write what the following abbreviations stand for.

MEC: _____

SDS: _____

EtO: _____

Four "Rs": _____

Assignment 9-4: Short Answer

1. List and describe four types of anesthesia.

   A. _____

   _____

   _____

   B. _____

   _____

   _____

C. _____

_____

_____

D. _____

_____

_____

2. List five common solutions used in minor surgery and explain their use.

A. _____

_____

B. _____

_____

C. _____

_____

D. _____

_____

E. _____

_____

3. Describe the function of a surgical wick.

_____

_____

_____

4. List and explain various ways to close the skin other than the use of sutures and staples.

A. _____

_____

_____

_____

B. _____

_____

_____

5. Describe the different types of disinfecting solutions and which microorganisms each one is capable of destroying, and explain under which conditions you would use each type.

A. _____

_____

B. _____

_____

_____

_____

C. _____

_____

_____

_____

_____

6. List three different types of wrapping materials and unique features of each type.

A. _____

_____

_____

_____

_____

_____

_____

B. _____

_____

_____

_____

_____

C. _____

_____

_____

_____

_____

_____

7. List the chain of events that must occur in order to achieve complete sterilization when using the autoclave as your means of sterilization.

A. _____

B. _____

C. _____

D. _____

E. _____

8. Compare and contrast the differences between medical and surgical asepsis and list examples of each.

A. _____

_____

_____

_____

_____

_____

B. _____

_____

_____

_____

_____

9. What is a biological indicator and what is the purpose of the indicator? How often should this test be performed?

_____

_____

_____

_____

_____

_____

10. Upon running a spore check on the autoclave, the results come back positive. What would be the next course of action?

_____

_____

_____

Assignment 9-5: Matching II

Match the instrument to its use.

Answer	Instrument	Use of instrument
_____	1. Speculum	A. Grasps suture needle during suturing
_____	2. Surgical knife	B. Grasps tissue
_____	3. Needle holder	C. Clamp off blood vessels
_____	4. Dressing forceps	D. Makes incisions, also referred to as a scalpel
_____	5. Hemostats	E. Cuts through tissue
_____	6. Uterine curette	F. Opens structures that are constricted
_____	7. Bandage scissors	G. Used to obtain tissue from the endocervical and uterine area
_____	8. Operating scissors	H. An instrument that is used to increase the viewing area of a body cavity for examination purposes.
_____	9. Dilators	I. Used to cut tape, gauze, bandages, and dressings
_____	10. Tissue forceps	J. Grasps tissue and packs wounds

CERTIFICATION PRACTICE

Assignment 9-6

Choose the best answer and place the corresponding letter in the blank.

____ 1. To determine if a pack is sterile, check the:

A. sterilization date.

B. sterilization indicator.

C. general condition of the wrapping material, confirming there are no signs of moisture, holes, or other defects.

D. All of the above

____ 2. Which of the following statements is true regarding labeling of a sterilization pack?

A. List the name of the item, date of sterilization, and first initial and last name of the person who prepared the pack for sterilization.

B. List the date of use.

C. Remove for use in a last-in first-out order.

D. All of the above

____ 3. The type of suture material that is used when suturing deeper layers of the skin or when suturing structures that are difficult to reach is called:

A. absorbable.

B. nonabsorbable.

C. glue.

D. cold spray.

____ 4. The most common gas used for sterilization because of its ability to kill all forms of microorganisms including bacterial endospores is:

A. oxygen.

B. nitrogen.

C. ethylene oxide.

D. carbon dioxide.

____ 5. The most dependable and cost effective method of sterilization used in medical clinics is:

A. autoclaving.

B. chemical.

C. dry heat.

D. gas.

____ 6. Which of the following steps would come last when sanitizing an instrument?

A. Sanitizing

B. Disinfecting

C. Rinsing

D. Wiping dry with a non-lint-producing material such as muslin cloth

____ 7. Which of the following is a skin cleanser used to prepare the skin prior to surgery (it also helps reduce bacteria that could potentially cause skin infection)?

A. Sterile saline

B. Betadine

C. Hydrogen peroxide

D. Tincture of benzoin

___ 8. An instrument used to grasp and hold tissue and other items is:

    A. a scalpel.

    B. bandage scissors.

    C. a retractor.

    D. forceps.

___ 9. Which of the following is used to pack wounds and acts as an antiseptic that inhibits the growth of microorganisms?

    A. Saline applicators

    B. Steri-strips

    C. Iodoform sterile packing material

    D. Wicks

___ 10. Which of the following is a topical aerosol product that causes temporary relief from pain by cooling the skin also known as "cold spray"?

    A. Silver nitrate

    B. Ethyl chloride

    C. Iodine

    D. Rubbing alcohol

SKILL APPLICATION CHALLENGE

Assignment 9-7: Labeling

1. Label the parts of the following instrument:

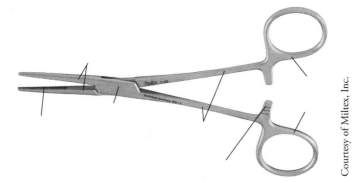

Courtesy of Miltex, Inc.

2. Identify the instruments below and record the name of each instrument in the blank.

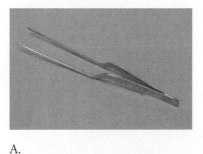

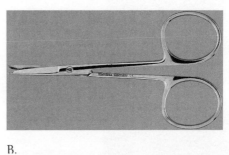

A. _____

B. _____

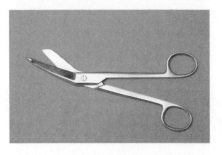

C. _____

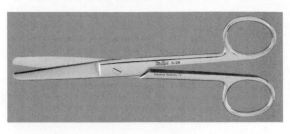

D. _____

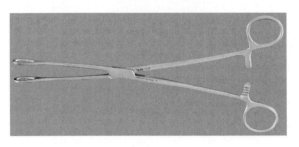

E. _____

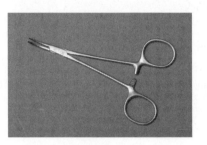

F. _____

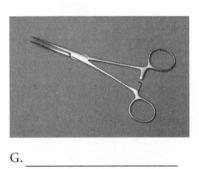

G. _____

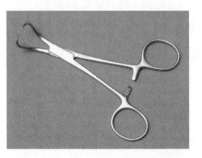

H. _____

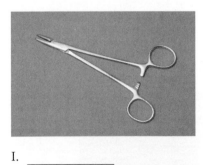

I. _____

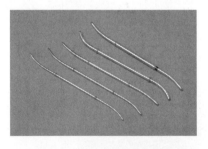

J. _____

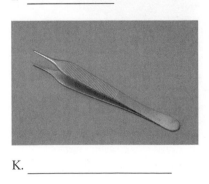

K. _____

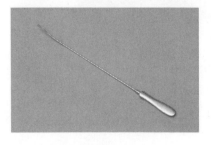

L. _____

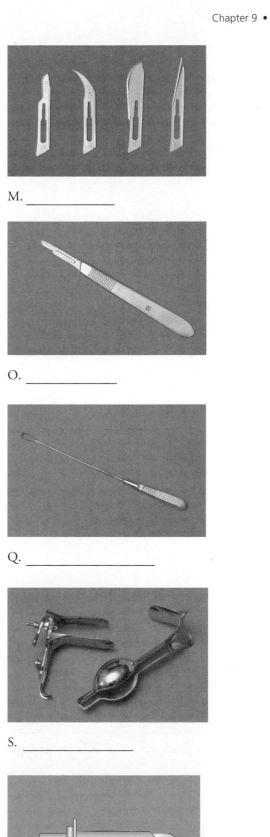

M. _____

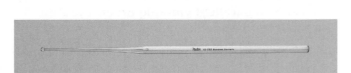

N. _____

O. _____

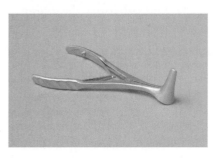

P. _____

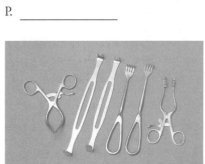

Q. _____

R. _____

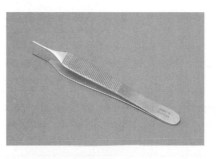

S. _____

T. _____

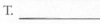

~10 cm

U. _____

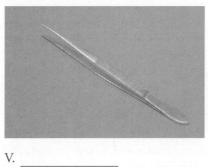

V. _____

Assignment 9-8: Ordering Exercise

The following sentences illustrate the steps that are taken to properly clean and maintain surgical instruments in order to minimize the risk of post-op infection to the patient and to keep the instruments in excellent working order. The steps are not in the correct order. In the blanks below, place the letter beside the number that represents the order in which each step is performed.

1. _____   A. Thoroughly rinse each instrument in distilled water or an approved rinsing solution.

2. _____   B. Dry each instrument with a muslin cloth or comparable material.

3. _____   C. Clean the area using an approved disinfectant.

4. _____   D. Thoroughly scrub each part of the instruments. Pay close attention to parts of the instruments that contain crevices, teeth, and serrations.

5. _____   E. Place pre-soaked instruments into basin filled with a solution of warm water and surgical soap.

6. _____   F. Inspect each instrument for any defects. Remove any instruments that are damaged.

7. _____   G. (Optional) Lubricate each instrument, especially on box locks and moving parts.

8. _____   H. Dry the lubricated instruments according to the instructions found on the lubricant label.

9. _____   I. Place each instrument on a waterproof drape until all instruments have been thoroughly sanitized and rinsed.

10. _____   J. Remove utility gloves, hang them upside down (by the finger tips) to dry, and wash hands.

11. _____   K. Wash your hands and apply utility gloves.

FIELD APPLICATION CHALLENGE

Assignment 9-9

Read the following Field Application Challenge and respond to the questions following the scenario.

You run a spore check with a load and send it to the lab. You continue to run the autoclave and sterilize six more laceration trays and three incision and drainage (I&D) trays between the time you ran the spore check and the time you receive the results. The report comes back as positive for spores. The chemical indicators in each pack have turned the appropriate color.

1. What will be the plan of action for using the autoclave from this point forward?

_____

_____

_____

_____

2. What should be done with any remaining sterile packs that were autoclaved at the same time the spore check was autoclaved or following the initial spore check?

_____

3. What should be done about the packs that were autoclaved at the time the spore check was performed or following the initial spore check and used on patients?

_____

_____

_____

JOURNALING EXERCISE

Assignment 9-10

The medical assistant must be familiar with how to properly clean, disinfect, and sterilize instruments to prevent patients from developing postoperative infections. What content within this chapter was most meaningful to you? Why? List some examples of how you might apply information contained in this chapter, and which professionalism keys would relate best to this topic.

C H A P T E R **10**

Assisting with Minor Office Surgeries and Wound Care Procedures

VOCABULARY REVIEW

Assignment 10-1: Misspelled Words

Underline the correctly spelled term.

1. Purulint	Purelent	Purulent
2. Exedate	Exodate	Exudate
3. Debribdement	Debridement	Debribment
4. Bandge	Bandage	Bandege
5. Serosangunious	Serosanguineous	Seronsangious
6. Sterile consceince	Sterile conscience	Stirele conscious
7. Sanguineous	Sangunious	Sangious
8. Absess	Abscess	Absecs
9. Asperation	Aspiration	Asperashun

Assignment 10-2: Definitions

Define the following terms.

1. Closed wound: _____

_____

2. Concentric circle: _____

_____

3. Dressing: _____

_____

_____

4. Open wound: _____

_____

5. Primary dressing: _____

_____

6. Secondary dressing: _____

_____

7. Subatmospheric pressure device: _____

8. Sterile conscience: _____

_____

9. Sebaceous cyst: _____

10. Electrocoagulation: _____

_____

CHAPTER REVIEW

Assignment 10-3: Matching

Match the item to be placed directly on the sterile field or placed on the side for an electrosurgical tray. Place the corresponding letter in the blank. Note: Answers may be used more than once.

_____ 1. Needle and syringe

_____ 2. Antiseptic solution/sterile saline

_____ 3. Cautery needles

_____ 4. Bovie pads

_____ 5. Electrosurgical unit

_____ 6. Specimen container

_____ 7. Sterile gauze pads

_____ 8. Triple antibiotic cream/ointment

_____ 9. Sterile gloves

_____ 10. Two sterile cups or basins

A. Items placed directly on the sterile field

B. Items placed on a side table

Assignment 10-4: Short Answer

1. Describe two different types of alternative treatments used to treat chronic wounds that will not heal.

A. _____

_____

_____

_____

_____

_____

_____

_____

B. _____

_____

_____

_____

_____

_____

_____

_____

_____

2. List the proper technique for preparing a Mayo stand for a surgical procedure.

_____

_____

_____

_____

_____

_____

_____

_____

_____

_____

_____

3. Describe the three stages of healing.

A. _____

_____

_____

_____

_____

_____

B. _____

_____

_____

_____

_____

_____

_____

C. _____

_____

_____

_____

_____

_____

4. Describe how a sterile conscience will help to reduce the patient's risk of developing a postop infection.

_____

_____

_____

_____

_____

_____

_____

CERTIFICATION PRACTICE

Assignment 10-5

Choose the best answer and place the corresponding letter in the blank.

_____ 1. Which of the following types of drape should be placed under the patient before cleansing the skin?

    A. Fenestrated drape

    B. Waterproof drape

    C. Sterile barrier

    D. Surgical towel

_____ 2. When bandaging, one needs to check for signs of poor circulation. All of the following are signs *except:*

    A. blueness around the nail beds.

    B. pallor.

    C. tingling sensation and numbness.

    D. itching.

_____ 3. Which of the following exudates contains serum only?

    A. Serous

    B. Sanguineous

    C. Serosanguineous

    D. Purulent

_____ 4. Which of the following exudates contains both serum and blood?

    A. Serous

    B. Sanguineous

    C. Serosanguineous

    D. Purulent

___ 5. Which of the following types of bandage is used when wrapping body parts that are uniform in size?

    A. Circular turn

    B. Spiral turn

    C. Reverse spiral turn

    D. Figure-eight bandage

___ 6. Which of the following types of bandage is used to immobilize a joint?

    A. Circular turn

    B. Spiral turn

    C. Reverse spiral turn

    D. Figure-eight bandage

___ 7. Which of the following bandaging techniques is used to anchor a bandage at the beginning or end of most bandaging applications?

    A. Circular turn

    B. Spiral turn

    C. Reverse spiral turn

    D. Figure-eight bandage

___ 8. A card that lists all of the specifics regarding physician preferences for procedures regularly performed is referred to as a:

    A. tickler card file.

    B. surgical procedure card file.

    C. surgery consent form.

    D. None of the above

___ 9. When setting up the surgical tray, it should be positioned so that the top of the tray is:

    A. 12 inches from the knees.

    B. even with the waist of the provider.

    C. countertop height.

    D. even with the waist of the preparer.

___ 10. You just finished setting up a sterile tray for an incision and drainage procedure. You are considered nonsterile during the procedure and will be assisting the physician as she needs items. The physician sticks her head in the room and tells you that she will be in just as soon as she performs a surgical scrub. You realize that you forgot to obtain the suture material, but the physician is almost scrubbed in and is ready for you to help her apply her PPE. You can't leave the room because you can't leave the tray unattended. What action would be best based in this scenario?

    A. Inform the physician that you are going to have to set up the tray again because you forgot an important item.

    B. Remain facing the tray, but work your way toward the door and yell down the hall for someone to bring the suture material to you.

    C. Once the physician has started the procedure and has taken ownership of the tray, inform the physician that you need to slip out to get the suture material.

    D. Ask the physician when she enters the room if she will get the suture material and just perform a new scrub.

SKILL APPLICATION CHALLENGE

Assignment 10-6: Preparing for Surgical Procedures

Fill in the table below with: (1) common patient instructions, (2) surgery room responsibilities, and (3) insurance responsibilities that are performed prior to, during, and following the surgical procedure. The first one has been completed for you. Note: Some tasks do not require an entry in all three columns. *Hint: Refer to Table 10-4 in your textbook.*

(1) Provide the patient with the following instructions:	(2) Surgery room responsibilities:	(3) Insurance responsibilities:
Any fasting or medication instructions	Block off the surgical suite in the appointment scheduler to prevent double booking	Notify the insurance company of the anticipated procedure

FIELD APPLICATION CHALLENGE

Assignment 10-7

Read the following Field Application Challenge and respond to the questions following the scenario.
This is your first day working with Dr. Janelle Speelman and you are assisting with a mole removal. You gather the supplies and set up a sterile tray for the procedure. The physician asks for 1% Lidocaine, and you hold the vial so that the physician can draw up the medication. The physician anesthetizes the patient and goes out of the room for a few minutes to allow time for the medication to take effect. While the physician is out of the room, you pick up the Lidocaine bottle to return it to its proper storage and notice that the label on the bottle reads 2% Lidocaine with epinephrine.

1. What should be your first course of action?

   A. Leave the surgery room and tell the physician about the mix-up.

   B. Immediately use computer or phone in surgery room to alert provider of the mix up.

   C. Tell the patient what happened.

   D. Privately tell the physician what happened upon her return to the surgery room.

2. Why did you choose this as your first course of action?

   _____

   _____

   _____

3. If after returning, the physician states that there is no problem and that she wants to go forward with the procedure, what will need to be done?

   A. Continue where you left off.

   B. Send someone new in to take your place.

   C. Set up an entirely new sterile tray and reprep the patient.

4. Why did you choose this response?

   _____

   _____

5. How can you make certain that nothing like this will ever happen again?

   _____

   _____

JOURNALING EXERCISE

Assignment 10-8

What content within this chapter was most meaningful to you? Why? After reading Davene's scenario regarding her experience receiving a cortisone injection in her shoulder and the medical assistant's demeanor, describe ways you can make the patient feel more at ease when she is nervous about having surgical procedures performed. What professionalism keys do you think would apply? Provide the rationale for your answer.

C H A P T E R **11**

Vital Signs and Measurements

VOCABULARY REVIEW

Assignment 11-1: Matching

Match the term with its definition and place the corresponding letter in the blank.

____ 1. Hyperpnea

____ 2. Dysrhythmia

____ 3. Afebrile

____ 4. Orthopnea

____ 5. Metabolism

____ 6. Baseline

____ 7. Calipers

____ 8. Pulse rhythm

____ 9. Pulse pressure

____ 10. Arrhythmia

A. Without fever

B. A known or initial value with which further determinations are compared

C. The interval timing between measured beats

D. Another name for dysrhythmia

E. The difference between the systolic and diastolic pressure

F. Irregularities in heart rhythm

G. Refers to breathing easiest while in a sitting or standing position

H. Occurs as nutrients are processed in the body; cells produce energy and heat is produced

I. An instrument used for measuring skinfolds to determine the percentages of body fat

J. Rapid and deep respirations

Assignment 11-2: Definitions

Define the following terms.

1. Diastole: _____

2. Korotkoff sounds: _____

3. Pulse volume: _____

4. Systolic pressure: _____

_____

_____

5. Vasodilation: _____

6. Metabolism: _____

_____

7. Bradycardia: _____

Assignment 11-3: Sentence Completion

Fill in the blanks below with Essential Terms from this chapter.

1. An excessively rapid heart rate of more than 100 beats per minute is known as _____.

2. A(n) _____ is the actual piece of equipment that measures the blood pressure (BP).

3. _____ is a decrease in the diameter of the cutaneous blood vessels, causing blood vessels to sink and trap more heat within the body.

4. Also known as the centigrade scale, _____ is the official scientific measurement of temperature.

5. _____ is the standard grade of measurement generally used for temperatures in the majority of medical offices in the United States.

6. A person who has an elevated body temperature is said to be _____.

7. _____ is breathing which is easiest while in a sitting or standing position.

8. The act of breathing is referred to as _____.

CHAPTER REVIEW

Assignment 11-4: Abbreviation Review

Write what each of the following abbreviations stands for.

1. BMI: _____

2. (C): _____

3. (F): _____

4. TPR: _____

5. BP: _____

6. CDC: _____

7. SLE: _____

8. CPR: _____

9. BPM: _____

10. O_2: _____

11. CO_2: _____

12. CHF: _____

13. COPD: _____

14. mmHg: _____

15. TIA: _____

16. MRI: _____

Assignment 11-5: Short Answer

1. Complete the information requested in the table below. Refer to the first line as an example.

Route	Location	Accuracy	Variables and Suggestions for Obtaining the Most Accurate Temperature and Avoiding Injury	Normal Temperature
Mouth/ oral cavity	Under the tongue, beside the frenulum linguae	Considered accurate if patient can close mouth completely and keep mouth closed throughout the procedure.	Should not be used when the patient has recently eaten, had something to drink, or smoked. Caution the patient about biting down on the thermometer.	98.6°F (37°C)
Rectal				
Aural/ tympanic membrane				
Axillary				
Temporal				

2. Identify the pulse points on the following figure.

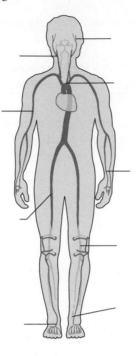

3. List the four standard vital signs and the normal adult (less than 60 years old) reading for each one.

_____

_____

_____

_____

4. List 12 factors that can cause changes in blood pressure. (*Hint:* Some factors are combined when referring to Table 11-9 in the textbook.)

_____

_____

CERTIFICATION PRACTICE

Assignment 11-6

Choose the best answer and place the corresponding letter in the blank.

____ 1. Which of the following measurements is not considered to be a vital sign?

A. Temperature

B. Pulse

C. Respiration

D. Height

____ 2. A pulse rate of 50 in an adult would be indicated as:

A. normal rate.

B. bradycardia.

C. tachycardia.

D. bradypnea.

___ 3. When taking a radial pulse on a patient you note some irregularity in the rhythm. For how long should you count the pulse?

    A. One full minute

    B. 30 seconds

    C. 45 seconds

    D. 15 seconds

___ 4. Blood pressure that is lower than normal would be classified as:

    A. hypertension.

    B. hypotension.

    C. orthostatic hypotension.

    D. Both A and B

___ 5. Which of the following can affect the pulse rate?

    A. Emotions

    B. Physical activity

    C. Medications

    D. All of the above

___ 6. At what location is the diaphragm of the stethoscope placed when taking an apical pulse?

    A. At the fourth intercostal space to the left of the sternum

    B. To the right at midsternum level

    C. Over the apex of the heart at the fifth intercostal space just to the left of the midclavicular line

    D. At the third intercostal space to the left of the sternum

___ 7. Which of the following is the best indicator of weight-related health?

    A. Desirable weight chart

    B. BSA

    C. BMI

    D. Provider's opinion

___ 8. A patient with a BMI of 35 would be considered:

    A. at an acceptable weight.

    B. obese.

    C. overweight.

    D. normal.

___ 9. In order for an adult heart rate to be considered tachycardia, it must be above:

    A. 100 BPM.

    B. 120 BPM.

    C. 115 BPM.

    D. 110 BPM.

___ 10. Calculate the pulse deficit if the radial pulse is 68 and the apical pulse is 80.

    A. 15

    B. 12

    C. 10

    D. 22

SKILL APPLICATION CHALLENGE

Assignment 11-7: Role Play

1. Choose another student to be your patient and obtain and record blood pressure readings after the following:

   A. Climbing a flight of stairs:

   B. Being seated for 10 minutes:

   C. Immediately upon standing:

   D. Immediately upon lying down:

2. Explain the possible reasons for the differences in the readings.

   _____

   _____

   _____

Assignment 11-8: Plotting Activities

1. Plot the following height measurements on the height bar by drawing a line at the correct mark and placing the corresponding letter on the line.

   A. 5 feet, 5 inches

   B. 5 feet, 4½ inches

   C. 5 feet, 3 inches

   D. 5 feet, 2¼ inches

   E. 5 feet, ½ inch

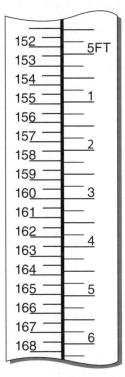

2. Plot the following weight measurements on the weight bar by drawing a line on the correct mark and placing the corresponding letter on the line.

   A. 11¼ pounds

   B. 12½ pounds

   C. 15 pounds

   D. 18¾ pounds

   E. 21¼ pounds

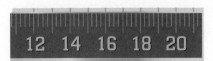

3. Plot the following blood pressure readings on the aneroid dial by placing a line on the correct mark for the systolic pressure (mark line with corresponding letter and an "S") and the correct mark for the diastolic pressure (mark the line with the corresponding letter of the reading and a "D").

A. 98/66

B. 104/78

C. 120/80

D. 146/88

E. 180/102

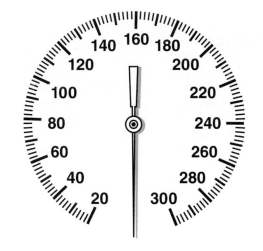

Assignment 11-9: Documentation Exercise

10/10/20XX 9:00 a.m. Mr. Anthony is a new patient and is here for a complete physical examination. You obtain his height (73 inches) and weight (175 pounds). He tells you that he is concerned about his blood pressure and wants to be certain that it is okay. Vital sign measurements include: temperature taken by the temporal artery method (99.6°F), pulse rate of 110, a respiration rate of 20, and a blood pressure rate of 138/86. Document the information into the following chart note.

FIELD APPLICATION CHALLENGE

Assignment 11-10

Read the following Field Application Challenge and respond to the questions following the scenario.

You have been asked to take a pulse and a blood pressure reading on 80-year-old Mrs. Leonard, who is very frail and thin. The provider is running ahead of schedule and is waiting on you so he can examine the patient. You are having to work rather quickly. You take the patient's pulse rate, which is 96 beats per minute. You notice that the patient's heart appears to skip a few beats. The patient's blood pressure is 152/94.

1. What type of blood pressure cuff would work best on this patient? _____

2. After reading about variables that can affect blood pressure readings in the chapter, what may be a contributor to the patient's pulse rate being so high?

_____

3. Would the patient be considered to have controlled blood pressure?

_____

4. The patient's heart rhythm would be termed as what?

_____

JOURNALING EXERCISE
Assignment 11-11

Obtaining accurate vital signs is an important role of the medical assistant. Physical changes that occur in the body from one visit to the next may be detected through a change in a patient's vital signs. What content within this chapter was most meaningful to you? Why? List some examples of how you might apply information contained in this chapter and which of the professionalism keys would be most beneficial. Practice taking and recording your vital signs daily for a week, and enter your readings and how they fit in a healthy lifestyle. Do you need to make changes or improvements?

C H A P T E R **1 2**

The Physical Exam

VOCABULARY REVIEW

Assignment 12-1: Misspelled Words

Underline the correctly spelled term.

1.	asculation	auscultation	ascultation
2.	examantion	escamination	examination
3.	inspecsion	inspectsion	inspection
4.	manipulation	manipulasion	manipulashun
5.	mestuation	mensuration	menestration
6.	observashun	obsurvation	observation
7.	palpitation	palpashun	palpation
8.	percussion	purcussion	percusion
9.	posture	potsure	pausture
10.	timpanny	tympany	timpany
11.	vertico	vertigo	vurtigo

Assignment 12-2: Matching

Match the term with its definition and place the corresponding letter in the blank.

_____ 1. Palpation

_____ 2. Posture

_____ 3. Inspection

_____ 4. Auscultation

A. Applying passive movement to a joint while using force

B. Position of the body

C. Disturbance in the equilibrium of the body and balance when a patient becomes dizzy

D. The process of measuring

___ 5. Vertigo

    E. The process of observing the patient for any signs of pathology that might indicate a disease or disorder, including physical, mental, and emotional signs

___ 6. Mensuration

    F. Touching the body to evaluate pain and tenderness, and the location and size of internal organs

___ 7. Manipulation

    G. Using the fingertips to tap the body slightly but sharply to determine position, size, and consistency of underlying structures or cavities

___ 8. Percussion

    H. Process of listening to sounds within the body with the aid of a stethoscope

___ 9. Tympany

    I. A process in which the body is inspected and systems are analysed to determine the presence or absence of disease

___ 10. Examination

    J. The process of watching or visualizing

___ 11. Observation

    K. A drum-like sound

CHAPTER REVIEW

Assignment 12-3: Abbreviation Review

Write what each of the following abbreviations stands for.

1. PPE: _____

2. LDL: _____

3. HEENT: _____

Assignment 12-4: Short Answer

1. List at least four techniques used during the physical examination.

    _____

2. Explain the technique of draping the patient in each position.

   a. Sitting: _____

    _____

   b. Supine: _____

   c. Prone: _____

   d. Dorsal recumbent: _____

    _____

   e. Sims': _____

    _____

    _____

   f. Semi-Fowler's: _____

    _____

   g. Full-Fowler's: _____

    _____

   h. Lithotomy: _____

_____

   i. Knee-chest: _____

_____

   j. Trendelenburg position: _____

_____

   k. Trendelenburg alternative: _____

_____

3. List at least five guidelines for preparing the exam room.

_____

   a. _____

_____

   b. _____

   c. _____

   d. _____

   e. _____

   f. _____

   g. _____

   h. _____

_____

   i. _____

_____

4. List at least five procedures that may be necessary before dismissing the patient.

_____

   a. _____

   b. _____

   c. _____

_____

   d. _____

   e. _____

   f. _____

   g. _____

CERTIFICATION PRACTICE

Assignment 12-5

Choose the best answer and place the corresponding letter in the blank.

____ 1. For an evaluation of the head, neck, and shoulders, which of the following positions would be used?

    A. Sitting

    B. Supine

    C. Dorsal recumbent

    D. Sims'

____ 2. In which of the following examination techniques are sounds evaluated by tapping the body with the fingers?

    A. Palpation

    B. Inspection

    C. Manipulation

    D. Percussion

____ 3. Which of the following components of the physical exam is either completely or partially performed by the medical assistant?

    A. General survey

    B. Vital signs

    C. Skin

    D. Both A and B

____ 4. Which of the following examination techniques would be used to evaluate the cardiovascular system?

    A. Auscultation

    B. Inspection

    C. Palpation

    D. All of the above

____ 5. The Sims' position would be used for which of the following types of exams?

    A. Rectal or prostate

    B. Abdominal

    C. Vaginal

    D. Genitalia

____ 6. A patient becomes very dizzy after getting down from the exam table. If at all possible the patient should be escorted back up onto the exam table and placed in which of the following positions?

    A. Prone

    B. Supine

    C. Trendelenburg

    D. Semi-Fowler's

____ 7. Of the following instruments, which one would be used to examine the ear?

    A. Aural speculum

    B. Otoscope

    C. Ophthalmoscope

    D. Pen light

___ 8. Which of the following would not be routinely used during a physical exam?

   A. Percussion hammer

   B. Stethoscope

   C. Hemostat

   D. Tongue depressor

___ 9. For which types of exams and procedures could the dorsal recumbent position be used?

   A. Abdominal

   B. Rectal

   C. Catheterization

   D. All of the above

___ 10. A patient presents with shortness of breath and chest pains; which position would assist the patient with breathing?

   A. Supine

   B. Prone

   C. Semi-Fowler's

   D. Lithotomy

SKILL APPLICATION CHALLENGES

Assignment 12-6: Role Play

Complete a tray setup for a complete physical examination. In the space below, list each instrument/supplies on your tray and the rationale for its use.

1. _____

2. _____

3. _____

4. _____

_____

5. _____

6. _____

_____

7. _____

8. _____

9. _____

10. _____

11. _____

12. _____

_____

13. _____

14. _____

15. _____

_____

16. _____

Assignment 12-7: Labeling

Identify the following patient positions and list one example for which the position is used.

	Position	Position Name	Example
1.	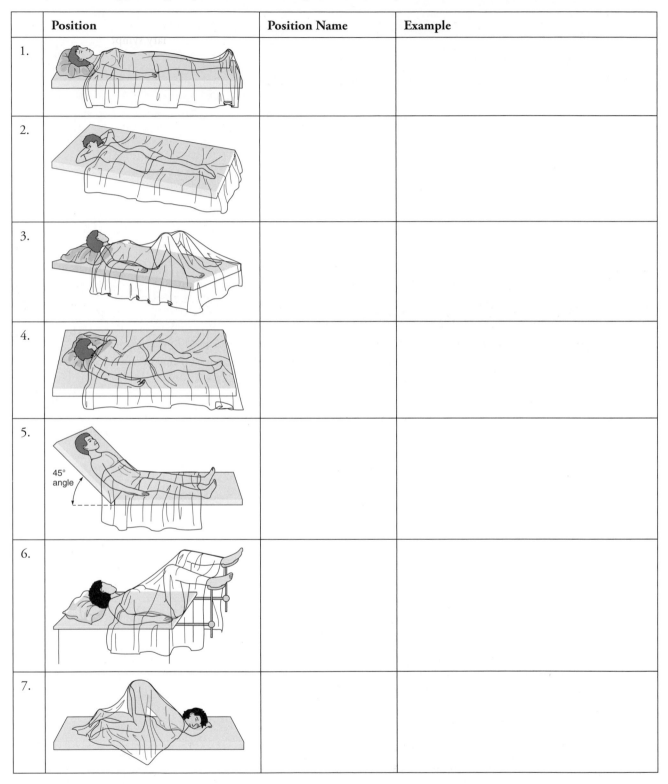		
2.			
3.			
4.			
5.			
6.			
7.			

FIELD APPLICATION CHALLENGE

Assignment 12-8

Read the following Field Application Challenge and respond to the questions following the scenario.
Mrs. Price is being seen in the office today for an assessment of her lower back pain and urinary symptoms. She appears to be very agitated and nervous. She is reluctant to get on the scale and later hesitates to give a urine specimen following the provider's examination.

1. What can you do as the medical assistant to convince the patient to step on the scale?

_____

_____

_____

_____

_____

2. How might you prompt the patient to give you the needed urine specimen?

_____

_____

_____

_____

_____

3. What can the medical assistant do to help reduce the patient's anxiety?

_____

_____

_____

_____

JOURNALING EXERCISE

Assignment 12-9

What content within this chapter was most meaningful to you? Why? List some examples of how you might apply information contained in this chapter, both during your training and after you enter the health care industry. Reflect on Davene's "Professionalism Mentor" tips on preparing for the physical exam. Think about what else you could do to ensure that the patient is as comfortable as possible during their examination. Write down two additional measures you would take to go above and beyond for your patient.

CHAPTER **13**

Eye and Ear Exams and Procedures

VOCABULARY REVIEW

Assignment 13-1: Matching

Match the term with its definition and place the corresponding letter in the blank.

_____ 1. Hyperopia

_____ 2. Auricle

_____ 3. Cerumen

_____ 4. Instillation

_____ 5. Glaucoma

_____ 6. Astigmatism

_____ 7. Conjunctiva

_____ 8. Snellen chart

_____ 9. Ophthalmic

_____ 10. Audiometer

_____ 11. Optician

_____ 12. Otoscope

_____ 13. Visual acuity

_____ 14. Tympanometer

_____ 15. Otic

A. Pertaining to the ear

B. Chart used to test distance visual acuity

C. Farsightedness; the ability to see only objects that are far away

D. A provider that is able to fills prescriptions for eyeglasses and contact lenses

E. Screening procedure used to detect errors in refraction

F. An electronic device with an attached probe that is placed snugly in the patient's ear

G. Instrument that measures hearing

H. Pertaining to the eye

I. Instrument used to examine the ear, during the physical examination

J. Inserting liquid, such as medication, into a body cavity such as the eye or ear

K. Ear wax

L. Abnormal curvature of the cornea causing blurred vision

M. A group of diseases that eventually may lead to destruction of the optic nerve, which is the nerve that allows us to see.

N. The outer ear

O. A thin layer over the cornea

Assignment 13-2: Sentence Completion

Fill in the blanks below with Essential Terms from this chapter.

1. A professional trained to identify and treat hearing or balance problems is the _____.

2. The medical doctor who specializes in diagnosis and treatment of diseases and disorders of the eye, prescribes medications, and performs various types of surgical procedures on the eye is a(n) _____.

3. The eye is a spherical organ that serves to allow vision. The _____ is the middle layer.

4. The _____ are found in the retina and are sensitive to bright light and help differentiate colors.

5. A foreign body or chemical can be flushed from the eye by performing a(n) _____.

6. A(n) _____ is a professional licensed to diagnose, prescribe, and treat eye disorders; can treat refractive disorders, but cannot perform surgery.

7. The instrument used to visualize the internal structures of the eye is the _____.

8. The _____ is an area in the posterior retina where incoming light waves focus, and light, color, and shapes are formed into nerve impulses.

9. The _____, commonly used for near vision assessment, consists of a series of readings with the type ranging in size from newspaper headline print to the small print commonly found in telephone directories.

10. The _____ is suspended by ciliary muscles that relax and contract to alter the shape of it.

11. _____ (nearsightedness) is the ability to see only objects that are close up.

12. The tympanic membrane vibrates from the incoming sound waves and passes that vibration along to the bones of the middle ear, or _____.

13. The _____ is a medical doctor who specializes in disorders of the ear, nose, and throat (ENT).

14. When referring to ear anatomy, the stapes rests against the membranous _____ of the cochlea, a snail-shaped structure of the inner ear.

15. _____ is farsightedness due to the aging process, caused by loss of elasticity of the lens.

16. _____ is a condition in which the lens and cornea do not bend light correctly, resulting in visual defects.

17. The _____ is the innermost layer of the eye.

18. Specialized cells called _____ and cones are found in the retina and are sensitive to dim light.

19. The _____ is the outermost lining of the eye's protective layers, also known as the white of the eye.

20. Intraocular pressure can be checked using an instrument called a(n) _____.

21. Sound waves pass through the auditory canal until they reach the eardrum, or _____.

CHAPTER REVIEW

Assignment 13-3: Abbreviation Review

Write what each of the following abbreviations stands for (Eyes).

1. O.D.: _____

2. OD: _____

3. OS: _____

4. OU: _____

5. DVA: _____

6. NVA: _____

Write what each of the following abbreviations stands for (Ears).

7. AD: _____

8. AOM: _____

9. AS: _____

10. AU: _____

11. ENT: _____

12. OE, OM, and OI: _____

13. TM: _____

Assignment 13-4: Matching

Match the degree of hearing loss to the associated problems

Degree of hearing loss:	Associated problems:
____ 1. Mild	A. Both speech and language deteriorate
____ 2. Moderate	B. Difficulty with speech. Does not hear most conversational speech
____ 3. Moderate–severe	C. May affect voice quality
____ 4. Severe	D. May affect language development, articulation, interaction with peers, and self-esteem
____ 5. Profound	E. May not hear soft speech

Assignment 13-5: Short Answer

1. Explain the difference between a conduction hearing loss and nerve deafness.

_____

_____

_____

_____

_____

_____

2. List three types of irrigation solutions used for eye injuries and conditions.

_____

3. List and describe four types of ear irrigation systems.

A. _____

_____

B. _____

_____

C. _____

_____

_____

_____

D. _____

_____

_____

_____

4. List the two types of gross hearing tests that utilize a tuning fork.

_____

5. Describe the medical assistant's role during visual acuity testing.

_____

_____

_____

_____

_____

_____

_____

_____

_____

_____

_____

_____

_____

_____

_____

_____

CERTIFICATION PRACTICE

Assignment 13-6

Choose the best answer and place the corresponding letter in the blank.

____ 1. Which of the following disorders is usually associated with increased ocular pressure?

    A. Cataract

    B. Stye

    C. Hyperopia

    D. Glaucoma

____ 2. Another name for the eardrum is the:

    A. auricle.

    B. pinna.

    C. tympanic membrane.

    D. eustachian tube.

____ 3. Choose the instrument that measures hearing acuity at different frequencies.

    A. Tympanometer

    B. Audiometer

    C. Tuning fork

    D. Weber test

____ 4. Irrigation fluid should be flushed through the eye from:

    A. the outer canthus to the inner canthus (corner).

    B. the inner canthus (corner) to the outer canthus.

    C. the middle of the eye.

    D. the upper eyelid.

____ 5. Interpret the following results of a visual acuity test: R. eye 20/10.

    A. The patient sees at 20 feet what most people are able to see from 10 feet.

    B. The patient sees at 10 feet what most people are able to see from 20 feet.

    C. The patient's vision is poor in the right eye.

    D. The patient's vision is excellent in the right eye.

____ 6. When screening a patient for any disorders or problems with the eyes, the medical assistant should ask which of the following questions?

    A. Are you experiencing any visual disturbances, double vision, or light sensitivity?

    B. Are you experiencing excessive tearing?

    C. Do you see blind spots, halos around objects, floaters, or flashes?

    D. All of the above

____ 7. Which of the following conditions may be indicated when a patient complains of an inability to see objects up close?

    A. Myopia

    B. Astigmatism

    C. Hyperopia

    D. Cataract

___ 8. Which of the following eye specialists would perform cataract surgery?

    A. Optometrist

    B. Optician

    C. Ophthalmologist

    D. General surgeon

___ 9. Which of the following degrees of hearing loss can affect language development?

    A. Mild

    B. Moderate

    C. Moderate–severe

    D. Severe

___ 10. When placing drops in a patient's eye(s), gently pull down on skin to expose the lower conjunctival sac and the patient is instructed to look:

    A. down.

    B. up.

    C. to the right.

    D. to the left.

SKILL APPLICATION CHALLENGE

Assignment 13-7: Documentation Exercise

Correctly chart the following information regarding a visual acuity screening using the Snellen chart as ordered by Dr. Leonard. The date is 10/10/20XX and it is 12:30 p.m. The patient read the line marked 20/40 with his right eye, 20/20 with his left eye, and 20/20 with both eyes. The patient was wearing eyeglasses and appeared to be squinting at times. Sign your name followed by the initials RMA.

Assignment 13-8: Research Activity

Research the topics of macular degeneration and retinal detachment and prepare a short report on these disorders. Include treatments used to correct or improve these conditions, including any new experimental treatments being used along with statistics on success.

FIELD APPLICATION CHALLENGE

Assignment 13-9

Read the following Field Application Challenge and respond to the questions following the scenario.
The provider orders an ear irrigation on a patient due to a buildup of cerumen. The medical assistant is in a hurry and places the irrigating solution into a bulb syringe without warming it. The patient begins to complain of pressure and dizziness during the irrigation, but the medical assistant reassures the patient that the procedure will be over within just a few minutes, and that it is common to feel a bit of pressure and dizziness, and continues the irrigation. There was no cerumen in the return basin.

1. What things did the medical assistant do incorrectly in the above scenario?

   _____

   _____

2. Why should the ear irrigation solution be warmed?

   _____

   _____

3. When the patient complained of pressure and dizziness what should the medical assistant have done?

   _____

   _____

JOURNALING EXERCISE

Assignment 13-10

What content within this chapter was most meaningful to you? Why? List some examples of how you might apply information contained in this chapter, both during your training and after you enter the health care industry. Reflect on Davene's "Professionalism Mentor" tips regarding routine or regular tasks. How would you avoid taking shortcuts when performing routine, regular, and daily tasks and procedures? Which of the professionalism keys do you think would most apply in this situation?

CHAPTER **14**

Cardiovascular Exams and Procedures

VOCABULARY REVIEW

Assignment 14-1: Matching I

Match the term with its definition and place the corresponding letter in the blank.

____ 1. Cardiac catheterization

____ 2. Dobutamine stress test

____ 3. Repolarization

____ 4. Baseline

____ 5. Bipolar leads

____ 6. Rhythm strip

____ 7. Cardiac cycle

____ 8. Stylus

____ 9. Cardioversion

____ 10. Electrolyte

A. The heated wire that produces the tracing on an ECG tracing

B. A procedure to reverse fibrillation of the heart

C. For patients who are unable to exercise on a treadmill due to physical limitations or age

D. A separate 12 inch recording of a particular lead, lead II generally appears at the bottom of a standard 12-Lead ECG. A rhythm strip assists the provider in detecting abnormalities in the patient's heart rhythm

E. Follows depolarization; returns the cells to a negative state. The resting phase of the cardiac cycle.

F. A solution that helps conduct the electrical current

G. A procedure in which a long catheter is threaded either from the groin region (femoral artery) or arm region (brachial artery) with the assistance of an X-ray camera (fluoroscopy) to look for occlusions in the blood vessels or heart

H. A flat, horizontal line separating ECG cycles

I. Leads on an ECG which record the electrical activity from two limb electrode at the same time (Leads I, II, and III)

J. Events that occur from the initiation of one heart beat to the onset of the next heart beat

Assignment 14-2: Matching II

Match the term with its definition and place the corresponding letter in the blank.

____ 1. Electrocardiogram

____ 2. Depolarization

____ 3. Precordial leads

____ 4. Normal sinus rhythm

____ 5. Isoelectric line

____ 6. Holter monitor

____ 7. Lead

____ 8. Artifact

____ 9. Augmented lead

____ 10. Amplitude

K. Unwanted interference on an ECG tracing

L. A lead on an ECG in which a single positive electrode is referenced against "null point" (a point with little or no significant electronic variation) between the remaining limb electrodes (aVR, aVL, and aVF)

M. A safe, noninvasive, and painless diagnostic tool to check the electrical activity of the heart

N. The straight line seen on the ECG strip

O. A discharge of electricity which causes the heart to contract during the cardiac cycle

P. The term used to describe an ECG that falls within normal limits (WNL). The normal adult heart rate ranges from 60 to 100 beats per minute (BPM).

Q. The height or amplitude of the beats on an ECG tracing or standardization

R. A portable ambulatory heart monitoring device that continuously looks at a patient's heart over a prolonged period of time (usually 24 hours but may be longer in some instances)

S. The chest leads in an ECG. Considered the unipolar leads and designated as V1-V6

T. A representation referenced on an ECG that transmits a recording of the electrical impulses coming from the heart at different angles

Assignment 14-3: Misspelled Words

Underline the correctly spelled term.

1. ahrrhythmia   arrhythmia   arrhythemia

2. cardioversion   cardeovertion   cardioveartion

3. difibrillation   difibrallation   defibrillation

4. interval   enterval   intervol

5. arthrectomy   orthrectomy   arthrectromy

6. standardization   standardazation   standardizasion

7. stylis   stilus   stylus

8. isoelectric   iso-electric   isoeelectric

CHAPTER REVIEW

Assignment 14-4: Abbreviation Review

Write what each of the following abbreviations stands for.

1. MI: _____

2. PAC: _____

3. EKG: _____

4. ECG: _____

5. PVC: _____

6. PAT: _____

7. BPM: _____

8. VT: _____

9. VF: _____

10. Afib: _____

Assignment 14-5: Short Answer

1. Trace the circulation of blood through the heart to the tissues of the body by completing the chart below. The first structure(s) is provided for you.

A. Superior and inferior vene cava.	H.
B.	I.
C.	J.
D.	K.
E.	L.
F.	M.
G.	N.

2. Trace the heart's electrical system by filling in the diagram below.

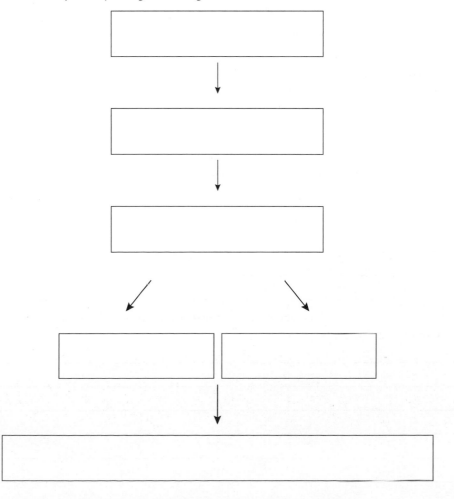

3. The SA node generates impulses through the muscle fibers of the _____. The most serious of the cardiac arrhythmias, _____ is characterized by uncoordinated beats that cause a quivering or twitching of the ventricles.

4. Why is cardiac defibrillation sometimes necessary?

   _____

   _____

   _____

   _____

5. Describe the following miscellaneous cardiac diagnostic tests.

   a. Holter monitor: _____

   _____

   b. Treadmill stress test: _____

   _____

   _____

   _____

   c. Echocardiography: _____

   _____

   d. Cardiac catheterization: _____

   _____

   _____

   _____

   e. Noninvasive heart scan: _____

   _____

   _____

   _____

6. Explain the purpose of the graphing lines on the ECG paper.

   _____

   _____

   _____

   _____

7. As the body ages, arteries which were elastic and pliable lose elasticity, dilate, and elongate. Describe what happens to the heart over the life span.

   _____

   _____

   _____

   _____

   _____

_____

_____

_____

_____

_____

Assignment 14-6: Matching

Match the term with its definition and place the corresponding letter in the blank.

____ 1. Heart

____ 2. Pericardium

____ 3. Apex

____ 4. Atria

____ 5. Ventricles

____ 6. Base

____ 7. Septum

____ 8. Epicardium

____ 9. Myocardium

____ 10. Endocardium

A. The rounded tip at the bottom of the heart that lies just above the diaphragm

B. The top of the heart, approximately at the level of the third rib

C. A muscular pumping organ that is located within the mediastinum

D. The thick middle layer of the heart; composed of specialized cardiac muscle cells and is responsible for the contraction of the heart muscle

E. The smooth outer layer of the heart; the main coronary arteries are located on the surface

F. The two upper chambers of the heart

G. The inner layer of the heart; composed of thick connective tissue as well as stretch sensors which only now are being understood

H. The structure that separates the heart (located in the middle of the heart)

I. The outer layer surrounding the heart; composed of tough fibrous connective tissue and serves to prevent the heart from overstretching as well as providing a small layer of fluid to allow the heart to move more freely

J. The two lower chambers of the heart

CERTIFICATION PRACTICE

Assignment 14-7

Choose the best answer and place the corresponding letter in the blank.

____ 1. What is referred to as the "primary pacemaker" of the heart's intrinsic conduction system?

    A. AV node

    B. SA node

    C. Bundle of His

    D. Purkinje fibers

____ 2. Which of the following waves appears after the T wave of the cardiac cycle?

    A. P wave

    B. R wave

    C. S wave

    D. U wave

____ 3. Which of the following statements is true regarding the isoelectric line?

    A. It is a straight line seen on the ECG strip.

    B. It is referred to as the baseline.

    C. It is used as a reference point when vertically centering the tracing.

    D. All of the above

____ 4. How many sensors are placed on the body when recording a 12-lead ECG?

    A. 12

    B. 10

    C. 8

    D. 7

____ 5. What occurs during depolarization?

    A. Discharge of electrical energy (impulses)

    B. The heart is recharging

    C. The heart is resting

    D. None of the above

____ 6. Large squares on the ECG paper measure:

    A. 1 mm × 1 mm.

    B. 2 mm × 2 mm.

    C. 0.5 mm × 0.5 mm.

    D. 5 mm × 5 mm.

____ 7. What do the horizontal lines on the ECG paper measure?

    A. Amplitude

    B. Timing of the impulses

    C. Interval between complexes

    D. Height of the complexes

____ 8. The purpose of including this in an ECG is to detect abnormalities in the patient's heart rhythm that may not be detectable in the standard leads due to the shorter representations of each lead.

    A. Standardization

    B. Markings

    C. Rhythm strip

    D. None of the above

____ 9. The letters aV on leads aVR, aVL, and aVF stand for which of the following?

    A. Anion volt

    B. Assisted voltage

    C. Augmented voltage

    D. Allocated voltage

____ 10. What is the location of lead V4?

    A. Fourth intercostal space at the left of the sternum

    B. Fifth intercostal space at the midclavicular line

    C. Fifth intercostal space at the midaxillary line

    D. Fourth intercostal space to the right of the sternum

SKILL APPLICATION CHALLENGE
Assignment 14-8: Labeling

1. Label the different types of interference.

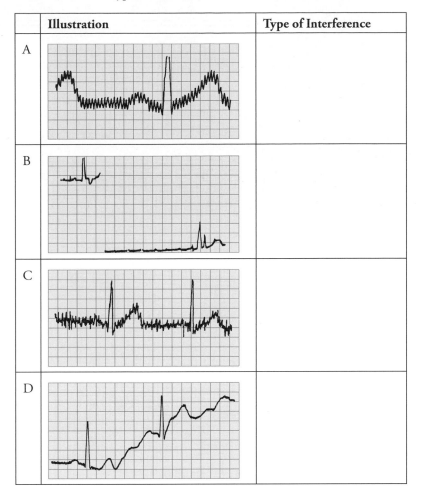

	Illustration	Type of Interference
A		
B		
C		
D		

2. On the diagram below, draw a circle where each chest lead should be placed.

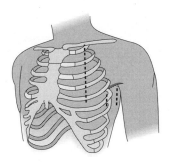

3. On the diagram below, draw squares where each limb lead should be placed.

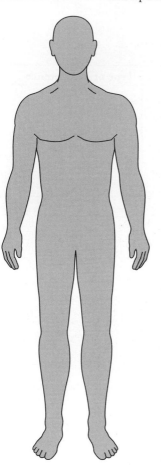

4. Label the following ECG cycle.

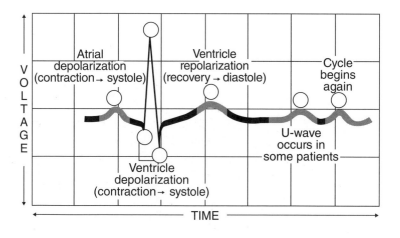

FIELD APPLICATION CHALLENGE

Assignment 14-9

Read the following Field Application Challenge and respond to the questions following the scenario.
The medical assistant is performing an ECG on a 79-year-old male who has a history of cardiac arrhythmias. The provider orders a standard 12-lead tracing along with a rhythm strip. The waves are barely visible on the tracing and there appears to be an interrupted baseline only in leads I, II, and AVR.

1. What can be done to the ECG unit to increase the amplitude of waves that are very small and difficult to read?

_____

2. Which lead wire(s) may have a problem based on the scenario above?

_____

_____

_____

3. What may be the cause of the interrupted baseline?

_____

4. What professionalism keys would be important in this situation? How could you display "professionalism" in this scenario?

_____

_____

_____

JOURNALING EXERCISE

Assignment 14-10

What content within this chapter was most meaningful to you? Why? List some examples of how you might apply the professionalism keys to information contained in this chapter, both during your training and after you enter the health care industry.

Keep a separate journal and conduct a self-assessment on your cardiology fitness by documenting, analyzing, and evaluating the following for one week:

1. The total fats consumed each day.

2. Separate the types of fat consumed each day.

3. Research saturated fats and trans fats. Describe the difference and the effect on cardiac health. Are you consuming too much?

4. Research omega-3 fatty acids. Describe the benefits these fatty acids have on cardiac health. Are you getting enough?

5. Evaluate your current diet and create a plan to eat more heart healthy.

6. Record how much time and what type of physical exercise you participate in each day.

7. Analyze the stress you feel in your day-to-day life, and develop a plan to reduce stress.

CHAPTER **15**

Pulmonary Examinations and Procedures

VOCABULARY REVIEW

Assignment 15-1: Misspelled Words

Underline the correctly spelled term.

1. Dispnea   Dipsnea   Dyspnea

2. Pulmonology   Polmonology   Pulmonlogy

3. Spirmetry   Sprometry   Spirometry

4. Thoracenteses   Thoracentesis   Thrococentsis

5. Tubirculosis   Tuberculosis   Teberculosis

Assignment 15-2: Matching

Match the term with its definition and place the corresponding letter in the blank.

____ 1. Bronchoscopy

____ 2. Carcinogen

____ 3. Pleural effusion

____ 4. Hypoxic

____ 5. Induration

____ 6. Inhaler

____ 7. Mantoux skin test

____ 8. Nebulizer

____ 9. Peak flow meter

A. Maximum amount of air the patient can inhale and exhale

B. A common screening test for tuberculosis

C. Handheld portable device that delivers oxygen directly into the lungs

D. Small handheld device that measures the fastest speed air can be blown out of the lungs; is also a great tool for the patient to monitor lung ailments such as asthma while at home

E. A procedure used to examine bronchial tubes and related structures

F. Cancer-causing agent

G. Units that change liquid medications into an aerosol mist so that they can be inhaled through a mouthpiece or facemask

H. Buildup of excess fluids in the pleural space

I. A noninvasive test that checks lung function

____ 10. Pulmonary function test   J.   Describing a patient who has a low oxygen level

____ 11. Pulmonologist   K.   A degree of hardening of normally soft tissue in the area

____ 12. Sputum   L.   A physician who specializes in respiratory care

____ 13. Vital capacity   M.   Fluid or matter that is produced in the lungs and bronchi

CHAPTER REVIEW

Assignment 15-3: Abbreviation Review

Write what each of the following abbreviations stands for.

1. MDI: _____

2. PEF: _____

3. PPD: _____

4. TB: _____

5. VC: _____

6. Bi-PAP: _____

7. O_2: _____

8. CO_2: _____

9. COPD: _____

10. C-PAP: _____

11. CXR: _____

12. ABGs: _____

Assignment 15-4: Short Answer

1. What factors may increase the patient's risk for lung cancer?

   _____

   _____

   _____

2. What is a common screening test for tuberculosis?

   _____

3. Arterial blood gases, ABGs, are ordered and studied for what two general purposes?

   A. _____

   B. _____

4. Results of the ABGs will measure what three items?

   A. _____

   B. _____

   C. _____

5. Where are arterial blood gases drawn from?

   _____

6. Why should ABG levels be performed on smokers, in addition to pulse oximetry testing?

_____

_____

_____

_____

_____

7. List at least five benefits that come with smoking cessation.

_____

_____

_____

_____

_____

8. The body has two lungs, contained within the rib cage. Each lung is divided into lobes. The right lung has _____, while the left has _____.

9. The _____ is a hollow tube reinforced with cartilaginous rings to keep it open.

10. When the pressure of the air outside of the body becomes greater than that in the lungs, the _____, a thin, dome-like muscle that divides the chest from the abdominal cavity, contracts, pulling the bases of the lung down with it, causing further decreased pressure in the lungs.

CERTIFICATION PRACTICE

Assignment 15-5

Choose the best answer and place the corresponding letter in the blank.

_____ 1. A test that uses spirometry before and after strenuous activity such as walking on a treadmill or riding a stationary bike is called a(n):

A. exercise challenge test.

B. PEF.

C. PFT.

D. peak flow meter.

_____ 2. Which of the following contagious infections is not spread through direct or indirect contact with infected individuals?

A. Influenza

B. Tuberculosis

C. Asthma

D. Pneumonia

_____ 3. Which of the following tests is considered to be more accurate when measuring oxygen saturation?

A. Pulse oximetry

B. ABGs

C. Spirometry

D. PFT

___ 4. Which of the following roles should the medical assistant assume when performing spirometry testing?

    A. Teacher

    B. Coach

    C. Nurse

    D. Friend

___ 5. Which of the following radiological exams is typically performed for routine screening as well as for diagnostic purposes to view the lung?

    A. Chest X-ray

    B. CT scan

    C. MRI

    D. Bronchoscopy

___ 6. All of the following are common medications used in a nebulizer *except*:

    A. anticholinergics.

    B. bronchodilators.

    C. antibiotics.

    D. corticosteroids.

___ 7. All of the following are symptoms for TB *except*:

    A. night sweats.

    B. tachycardia.

    C. cough with bloody sputum.

    D. tonsillitis.

___ 8. The leading cause of cancer death for both males and females according to the American Cancer Society is:

    A. colon cancer.

    B. lung cancer.

    C. breast cancer.

    D. prostate cancer.

___ 9. Normal PFTs should fall within what percentage of the predicted value?

    A. 35%

    B. 45%

    C. 75%

    D. 85% or higher

___ 10. The following are all guidelines for using a peak flow meter *except*:

    A. The pointer on the flow meter should start on the number 10.

    B. Remove all food or gum from mouth before starting the test.

    C. Breathe out as hard and fast as possible.

    D. Record the highest reading of three attempts.

COMPLETING SPECIAL FORMS

Assignment 15-6: Completing a Lab Requisition Form for a Sputum Culture

Work Form Necessary: FORM 15-1

Directions: Using the scenario information below, complete the lab requisition form (Work Form 15-1).
Sandy B. Bell needs to have a sputum culture done today, July 7, 20XX. Her provider, Dr. Thomas Weston, thinks that she may have pneumonia.

Patient's address: 111 Guthrie Road, Douglasville, NY 01234

Patient's DOB: 08-11-55

Patient's telephone number: (123) 858-9989

Provider's number: 25698745

Provider's address: Douglasville Medicine Associates, 5076 Brand Blvd, Douglasville, NY 01234

Provider's telephone number: (123) 456-7890

Test code: 45213

Test name: Sputum Culture

Specimen type: Sputum

Tube type/collection container: Nonsterile specimen container

ICD-10: J15.9

CPT: 87070

FIELD APPLICATION CHALLENGE

Assignment 15-7

Read the following Field Application Challenge and respond to the questions following the scenario.
It is Monday morning and Maria Santias calls to state that she is not feeling well. While on the phone with her, you hear her wheezing. Maria states that she is having trouble breathing. She has a history of asthma and has an asthma inhaler at home. She states that she took the recommended number of puffs from her inhaler but has not gotten any relief.

1. Based on this information, what should you have Mary do?

   _____

   _____

2. Document the phone call and your instructions to the patient on the following chart note. Use today's date and your name and credentials in the closing signature.

JOURNALING EXERCISE

Assignment 15-8

What content within this chapter was most meaningful to you? Why? List some examples of how you might apply information contained in this chapter, both during your training and after you enter the health care industry. Reflect on Davene's "Professionalism Mentor" tips regarding difficulties a patient suffering with pulmonary disease may have. Perhaps you have a family member or know of someone who has COPD or asthma. Which of the professionalism keys would apply when treating a patient struggling to breathe? List some examples.

Work Form 15-1

<table>
<tr><td colspan="2" align="center">

ABC Laboratory

</td></tr>
<tr>
<td>**Patient's Name**</td>
<td>**Patient's Address**</td>
</tr>
<tr>
<td>**Patient's Date of Birth:**</td>
<td>**Patient's Telephone Number**</td>
</tr>
<tr>
<td>

Provider Name:

Provider Number:
</td>
<td>**Provider Address & Phone:**</td>
</tr>
</table>

Testing Information

Test Date:	
Test Code:	
Test Name:	
Specimen Type:	
Tube Type/ Collection Container:	
ICD-10 Code:	
CPT Code(s):	

C H A P T E R **16**

Gastrointestinal Exams and Procedures

VOCABULARY REVIEW

Assignment 16-1: Matching

Match the term with its definition and place the corresponding letter in the blank.

_____ 1. Hepatologist

_____ 2. Proctologist

_____ 3. Anorexia of aging

_____ 4. Proctoscope

_____ 5. Aspiration

_____ 6. Gastroenterologist

_____ 7. Colostomy

_____ 8. Anoscope

_____ 9. Endocrinologist

_____ 10. Etiology

_____ 11. Gastritis

_____ 12. Fissure

_____ 13. Rectoscope

_____ 14. Polyps

_____ 15. Hemorrhoids

_____ 16. Fistula

_____ 17. Stoma

A. Examination of the sigmoid colon with a lighted scope

B. Inflammation of the stomach lining, caused by an irritant (alcohol) or from an infection from a bacteria or a virus, leading to stomach pain

C. A provider who specializes in treating diseases and disorders of the liver

D. The loss of appetite for food in the later years of life

E. The abnormal connection between two surfaces

F. Inhaling a foreign substance into the upper respiratory tract

G. The cause of disease

H. Creating an opening to the outside of the body

I. A type of speculum used to visualize the anus

J. A mushroom-like growth from the surface of the mucous membrane

K. Instrument used to visually inspect the anus and rectum

L. An instrument to examine the rectum

M. When the colon is attached to the abdomen, creating an opening to the outside of the body

N. A doctor who specializes in treating gastrointestinal disorders

O. Painful, swollen, and bleeding veins in the anal region

P. A linear ulcer located on the edge of the anus

Q. A physician who diagnoses and treats diseases of the endocrine system, which includes the pancreas and the treatment of diabetes

___ 18. Sigmoidoscopy

R. A provider who specializes in treating diseases and disorders of the colon, rectum, and anus

___ 19. Colonoscopy

S. Examination of the colon with a lighted scope

Assignment 16-2: Vocabulary Builder

Find the words below that are misspelled; circle them and then correctly spell them in the spaces provided. Then fill in the blanks in the following sentences with the correct vocabulary terms from the list.

hemotemesis   hematochezia   dietician

idiopathic   illeostomy   peristalosis

_____   _____   _____

_____   _____   _____

GI diseases and disorders are quite common, especially as the body ages. Signs and symptoms include nausea, vomiting, stomach cramping, diarrhea, heartburn, loss of appetite, weight loss, indigestion, fatigue, (1) _____ (vomiting blood), and bright red blood in the feces or black stools. (2) _____ is the term used when bleeding originates in the lower GI tract (colon, rectum, and anus) and is generally associated with bright red blood. A(n) (3) _____ is a professional who counsels patients on the special diets that are required for specific diseases. Sometimes a condition is (4) _____, meaning there is no known cause. When a complete colectomy (removal of the entire colon) is performed, the ileum may be used as the site in which a stoma is created. This procedure is referred to as a(n) (5) _____. (6) _____ is a series of wave-like contractions of the smooth muscles, moving food forward in the digestive system.

CHAPTER REVIEW

Assignment 16-3: Abbreviation Review

Write what each of the following abbreviations stands for.

1. GI: _____

2. EGD: _____

3. ERCP: _____

4. C-Diff: _____

5. O&P: _____

6. EUS: _____

7. NSAID: _____

8. GERD: _____

9. IBS: _____

Assignment 16-4: Short Answer

1. Medical assistants are often assigned the responsibility of screening patients over the phone or prior to provider examination in the office. The degree of screening will be established by office protocol, but, in general, medical assistants should be able to ask a series of questions related to the patient's symptoms. List four questions you should ask patients exhibiting gastrointestinal symptoms.

   1. _____
   2. _____
   3. _____
   4. _____
   _____

2. Describe the following procedures that are performed by a gastroenterologist.

   A. Sigmoidoscopy: _____
   _____
   _____

   B. Capsule endoscopy: _____
   _____
   _____
   _____

   C. 24-hour pH monitoring: _____
   _____
   _____

   D. Hydrogen breath test: _____
   _____
   _____
   _____

   E. Colonoscopy: _____
   _____
   _____
   _____
   _____

   F. Esophagogastroduodenoscopy (EGD): _____
   _____

   G. Endoscopic retrograde cholangiopancreatography (ERCP): _____
   _____

   H. Enteroscopy: _____
   _____

   I. Endoscopic ultrasound (EUS): _____
   _____

3. Describe common gastrointestinal conditions and treatments and/or causes.

A. Constipation: _____

_____

_____

B. Crohn's disease: _____

_____

_____

_____

_____

_____

_____

C. Diarrhea: _____

_____

_____

_____

_____

_____

D. Gastritis: _____

_____

_____

E. Gastroenteritis: _____

_____

_____

F. Hiatal hernia: _____

_____

G. Irritable bowel syndrome: _____

_____

_____

_____

H. Pancreatitis: _____

_____

CERTIFICATION PRACTICE

Assignment 16-5

Choose the best answer and place the corresponding letter in the blank.

____ 1. Which of the following would be a role of the medical assistant working in a gastroenterology practice?

A. To provide patient education regarding a colonoscopy

B. To perform fecal occult blood testing

C. To assist the provider during a sigmoidoscopy by handing instruments, suctioning, and giving support to the patient during the procedure

D. All of the above

Chapter 16 • *Gastrointestinal Exams and Procedures*   **145**

____ 2. Which lab test would a provider order to test for liver function?

     A. Comprehensive GI function panel

     B. Complete Blood Count

     C. Lipid panel

     D. Protein, bilirubin, alkaline, phosphatase, gamma-globulin

____ 3. When instructing a patient regarding preparation for collecting a fecal occult blood test sample, you would include all of the following *except*:

     A. Avoid red and processed meats and liver; no turnips, broccoli, cauliflower, or melons, for three days prior to collection.

     B. Do not consume alcoholic beverages for three days prior to collection.

     C. Avoid NSAIDs or Aspirin for seven days prior to collection.

     D. Collect samples on three different days.

____ 4. When instructing a patient on how to collect a fecal sample for occult, all of the following are true *except*:

     A. The patient may use a tongue depressor to collect a small portion of the stool.

     B. Instruct the patient to collect the sample in a wide-mouth jar.

     C. Stress the importance of not contaminating the specimen with urine.

     D. The patient should urinate in the commode before setting up the collection (toilet) hat.

____ 5. Which of the following are considered risk factors for colon cancer?

     A. A family history of colon cancer

     B. A personal history of colon polyps

     C. A diet high in red and processed meats.

     D. All of the above

____ 6. All of the following are the structures of the digestive system in which food and wastes travel *except*:

     A. oral cavity.

     B. esophagus.

     C. kidney.

     D. rectum.

____ 7. The digestive tube has several different names: _____, the GI tract, and the digestive tract.

     A. the alimentary canal

     B. the parietal tract

     C. the peristalsis canal

     D. the peritoneum tract

____ 8. When someone suffers from _____, stomach acid backs up into the esophagus, due to a defect in the sphincter muscle between the stomach and the esophagus. Patients may complain of heartburn or chest pain.

     A. ulcerative colitis

     B. Crohn's disease

     C. ascites

     D. gastroesophageal reflux disease (GERD)

____ 9. The term _____ refers to stool that is black and tarry and is often the result of blood entering the stool from the upper GI tract (stomach and small intestines).

     A. melena

     B. hematochezia

     C. occult reflux

     D. fissures

___ 10. The lab test "Comprehensive GI function panel":

   A. detects abnormalities in the total blood profile, such as a low hematocrit, which could indicate blood loss.

   B. monitors the GI level in the blood.

   C. tests liver function.

   D. measures inflammatory, digestive, and immune markers, to detect abnormal GI function.

SKILL APPLICATION CHALLENGE
Assignment 16-6: Research Activity

1. Construct a three-day diet that contains high-fiber content for a patient suffering from IBS. Include breakfast, lunch, dinner, and snacks.

2. Using the Internet, look for resources, information, and ideas, then design informational pamphlets to be given to patients that explain the following procedures and include special preparation instructions:

   A. Fecal occult blood test

   B. Sigmoidoscopy

   C. Colonoscopy

   D. EGD

FIELD APPLICATION CHALLENGE
Assignment 16-7

Read the following Field Application Challenge and respond to the questions following the scenario.

A 55-year-old male is sent to your office to have a colonoscopy. He is a heavy drinker and smoker who also consumes spicy foods on a daily basis. He is quite anxious about having the procedure performed. His father and younger brother were both diagnosed with colorectal cancer. His father died, but the brother was just recently diagnosed and is taking chemotherapy.

1. List the risk factors the patient has for developing cancer.

_____

_____

_____

_____

_____

_____

_____

2. How might you calm the patient's fears about the procedure?

_____

_____

JOURNALING EXERCISE
Assignment 16-8

What content within this chapter was most meaningful to you? Why? List some examples of how you might apply information contained in this chapter, both during your training and after you enter the health care industry. Reflect on Davene's "Professionalism Mentor" tips regarding the sometimes embarrassing topic and GI procedures the patient may need. If you were a patient requiring a sigmoidoscopy for the first time, how would you feel? Which of the professionalism keys would you want your health care professional to apply in this setting? Can you demonstrate how you, as a medical assistant, would exhibit professionalism? List some examples.

CHAPTER **17**

Women's Health Issues: Obstetrics and Gynecology

VOCABULARY REVIEW

Assignment 17-1: Matching

Match the term with its definition and place the corresponding letter in the blank.

_____ 1. Abortion

_____ 2. Braxton-Hicks

_____ 3. Amniocentesis

_____ 4. Dysmenorrhea

_____ 5. Colposcopy

_____ 6. Menarche

_____ 7. Ectopic

_____ 8. Effacement

_____ 9. Gravida

_____ 10. Meconium

_____ 11. Eclampsia

_____ 12. Toxemia

_____ 13. Parturition

_____ 14. Puerperium

_____ 15. Trimester

A. Another term for preeclampsia

B. Another name for labor

C. Term for the three-month intervals that a pregnancy is divided into

D. Another name for the postpartum period

E. A woman's first menstrual cycle

F. A progression of preeclampsia in which all of the same symptoms are present as seen in preeclampsia but with the addition of seizures or convulsions or coma

G. Total number of pregnancies including the present one

H. Pregnancy occurs outside the uterus; tubal pregnancy

I. Earliest stools of the newborn

J. Thinning of the cervix

K. Examination of the vagina and cervix with the aid of a lighted scope

L. Difficult or painful menstruation

M. Removal or expulsion of an embryo or fetus from the uterus, resulting in death

N. Intermittent and painless uterine contractions that usually occur 10 to 20 minutes apart (false labor)

O. Procedure to withdraw amniotic fluid from the amniotic sac for testing purposes (usually testing for chromosomal abnormalities)

Assignment 17-2: Sentence Completion

Fill in the blanks below with Essential Terms from this chapter.

1. _____ is the expansion of the cervix during labor to facilitate delivery of the fetus.

2. _____ is the period of time from conception to birth.

3. A(n) _____ is also known as a spontaneous abortion.

4. The vaginal discharge of blood, mucous, and tissue coming from the uterus following delivery is known as _____ .

5. The period of time before birth is called the _____ period.

6. _____ begins when estrogen production by the ovaries gradually decreases and normally lasts from one to two years.

7. A(n) _____ is a procedure in which a surgical incision is made through the abdominal wall and into the uterus to remove the fetus and placenta.

8. _____ refers to the number of live births that a patient has had.

CHAPTER REVIEW

Assignment 17-3: Abbreviation Review

Write what each of the following abbreviations stands for.

1. AUB: _____

2. STD: _____

3. STI: _____

4. OB-GYN: _____

5. BSE: _____

6. HRT: _____

7. LH: _____

8. FSH: _____

9. FDA: _____

10. SSRI: _____

11. SNRI: _____

12. CNM: _____

13. CPM: _____

14. PCR: _____

15. GBS: _____

16. HPV: _____

17. CDC: _____

18. NCI: _____

19. TBS: _____

20. ACS: _____

21. D&C: _____

22. LEEP: _____

23. hCG: _____

24. EDD: _____

25. EDC: _____

26. FAS: _____

Assignment 17-4: Short Answer

1. Provide the recommended schedule for prenatal and postpartum visits.

   _____

   _____

   _____

2. Describe at what points ultrasound testing is performed during pregnancy and what is evaluated during each ultrasound.

   _____

   _____

   _____

   _____

   _____

   _____

3. List and explain the stages of labor.

   1. _____

   _____

   _____

   2. _____

   _____

   _____

   _____

   _____

   _____

   _____

   _____

   3. _____

   _____

   _____

   _____

4. Discuss the importance of the postpartum exam and what is performed during the exam.

_____

_____

_____

_____

_____

_____

_____

_____

_____

_____

_____

_____

_____

5. List and describe the components of the GYN exam.

1. _____

2. _____

3. _____

4. _____

5. _____

CERTIFICATION PRACTICE

Assignment 17-5

Choose the best answer and place the corresponding letter in the blank.

_____ 1. Which of the following medical terms is used when a patient is in labor?

    A. Parity

    B. Puerperium

    C. Parturition

    D. Postpartum

_____ 2. A pregnant patient is considered to be full term at:

    A. 10 months.

    B. 9 months.

    C. 35 weeks.

    D. 37 to 42 weeks.

_____ 3. Which of the following hormones is responsible for strong uterine contractions?

    A. Estrogen

    B. Oxytocin

    C. Insulin

    D. Progesterone

____ 4. A patient is in the office today for her yearly GYN exam. You take her blood pressure and weight and update her medical history. You give her disrobing instructions and then leave the room. Which of the following additional steps should have been performed to promote patient comfort during the exam?

    A. Asking the patient to empty her bladder

    B. Telling the patient to sit in the chair until the provider comes in

    C. Asking the patient if she is warm enough

    D. Asking the patient if she has any questions

____ 5. Which of the following statements about breast cancer is true?

    A. Only women with a family history of the disease are at risk.

    B. If the BRCA genes mutate, a women's risk for developing breast or ovarian cancer, or both, is greatly increased.

    C. You are only at risk if you have a palpable lump in your breast.

    D. None of the above

____ 6. Which of the following advantages of the liquid prep method makes it more desirable than conventional Pap tests?

    A. Only a small portion of cells are used.

    B. It eliminates debris and evenly distributes a thin layer of cells on the slide.

    C. It needs to be performed five days after the LMP.

    D. The test is less expensive.

____ 7. Which of the following abnormalities might the provider be looking for during a rectal exam?

    A. Hemorrhoids

    B. Fistulas

    C. Fissures

    D. All of the above

____ 8. The alpha-fetoprotein (AFP) test is performed to detect which of the following defects?

    A. Gestational diabetes

    B. Fetal gender

    C. Fetal blood type

    D. Neural tube defects

____ 9. Which of the following is a mild form of diabetes that develops in the second or third trimester and resolves when the pregnancy ends?

    A. Type 1

    B. Type 2

    C. Diabetes mellitus

    D. Gestational

____ 10. The correct term for the vaginal discharge that can last for up to six weeks after delivery is:

    A. Lochia rubra.

    B. Lochia alba.

    C. Lochia serosa.

    D. Lochia melanin.

SKILL APPLICATION CHALLENGES

Assignment 17-6: Application Activity

Using Naegle's Rule, calculate the following estimated delivery dates (EDDs).

    1. LMP: 01-11-2016   EDD: _____

    2. LMP: 05-06-2017   EDD: _____

    3. LMP: 02-17-2018   EDD: _____

Assignment 17-7: Documentation Exercise

Interpret the following documentations.

1. G4T2P1A1L3 _____

   _____

2. G6T6P0A0L4 _____

   _____

3. G0 _____

Assignment 17-8: Research Activity

1. Look up the latest methods of birth control and prepare a PowerPoint or YouTube presentation that illustrates the advantages and disadvantages of each type.

2. Research the topic of new advances in intrauterine surgery to correct fetal abnormalities and write a paper which includes photos to present to the class.

3. Interview an OB-GYN specialist in your area and gather statistics on how many babies the physician has delivered, whether or not the physician's practice uses a midwife, how many multiple births the physician has performed, how many C-sections, etc. Include any interesting information provided by the physician about difficult or unusual births.

FIELD APPLICATION CHALLENGE

Assignment 17-9

Read the following Field Application Challenge and respond to the questions following the scenario.

A 28-year-old female at 20 weeks gestation is in the office today for an ultrasound (Doppler Fetal Heart Tones [Doptones]). She is very excited about the procedure and is anxious to find out the baby's sex but she also states that she is a bit nervous because she has not felt any movement over the past couple of days. You set the patient up for her exam and leave the room to alert the physician about the information provided by the patient. The physician asks you to remain in the exam room during the ultrasound just in case there are any problems. Upon ultrasound examination, the physician cannot see any signs that the heart is beating nor were there any heart tones picked up by the fetal monitor.

1. What do these findings mean?

   _____

2. The physician leaves the room after explaining to the patient the progression plan that will be followed from this point forward. The physician was very caring and nurturing but the patient falls apart emotionally after the physician leaves the room. What can you do to assist the patient during this difficult encounter?

   _____

   _____

   _____

JOURNALING EXERCISE

Assignment 17-10

What content within this chapter was most meaningful to you? Why? Write down some of the conditions and procedures you may see while working with the OB/GYN patient. As Davene suggested, try to imagine how they may be feeling so that when you interact with them, your actions will demonstrate your professionalism. Cite specific examples of displaying professionalism to the conditions and procedures you noted above.

CHAPTER **18**

Urology and Male Reproductive Exams and Procedures

VOCABULARY REVIEW

Assignment 18-1: Matching

Match the term with its definition and place the corresponding letter in the blank.

____ 1. Benign prostatic hypertrophy

    A. The provider places a gloved finger into the patient's rectum to examine the prostate for enlargement, lumps, and other abnormalities

____ 2. Catheterization

    B. Insertion of a lighted scope into the bladder

____ 3. Circumcision

    C. Dialysis in which the patient is hooked up to a dialysis unit through tubes that connect to the patient's blood vessels

____ 4. Cystoscopy

    D. The study of the urinary system and male reproductive system

____ 5. Dialysis

    E. A catheter that includes a balloon so that the catheter can stay in place for prolonged periods of time

____ 6. Digital rectal exam

    F. Enlarged prostate that is not related to cancer of the prostate

____ 7. Erectile dysfunction (ED)

    G. Removal of the foreskin of the penis

____ 8. Foley catheter

    H. Filtering waste products from the blood with the aid of a machine

____ 9. Hemodialysis

    I. The insertion of a sterile tube directly into the bladder through the urethra to obtain a sterile specimen

____ 10. Urology

    J. The inability to achieve or maintain an erection during sexual relations

Assignment 18-2: Sentence Completion

Fill in the blanks below with essential terms from this chapter.

1. _____ is an infection in the bladder.

2. _____ is defined as difficult or painful urination.

3. _____ is the need to urinate frequently at the time of sleep.

4. Excessively large amounts of urine is known as _____.

5. The _____ is a procedure performed on males who have BPH.

6. _____ is a surgical procedure in which the vas deferens is cut, clamped, or sealed to prevent the sperm from entering the ejaculate and should be considered to be a permanent form of birth control.

7. _____ is an infection in the prostate.

8. The term _____ means no urine is being formed by the kidneys.

9. _____ (outside the body) shockwaves produce pressure waves that pass through the body to the kidney stone.

10. A physician specializing in the treatment of diseases and disorders of the kidneys is called a(n) _____.

CHAPTER REVIEW

Assignment 18-3: Abbreviation Review

Write what each of the following abbreviations stands for.

1. TURP: _____

2. TRUS: _____

3. TSE: _____

4. BUN: _____

5. CAPD: _____

6. IVP: _____

7. BPH: _____

8. ED: _____

9. KUB: _____

10. UTI: _____

Assignment 18-4: Short Answer

1. What is the medical assistant's role in diagnostic examinations of the urinary system?

   _____

   _____

   _____

   _____

2. List and describe three types of access for hemodialysis.

   A. _____

   _____

   B. _____

   _____

   C. _____

   _____

3. What blood tests are performed to determine the health/function of the kidneys?

   _____

4. Name the two common types of catheters and describe when each would be used.

A. _____

_____

_____

B. _____

_____

_____

5. List some criteria that must be met prior to receiving a kidney transplant.

_____

_____

_____

_____

CERTIFICATION PRACTICE

Assignment 18-5

Choose the best answer and place the corresponding letter in the blank.

____ 1. Which of the following types of hemodialysis access is considered the most durable?

A. Graft

B. Fistula

C. Venous catheter/port

D. Peritoneal

____ 2. The only definitive diagnosis of prostate cancer is made through a:

A. blood test (PSA).

B. biopsy.

C. TURP.

D. vasectomy.

____ 3. The process that involves the insertion of a sterile tube directly into the bladder through the urethra using strict sterile technique is called:

A. catheterization.

B. cystoscopy.

C. IVP.

D. ultrasound.

____ 4. A procedure during which the provider can examine both the urethra and bladder is called:

A. catheterization.

B. cystoscopy.

C. IVP.

D. ultrasound.

____ 5. Which of the following procedures is used to treat the symptoms of BPH?

A. Vasectomy

B. TURP

C. TSE

D. ED

___ 6. The immediate need to urinate is referred to as:

     A. polyuria.

     B. frequency.

     C. oliguria.

     D. urgency.

___ 7. A radiographic procedure in which contrast dye is injected into the patient through an IV to examine the internal structures of the kidneys, ureters, and bladder is called:

     A. cystoscopy.

     B. IVP.

     C. KUB.

     D. None of the above

___ 8. A word meaning a narrowing of the urethra is:

     A. stricture.

     B. stasis.

     C. narrosis.

     D. stent.

___ 9. The term that means crushing of kidney stones is:

     A. lithostasis.

     B. lithotomy.

     C. lithotripsy.

     D. triptolithiasis.

___ 10. Women are often prone to cystitis (infection in the bladder). Symptoms of cystitis include urinary frequency, urgency, and dysuria. Which of the following educational tips would *not* be helpful for preventing future infections?

     A. Stay away from cotton underwear; use nylon instead.

     B. Drink plenty of fluids.

     C. Woman should wipe from front to back.

     D. Urinate frequently and empty entire bladder.

SKILL APPLICATION CHALLENGES

Assignment 18-6: Labeling

1. Label the parts of the male urinary system.

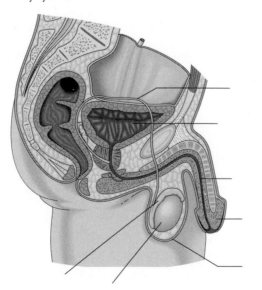

2. Label the parts of the female urinary system.

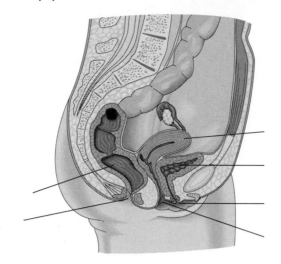

3. Label the parts of the female external genitalia.

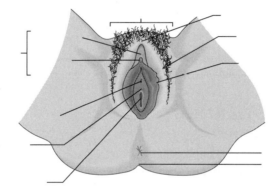

Assignment 18-7: Research Activity

Look up the term "kidney transplant" using your preferred Internet browser.

1. On the lines below, make a list of people that may be potential donors for someone needing a kidney.

   A. _____

   B. _____

   C. _____

2. How long is a patient's stay in the hospital following a kidney transplant?

   _____

   _____

3. What is the length of time a kidney may be out of the donor's body before placing it into recipient's body? How is the kidney preserved?

_____

_____

_____

_____

_____

_____

_____

_____

4. What types of patients would not be considered as suitable for a kidney transplant?

_____

_____

_____

Assignment 18-8: Research Activity

Mr. Honeycutt is diagnosed with an enlarged prostate. The provider asks you to provide education to the patient regarding his condition. Using an Internet browser, create a list of websites that will assist the patient in learning about his condition. Try to include at least one reference that includes an animation. Make a list of websites the patient can go to and provide reference information beside each website that describes what the patient should click on once they get to the website as well as the outstanding features of each website. Items of interest for this presentation include: how the size of the prostate affects urine flow; tests that are performed initially and for monitoring purposes thereafter; and procedures that can be performed to correct the condition.

FIELD APPLICATION CHALLENGE

Assignment 18-9: Case Study

Part I: A patient calls on the phone complaining of excruciating pain in his lower back and abdomen on the left side. The pain came on suddenly and the patient now has blood in his urine. The symptoms started approximately one hour ago. Answer the following questions based on this scenario.

1. What might be a likely cause of the patient's symptoms?

_____

_____

_____

_____

2. What would be typical instructions for a patient with the above symptoms and what forms of treatment are available if the patient does, in fact, have a kidney stone?

_____

_____

_____

_____

_____

_____

_____

_____

_____

4. Name the two common types of catheters and describe when each would be used.

   A. _____

   _____

   _____

   B. _____

   _____

   _____

5. List some criteria that must be met prior to receiving a kidney transplant.

   _____

   _____

   _____

   _____

CERTIFICATION PRACTICE

Assignment 18-5

Choose the best answer and place the corresponding letter in the blank.

_____ 1. Which of the following types of hemodialysis access is considered the most durable?

    A. Graft

    B. Fistula

    C. Venous catheter/port

    D. Peritoneal

_____ 2. The only definitive diagnosis of prostate cancer is made through a:

    A. blood test (PSA).

    B. biopsy.

    C. TURP.

    D. vasectomy.

_____ 3. The process that involves the insertion of a sterile tube directly into the bladder through the urethra using strict sterile technique is called:

    A. catheterization.

    B. cystoscopy.

    C. IVP.

    D. ultrasound.

_____ 4. A procedure during which the provider can examine both the urethra and bladder is called:

    A. catheterization.

    B. cystoscopy.

    C. IVP.

    D. ultrasound.

_____ 5. Which of the following procedures is used to treat the symptoms of BPH?

    A. Vasectomy

    B. TURP

    C. TSE

    D. ED

___ 6. The immediate need to urinate is referred to as:

A. polyuria.

B. frequency.

C. oliguria.

D. urgency.

___ 7. A radiographic procedure in which contrast dye is injected into the patient through an IV to examine the internal structures of the kidneys, ureters, and bladder is called:

A. cystoscopy.

B. IVP.

C. KUB.

D. None of the above

___ 8. A word meaning a narrowing of the urethra is:

A. stricture.

B. stasis.

C. narrosis.

D. stent.

___ 9. The term that means crushing of kidney stones is:

A. lithostasis.

B. lithotomy.

C. lithotripsy.

D. triptolithiasis.

___ 10. Women are often prone to cystitis (infection in the bladder). Symptoms of cystitis include urinary frequency, urgency, and dysuria. Which of the following educational tips would *not* be helpful for preventing future infections?

A. Stay away from cotton underwear; use nylon instead.

B. Drink plenty of fluids.

C. Woman should wipe from front to back.

D. Urinate frequently and empty entire bladder.

SKILL APPLICATION CHALLENGES

Assignment 18-6: Labeling

1. Label the parts of the male urinary system.

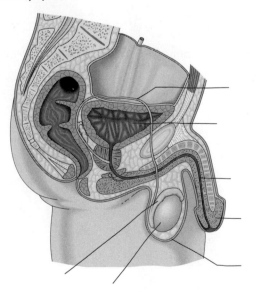

2. Label the parts of the female urinary system.

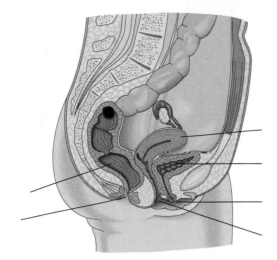

3. Label the parts of the female external genitalia.

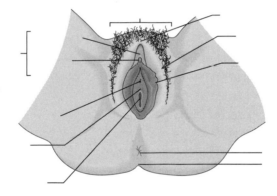

Assignment 18-7: Research Activity

Look up the term "kidney transplant" using your preferred Internet browser.

1. On the lines below, make a list of people that may be potential donors for someone needing a kidney.

   A. _____

   B. _____

   C. _____

2. How long is a patient's stay in the hospital following a kidney transplant?

   _____

   _____

3. What is the length of time a kidney may be out of the donor's body before placing it into recipient's body? How is the kidney preserved?

_____

_____

_____

_____

_____

_____

_____

4. What types of patients would not be considered as suitable for a kidney transplant?

_____

_____

_____

Assignment 18-8: Research Activity

Mr. Honeycutt is diagnosed with an enlarged prostate. The provider asks you to provide education to the patient regarding his condition. Using an Internet browser, create a list of websites that will assist the patient in learning about his condition. Try to include at least one reference that includes an animation. Make a list of websites the patient can go to and provide reference information beside each website that describes what the patient should click on once they get to the website as well as the outstanding features of each website. Items of interest for this presentation include: how the size of the prostate affects urine flow; tests that are performed initially and for monitoring purposes thereafter; and procedures that can be performed to correct the condition.

FIELD APPLICATION CHALLENGE

Assignment 18-9: Case Study

Part I: A patient calls on the phone complaining of excruciating pain in his lower back and abdomen on the left side. The pain came on suddenly and the patient now has blood in his urine. The symptoms started approximately one hour ago. Answer the following questions based on this scenario.

1. What might be a likely cause of the patient's symptoms?

_____

_____

_____

_____

2. What would be typical instructions for a patient with the above symptoms and what forms of treatment are available if the patient does, in fact, have a kidney stone?

_____

_____

_____

_____

_____

_____

_____

_____

_____

_____

Part II: You decide to develop the complaint a bit by asking the patient about his urinary history. The patient denies a history of any urinary tract or kidney problems. Because of the distress the patient is in, you decide to interrupt Dr. Roy to discuss the situation. Dr. Roy asks you to instruct the patient to go to the ER and directs you to call the ER to let them know that he is on his way. Using all of the information presented in Parts I and II, create a chart note that describes the call and the instructions given to the patient (use today's date, the current time, and list yourself as the medical assistant).

JOURNALING EXERCISE

Assignment 18-10

What content within this chapter was most meaningful to you? Why? List some examples of how you might apply information contained in this chapter, both during your training and after you enter the health care industry. Review Davene's "Professionalism Mentor" scenario regarding the need to be open, honest, and display compassion. What are some ways you can initiate and guide discussions with patients that can help to alleviate some of the uneasiness associated with sensitive health questioning?

C H A P T E R **19**

Other Specialty Procedures

VOCABULARY REVIEW

Assignment 19-1: Matching

Match the term with its definition and place the corresponding letter in the blank.

____ 1. Acupressure

____ 2. Acupuncture

____ 3. Allergen

____ 4. Epidermis

____ 5. Homeopathy

____ 6. Subcutaneous

____ 7. Wheal

____ 8. Urticaria

____ 9. Immunotherapy

____ 10. Melanocytes

A. Pigment-containing cells

B. Outer skin layer

C. A method used to stimulate acupoints; uses a firm pressure to massage the acupoints

D. A substance that causes an allergic reaction. Type I hypersensitivity

E. Also known as hives

F. A form of traditional Chinese medicine with at least 2,500 years of practice where thin needles are placed at specific points along 14 energy pathways or meridians to release the flow of the body's vital energy (*chi*)

G. The prevention or treatment of disease that stimulates the immune response

H. Under the skin

I. A 200-year-old system of medicine based on the Law of Similars: If a dose of a substance can cause a symptom, that same substance in minuscule amounts can cure the symptom

J. A small blister formed from the fluid raising the skin

Assignment 19-2: Vocabulary Builder

Find the words below that are misspelled; circle them and then correctly spell them in the spaces provided. Then fill in the blanks in the following sentences with the correct vocabulary terms from the list.

accupuncturist   anafylaxis   angioedema

Ayurveda   epinefrine   kinesiology

_____   _____   _____

_____   _____   _____

Serious allergic reactions include urticaria (also known as hives), (1) _____ (swelling under the skin), and (2) _____ leading to respiratory compromise and possibly death. A provider who inserts very thin needles through a patient's skin in varying depths at specific points on the body is known as a(n) (3) _____ . (4) _____ is the traditional medicine of India that emphasizes re-establishing balance in the body through diet, lifestyle, exercise, cleansing of the body, and on the health of the mind, body, and spirit. (5) _____ is the only medication that can reverse the symptoms of anaphylaxis. (6) _____ is the study of the principles of mechanics and anatomy in relation to human movement.

CHAPTER REVIEW

Assignment 19-3: Abbreviation Review

Write what each of the following abbreviations stands for.

1. CAM: _____

2. MAST: _____

3. OMT: _____

4. RAST: _____

5. OFC: _____

6. D.O.: _____

7. NCCIH: _____

Assignment 19-4: Short Answer

1. Medical assistants should be well educated about all procedures offered in the office. The role of the medical assistant will vary from one practice to another. Identify four roles the medical assistant will have when assisting with anti-aging procedures.

    A. _____

    B. _____

    C. _____

    D. _____

2. Whole medical systems cut across all four CAM domains. Treatments can be focused on one of the four types of CAM therapy. List and give examples of the four types of therapy.

A. _____
_____
_____
_____
_____
_____
_____
_____
_____
_____
_____
_____
_____

B. _____
_____
_____
_____
_____
_____
_____
_____
_____
_____
_____
_____
_____
_____
_____
_____
_____
_____
_____
_____
_____

C. _____
_____
_____
_____

D. _____
_____
_____
_____
_____
_____
_____
_____

_____

_____

_____

3. Identify the common triggers and type (if noted) of each of the allergies listed:

A. Food allergy: _____

_____

B. Skin allergy: _____

_____

_____

_____

C. Dust allergy: _____

_____

D. Insect sting: _____

_____

E. Pet allergy: _____

F. Eye allergy: _____

_____

_____

G. Drug allergy: _____

_____

H. Latex allergy: _____

_____

I. Mold allergy: _____

J. Sinus allergy: _____

_____

CERTIFICATION PRACTICE

Assignment 19-5

Choose the best answer and place the corresponding letter in the blank.

____ 1. _____ is a growing trend where providers and health care systems are integrating various practices into treatment and health promotion.

    A. Complementary and alternative medicine

    B. Traditional Chinese medicine

    C. Osteopathic manipulative therapy

    D. Integrative health care

____ 2. Sometimes called hypersensitivity, a(n) _____ is a reaction by the immune system.

    A. wheal

    B. chelation

    C. antigen

    D. allergy

___ 3. _____ is a serious allergic reaction with excessive release of histamine, which compromises the pulmonary and circulatory systems, and can lead to death if not properly treated.

   A. Angioedema

   B. Anaphylaxis

   C. Contact dermatitis

   D. Kinesiology

___ 4. What size needle is used to administer an intradermal injection?

   A. A fine-gauge needle, usually .01 to .02 in thickness.

   B. A fine-gauge needle, usually 26 G and ⅜ to ⅝ inches long.

   C. An 18 gauge needle, usually .01 to .03 in thickness.

   D. An 18 gauge needle, between ⅜ to ¾ inches long.

___ 5. Which test determines if you have contact dermatitis?

   A. Wheal

   B. Skin patch

   C. Skin prick

   D. Blood test

___ 6. To reduce the possibility of a local or systemic reaction when administering allergy shots, the medical assistant should:

   A. remove the needle that was used to draw up the injection and replace it with a brand new needle before administering the injection.

   B. use a 45° angle rather than a 90° angle to reduce the potential for back flow of allergy serum onto the skin.

   C. use the same needle that was used to draw up the injection to avoid cross-contamination.

   D. All of the above

___ 7. A surgical specialist who deals with the repair, reconstruction, or replacement of physical defects of form or function involving the skin, musculoskeletal system, craniomaxillofacial structures, extremities, breast and trunk, and external genitalia is a(n):

   A. plastic surgeon.

   B. cosmetic dermatologist.

   C. cosmetic dentist.

   D. All of the above

___ 8. Another noninvasive laser therapy that is said to help reverse the visible signs of aging that generates tiny microscopic wounds in the dermal layer of the skin, stimulating the body's own healing process and collagen production is known as:

   A. laser resurfacing.

   B. Fraxel Restore.

   C. chemical peel.

   D. microdermabrasion.

___ 9. _____ is a parallel branch of American medicine with a distinct philosophy and approach to patient care, practicing a "whole person" approach.

   A. Osteopathic medicine

   B. Chiropractic

   C. Homeopathy

   D. Naturopathic medicine

____ 10. The most common CAM therapy utilized by patients is:

    A. chiropractic.

    B. acupuncture.

    C. diet.

    D. herbs and nutritional supplements.

SKILL APPLICATION CHALLENGE

Assignment 19-6: Research Activity

1. Research the following websites (www.acaai.org, www.cdc.gov, www.nih.gov, and www.aafa.org) and provide a description of and construct a list of common triggers and treatments for:

    A. Asthma

_____

_____

_____

_____

_____

_____

_____

_____

_____

    B. Anaphylaxis

_____

_____

_____

_____

_____

_____

_____

_____

_____

_____

FIELD APPLICATION CHALLENGE
Assignment 19-7

Read the following Field Application Challenge and respond to the questions following the scenario.
Patient Jesse Monroy, a 36-year-old male, comes to the office today to see Dr. Richard Krebs, M.D. for a follow-up visit. Dr. Krebs is an orthopedic specialist who also embraces CAM. Jesse has been suffering from mid-back (thoracic) pain ever since his neck and spinal fusions last year. There is an order from Dr. Krebs to take X-rays of Jesse's cervical, thoracic, and lumbar spine.

1. What are your responsibilities when you take the patient back for his examination today?

_____

_____

2. When you take his chief complaint he asks about chiropractic being an option for him. How would you respond to his question?

_____

_____

_____

Upon examining the X-rays, Dr. Krebs notes that he sees good alignment and fusion at the C6-7 and L5-S1 levels, and nothing of concern in the thoracic area. He reviews your notes about the patient's interest in chiropractic (CAM) and recommends a referral to Dr. Sandra Skates, D.O., who practices OMT and acupuncture, for six weeks of treatment two times per week (the order), and to return to the office for a follow-up in two months.

3. What steps will you take at the end of the visit?

_____

_____

_____

_____

_____

JOURNALING EXERCISE
Assignment 19-8

What content within this chapter was most meaningful to you? Why? List some examples of how you might apply information contained in this chapter, both during your training and after you enter the health care industry. Reflect on Davene's "Professionalism Mentor" scenario regarding a patient's desire to explore alternative treatment to help with his neck pain. As Davene said, we always need to consider the patient's ideas and suggestions and work together as a team. What professionalism keys would you have included here? Why? Give an example of how you would demonstrate professionalism.

C H A P T E R **20**

Diet and Nutrition

VOCABULARY REVIEW

Assignment 20-1: Matching

Match the term with its definition and place the corresponding letter in the blank.

____ 1. Bariatrics

A. A protein found in grains such as wheat, rye, triticale (a cross between wheat and rye), and barley

____ 2. Bulimia nervosa

B. A hormone secreted by the beta cells of the pancreatic islet in response to high levels of glucose in the blood stream

____ 3. Electrolyte

C. A branch of medicine concerned with the prevention and control of obesity and associated diseases

____ 4. Gluten

D. Having too much body fat for the height, gender, and age of the individual

____ 5. Glycemic index (GI)

E. Unhealthy substances made through the hydrogenation of oils, turning oils into fats that are solid at room temperature

____ 6. Insulin

F. Measures how quickly carbohydrate foods raise the blood glucose level

____ 7. Obesity

G. Involves a dangerous pattern of eating or binging followed by purging

____ 8. Transfats

H. The inability of the GI tract to absorb some nutrients

____ 9. Metabolism

I. Mineral salts dissolved in water that carry an electrical current

____ 10. Malabsorption syndrome

J. Includes all of the processes involved in the body's use of nutrients

Assignment 20-2: Grammar Challenge

Select/underline the correct word.

1. A healthy infant doubles (its, it's) birth weight in three months and triples it by the first birthday.

2. (Where, Wear) can you find additional information about nutrition?

3. Fasting causes the body to conserve energy by increasing the breakdown of stored fats, resulting in ketones, which (effect, affect) the brain by decreasing appetite, slowing the rate of metabolism, and further decreasing the rate of weight loss.

4. Being overweight or obese is the result of a daily calorie intake that is higher (then, then) the body requires and exercise (which, that) is insufficient to offset the higher number of calories consumed.

5. Surgery (might, may) be considered for those who have failed weight loss and exercise programs and remain obese.

6. (There, they're, their) are (too, to, two) types of nutritional deficiencies: primary and secondary.

7. Providers who do not feel qualified to counsel patients about (there, they're, their) diet may share some general dietary information, but will (than, then) send the patient to a licensed dietician or nutritionist for specific dietary instructions.

8. (Their, They're, There) are (too, to, two) types of vitamins: fat-soluble, which includes A, D, E, and K, and water-soluble, which includes the B complex and C vitamins.

CHAPTER REVIEW

Assignment 20-3: Abbreviation Review

Write what each of the following abbreviations stands for.

1. BMI: _____

2. DASH: _____

3. GI (not referring to provider): _____

4. GI (referring to system): _____

5. RDN: _____

6. USDA: _____

7. FBS: _____

8. RDA: _____

9. mEq: _____

10. mcg: _____

11. mg: _____

Assignment 20-4: Short Answer

1. Compare and contrast the eating disorders anorexia nervosa, bulimia nervosa, compulsive overeating, and night eating syndrome.

    A. Anorexia nervosa: _____
    _____
    _____
    _____

    B. Bulimia nervosa: _____
    _____
    _____

    C. Compulsive overeating: _____
    _____
    _____

    D. Night eating syndrome: _____
    _____
    _____
    _____

2. Explain the importance of good nutrition as it relates to health and disease.
    _____
    _____
    _____
    _____

3. List five different food groups in the "ChooseMyPlate" food plan with examples of foods in each group (you may visit the website www.choosemyplate.gov to view information that is in addition to the text provided). Also include information regarding "oils" (not a food group, but they provide essential nutrients).

    A. Fruits: _____
    _____
    _____

    B. Vegetables: _____
    _____
    _____
    _____
    _____
    _____
    _____

    C. Grains: _____
    _____
    _____
    _____
    _____
    _____

D. Protein Foods: _____

_____

_____

_____

E. Dairy: _____

_____

_____

_____

_____

F. Oils: _____

_____

_____

_____

_____

_____

CERTIFICATION PRACTICE

Assignment 20-5

Choose the best answer and place the corresponding letter in the blank.

____ 1. The digestive structure that is responsible for digestive enzymes and the break down of fats, proteins, and carbohydrates into their basic components, which can then be absorbed and used by the body is the:

A. small intestine.

B. large intestine.

C. pancreas.

D. stomach.

____ 2. Which digestive structure produces insulin?

A. Stomach

B. Small intestine

C. Large intestine

D. Pancreas

____ 3. _____ are the main source of energy for the body when converted to glucose. When consumed in excess, they are converted into fat and stored in the adipose tissues.

A. Carbohydrates

B. Proteins

C. Lipids

D. Minerals

___ 4. The part of plant foods that is not digested, which is found in whole grains, vegetables, and fruits and is essential for the normal functioning of the gastrointestinal system is the:

    A. electrolytes.

    B. fiber.

    C. carbohydrates.

    D. proteins.

___ 5. Pasta would be an example from which of the following food groups?

    A. Carbohydrates

    B. Fats

    C. Dairy

    D. Grains

___ 6. Which of the following would not be a health benefit from the vegetable food group?

    A. Potassium

    B. Vitamin A

    C. Iron transport

    D. Vitamin C

___ 7. Which food group is high in fiber, decreases cholesterol, and helps reduce constipation?

    A. Grains

    B. Fruits and vegetables

    C. Milk and dairy

    D. Meats and oils

___ 8. Which mineral is the essential component of hemoglobin in the red blood cells, to transfer oxygen from the lungs to the tissues?

    A. Calcium

    B. Iron

    C. Sodium

    D. Magnesium

___ 9. Which food group's lead nutrients include folate, iron, and magnesium?

    A. Grains

    B. Fruits and vegetables

    C. Dairy

    D. Meats and oils

___ 10. Which of the following vitamins is a group of fat-soluble compounds with antioxidant activities that protect the cells from the damaging effects of the free radicals?

    A. Vitamin A

    B. Vitamin E

    C. B Complex

    D. Vitamin C

SKILL APPLICATION CHALLENGE
Assignment 20-6: Research Activity

1. Mrs. Hennessey is diagnosed with type 2 diabetes and has been struggling with her weight and blood glucose levels. The provider asks you to provide a health coaching session with the patient regarding her condition and to help her construct a diabetic diet and exercise plan. Using the Internet, create a list of websites that will assist the patient in learning about her condition. Try to include at least one reference that includes an animation. Make a list of websites the patient can go to and provide reference information beside each website that describes what the patient should click on once they get to the website as well as the exceptional features of each website. Items of interest for this presentation include: how the portion size of meals in addition to the variety of food groups is essential for managing her diabetes.

2. Research the topic of "Foodborne Illness." Identify the various types of foodborne illness, providing a description and symptoms. Now create a plan to protect yourself.

FIELD APPLICATION CHALLENGE
Assignment 20-7

Read the following Field Application Challenge and respond to the questions following the scenario.
Jackson Hewitt is a 38-year-old sales manager at a major marketing firm who has recently been diagnosed with high cholesterol, hypertension, and had blood glucose readings that are "pre-diabetic." Due to his high pressure job, he works long hours, exercises infrequently, and often grabs a fast-food meal on the run. His father died at the age of 52 from heart disease, and he says he is committed to making the necessary lifestyle changes to improve his health.

1. What basic nutritional information do you think he needs and what is a good website to view a daily food plan?

_____

_____

_____

_____

_____

2. Why would it be valuable to have him keep a food and exercise diary for a week?

_____

_____

_____

_____

_____

_____

_____

_____

_____

_____

3. How would you approach the subject of how to handle a high-stress job, long hours, and lack of exercise? How would your health coaching skills and professionalism keys factor in to the discussion?

_____

_____

_____

_____

_____

_____

_____

_____

_____

_____

JOURNALING EXERCISE

Assignment 20-8

What content within this chapter was most meaningful to you? Why? After reading Davene's mentoring statement, how do you personally feel about the subject of weight? Do you yourself want to lose weight and be in better health? Or do you follow a good diet and exercise regime and see people who are overweight and unhealthy as lazy and a drain on the system? While you must always withhold judgment, what are some phrases that you can use when reviewing diet and nutrition with your patients that won't make them feel like you are judging them? Jot down some ideas on what phrases you would use when speaking to your patient.

CHAPTER **21**

Evaluation and Care of the Pediatric Patient

VOCABULARY REVIEW

Assignment 21-1: Sentence Completion

Fill in the blanks below with Essential Terms from this chapter.

1. _____ is the name for an eating disorder in which an individual limits food intake or does not eat at all to the point of starvation.

2. Height or body type that occurs within a family is called _____.

3. A child in the first year of his life is called a(n) _____.

4. _____ is a condition in which the head is abnormally small.

5. _____ is an area of growth that includes reflexes, gross motor skills, and fine motor skills.

6. Activities that indicate acceptable growth and development patterns are known as _____.

7. The term _____ refers to a child in his first month of life.

8. _____ patients can range from the newborn to the young adult.

9. A teenager is the same as a(n) _____.

10. The term that refers to the initial period following birth is _____.

Assignment 21-2: Misspelled Words

Underline the correctly spelled term.

1. adolesent   adolescent   addolescent
2. circumcision   circumsion   circumscition
3. macrocephale   macrochephaly   macrocephaly
4. familial   famielial   famileal
5. buliemia nervosa   bulemia nervosa   bulimia nervosa
6. toddeler   toddler   toddelor
7. immunizaitions   immunizations   immunizasions
8. neonat   neonate   kneonate
9. puberty   peuberty   pubuerty
10. head circumfrance head circumferance head circumference

CHAPTER REVIEW

Assignment 21-3: Abbreviation Review

Write what each of the following abbreviations stands for.

1. PKU: _____
2. SIDS: _____
3. BPM: _____
4. IMZ: _____
5. CDC: _____
6. GACVS: _____
7. MMR: _____
8. HPV: _____
9. ACIP: _____
10. LAIV: _____
11. BMI: _____
12. BDI: _____
13. PCV13: _____

Assignment 21-4: Short Answer

1. Explain the importance of correctly plotting height, weight, and head circumference measurements on the pediatric patient.

_____

_____

2. Fill in the average heart rate and respiratory rate for each of the pediatric ages listed. The first one has been completed for you.

Age	Average Heart Rate	Average Respiratory Rate
Newborn to 3 months	80–160 BPM	30–60/min
3 months to 2 years		
Toddler (age 2–3 years)		
Children (age 2–10 years)		
Age 10 and above		

3. List and describe six reflexes that are tested in the newborn.

A. _____

B. _____

C. _____

D. _____

E. _____

F. _____

4. Explain how weight is calculated after an infant is weighed in a diaper and a t-shirt.

_____

_____

CERTIFICATION PRACTICE

Assignment 21-5

Choose the best answer and place the corresponding letter in the blank.

____ 1. Which of the following age classifications would be given to a child who is 2½ years old?

A. Child

B. Infant

C. Preschooler

D. Toddler

____ 2. Pediatric visual screenings begin at what age?

A. 18 months

B. 2 years

C. During infancy

D. 3 years

____ 3. Normal language milestones help identify:

A. intellectual development.

B. speech delay.

C. mental retardation.

D. learning disability

___ 4. The preferred location for the administration of an intramuscular injection in the young pediatric patient is:

  A. dorsogluteal.

  B. deltoid.

  C. gluteal.

  D. vastus lateralis.

___ 5. Which of the following signs could be an indication of childhood depression?

  A. Dangerous behavior

  B. Increased physical complaints

  C. Increased boredom

  D. All of the above

___ 6. Which of the following tests is required for newborns in most states?

  A. IRT

  B. Sickle cell test

  C. PKU

  D. Blood typing

___ 7. Which of the following could contribute to childhood obesity?

  A. Fast food

  B. Television or computers that have become the primary focus instead of some type of physical activity

  C. Genetics

  D. All of the above

___ 8. When taking vital signs on a patient that is four months old, the heart rate is 128 beats per minute. What action should be taken by the medical assistant?

  A. Record the information in the chart and notify the physician right away.

  B. Record the information in the chart and allow the physician to read it as he reviews the chart before entering the room. The pulse is normal for this age group.

  C. Notify the EMS.

  D. Gather heart monitor, oxygen, and IV equipment.

___ 9. What communication style is best when talking to the parents of a toddler?

  A. Alright, Mrs. Timmons, can you remove Connor's clothes down to his diaper?

  B. Alright, mommy, can you remove Connor's clothes down to his diaper?

  C. Alright, can you remove Connor's clothes down to his diaper?

  D. Alright, Connor's mommy, can you remove Connor's clothes down to his diaper?

___ 10. Which of the following abbreviations are connected with a disease that causes infants to stop breathing during periods of sleep?

  A. SADS

  B. SIDS

  C. SIDDS

  D. SADDS

SKILL APPLICATION CHALLENGE
Assignment 21-6: Research Activity

1. Using the Internet, research recent findings on the different forms of autism and present information to the class on your findings. Include an explanation of the different forms of autism along with available treatment options and the prognosis for each.

2. Using the Internet, gather statistics on the occurrence of heart attacks among high-school and college-age athletes. Present facts on possible screenings that would be advisable before a student participates in these activities.

COMPLETING SPECIAL FORMS
Assignment 21-7: Plotting Percentiles on a Growth Chart

Work Form Necessary: FORM 21-1

Directions: Complete the growth chart (Work Form 21-1) using the following information.

The child's name is Ashur Green. His chart number is 125655. His mother's stature is 62 inches and his father's stature is 66 inches. Measurements to be plotted are listed below.

Date	Age	Weight	Length	Head Circumference
10-10-15	Birth	9 pounds	20 inches	12 inches
01-12-16	3 months	12 pounds 3 ounces	21.5 inches	13.5 inches
04-11-16	6 months	15 pounds 6 ounces	24.75 inches	14 inches
07-11-16	9 months	22 pounds	26 inches	15 inches
10-12-16	12 months	26 pounds	28 inches	15.5 inches
04-15-17	18 months	30 pounds	30.5 inches	16 inches

FIELD APPLICATION CHALLENGE
Assignment 21-8

Read the following Field Application Challenge and respond to the questions following the scenario.

You are scheduled to give Mason Pendleton his four-month immunizations today. You give the paperwork and vaccination information statements (VIS) to Mason's mother and ask her to read over VIS forms while you prepare the vaccines. After reading them over, Mrs. Pendleton tells you that she does not want her son to receive the vaccines. When you ask her why, she responds by saying that she just watched a documentary on safety concerns regarding early infant immunizations and she just doesn't feel comfortable with having her son vaccinated.

1. What can you do to help Mason's mother feel reassured that it is in her son's best interest to be vaccinated?

_____

_____

_____

_____

_____

_____

_____

_____

_____

2. Should the medical assistant have drawn up the vaccination medication before the mother signed the release forms? Why or why not.

_____

_____

_____

3. Should the provider be alerted about the mother's hesitancy, even if she ends up allowing the child to be vaccinated? Explain your answer.

_____

_____

_____

4. If the child's mother declines the vaccinations, can the same vaccine be used on someone else? Why or why not.

_____

_____

JOURNALING EXERCISE

Assignment 21-9

Character traits necessary to work in pediatrics include patience, honesty, and a love for children. Communication skills and the needs of the patient will often fluctuate at each unique developmental level. Are you drawn to working in a pediatric practice? What content within this chapter was most meaningful to you? Why? List some examples of how you might apply information contained in this chapter to your career as a medical assistant. Which professionalism keys do you think would be most helpful when working with children?

Work Form 21-1

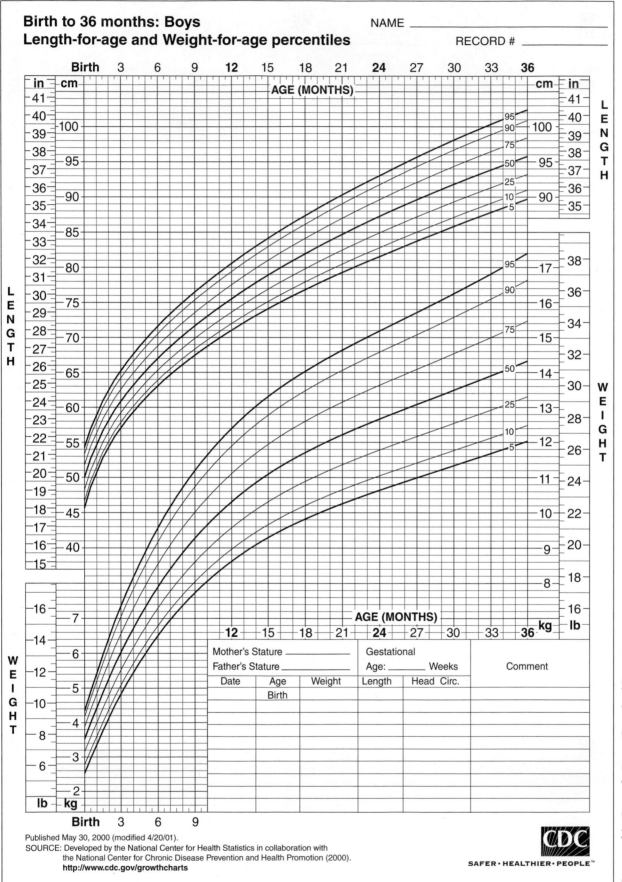

Birth to 36 months: Boys
Length-for-age and Weight-for-age percentiles

NAME _____

RECORD # _____

AGE (MONTHS)

	Date	Age	Weight	Length	Head Circ.	Comment
Birth						

Mother's Stature _____

Father's Stature _____

Gestational Age: _____ Weeks

Published May 30, 2000 (modified 4/20/01).
SOURCE: Developed by the National Center for Health Statistics in collaboration with
the National Center for Chronic Disease Prevention and Health Promotion (2000).
http://www.cdc.gov/growthcharts

CDC

SAFER • HEALTHIER • PEOPLE™

Courtesy of the Centers for Disease Control and Prevention

CHAPTER **22**

Orthopedics, Rehabilitation, and Physical Therapy

VOCABULARY REVIEW

Assignment 22-1: Matching

Match the term with its definition and place the corresponding letter in the blank.

_____ 1. Ambulation

_____ 2. Cartilage

_____ 3. Cryotherapy

_____ 4. Arthroscopy

_____ 5. Modalities

_____ 6. Orthopedist

_____ 7. Prosthesis

_____ 8. Rehabilitation

_____ 9. Sprain

_____ 10. Strain

_____ 11. Thermotherapy

_____ 12. Massage

_____ 13. Dislocation

_____ 14. Physical therapist

_____ 15. Ultrasound

A. The use of high-frequency sound waves used to create heat deep in soft tissues such as muscles and tendons

B. Use of dry or moist heat to promote healing and restore function

C. An artificial joint

D. Process of treatments designed to return a body part to its full function, following an illness or injury; helps patients find a workable solution to assist them with the activities of daily living

E. Trauma to ligaments; may also involve injury to the tendons and muscles

F. A medical doctor who specializes in the treatment of diseases and disorders of the bones and muscles (and can perform surgery)

G. Injury to a muscle or tendon caused by excessive use or overexertion

H. Physical agents, such as heat, cold, water, and exercise, to improve or restore lost function

I. Use of pressure, friction, and kneading to promote muscle relaxation

J. A specialist who helps to restore function, improve mobility, and decrease pain to an area that has been damaged by injury or disease

K. Ability to walk or move about freely

L. Visualization of a joint and joint capsule through a lighted instrument for treatment

M. A temporary displacement of a bone from its usual position within a joint

N. Connective tissue located between the articular surfaces of bones, joints, and vertebrae that acts as a shock absorber

O. The application of dry or moist cold to the affected area of the body

Assignment 22-2: Vocabulary Builder

Find the words below that are misspelled; circle them and then correctly spell them in the spaces provided. Then complete the following sentences with the correct vocabulary terms from the list.

alograft   atrophy   greenstick

kiphosis   ostoporosis   compression

_____   _____   _____

_____   _____   _____

Cartilage grafting involves transplanting cartilage from a healthy area into the joint that has little or no cartilage left. A patient's own tissue (autograft) or a donor graft (1) (_____) may be used to restore cartilage in joints where it has been lost. The shrinkage due to inadequate nutrition to the muscle is known as (2) _____. A (3) _____ fracture is when the bone is partially bent and partially broken (often seen in children). A (4) _____ fracture is when a piece of the broken bone is driven inward (sometimes seen in skull fractures). (5) _____ is the abnormal forward curvature of the spine. (6) _____ is a disease resulting in weak and brittle bone, occurring primarily in females.

CHAPTER REVIEW

Assignment 22-3: Abbreviation Review

Write what each of the following abbreviations stands for.

1. ROM: _____

2. PT: _____

3. RICE: _____

4. OT: _____

5. ACL: _____

6. ADLs: _____

7. DEXA: _____

8. TENS: _____

9: SERMs: _____

10. PTH: _____

11. CPK: _____

Assignment 22-4: Short Answer

1. Explain the differences between a sprain and a strain.

   _____

   _____

   _____

2. Describe the following types of fractures.

   A. Complete: _____

   B. Incomplete: _____

C. Complicated: _____

D. Greenstick: _____

E. Compression: _____

F. Hairline: _____

_____

G. Impacted: _____

H. Pathological: _____

I. Pott's: _____

J. Spiral: _____

K. Stress: _____

_____

L. Colles: _____

M. Comminuted: _____

N. Transverse: _____

O. Oblique: _____

3. Explain how to measure a patient for a cane, walker, and crutches.

A. Cane: _____

_____

B. Walker: _____

C. Crutches: _____

_____

_____

_____

4. Describe the following joint movement terms.

A. Abduction: _____

B. Adduction: _____

C. Circumduction: _____

D. Dorsiflexion: _____

E. Eversion: _____

F. Extension: _____

G. Flexion: _____

H. Hyperextension: _____

I. Inversion: _____

J. Plantar flexion: _____

K. Pronation: _____

L. Rotation: _____

M. Supination: _____

CERTIFICATION PRACTICE
Assignment 22-5
Choose the best answer and place the corresponding letter in the blank.

____ 1. Which of the following is not a risk factor for developing osteoporosis?

    A. Early menopause before age 45

    B. Sedentary lifestyle

    C. Smoking

    D. A diet low in B complex vitamins

____ 2. Which of the following tests visualizes the distribution of an IV-injected radioactive isotope that collects in the bones and joints?

    A. CT scan

    B. MRI

    C. Bone scan

    D. Discography

____ 3. Which of the following tests would be performed to detect a bone infection, cancer, or muscle atrophy?

    A. Arthroscopy

    B. Bone/muscle biopsy

    C. Electromyography

    D. Urine and blood tests

____ 4. A fracture may be treated with all but which of the following devices?

    A. Cast

    B. Splint

    C. Sterile gauze

    D. Pins and wires

____ 5. Viscosupplementation is a treatment used for severe knee pain associated with:

    A. osteoarthritis.

    B. bursitis.

    C. tendonitis.

    D. hairline fractures.

____ 6. Which of the following would be a reason for thermotherapy?

    A. To decrease bruising following an injury

    B. To relax muscles and alleviate muscle spasms

    C. To reduce swelling immediately following an injury

    D. To relieve pain immediately following an injury

____ 7. Examples of cryotherapy include all of the following *except:*

    A. ice bag.

    B. dry ice.

    C. chemical ice pack.

    D. commercial ice packs.

___ 8. When applying heat or cold packs to a muscle you should:

   A. always apply the packs directly over the skin.

   B. always keep in place for at least 30–60 minutes.

   C. always cover the pack so that there is a barrier between the pack and the patient's skin.

   D. always ask the patient to tense their muscle before applying the pack for better absorption.

___ 9. A physician who specializes in diagnosing and treating diseases and disorders of the nervous system, including the brain, spinal cord, and nerves is a(n):

   A. neurologist.

   B. neurosurgeon.

   C. orthopedist.

   D. physiatrist.

___ 10. A nonphysician who helps to restore function, improve mobility, and decrease pain to an area that has been damaged by injury or disease using physical agents or modalities is a(n):

   A. occupational therapist.

   B. physical therapist.

   C. occupational therapy assistant.

   D. physical technician.

SKILL APPLICATION CHALLENGE
Assignment 22-6: Labeling

1. Label the types of fractures illustrated below.

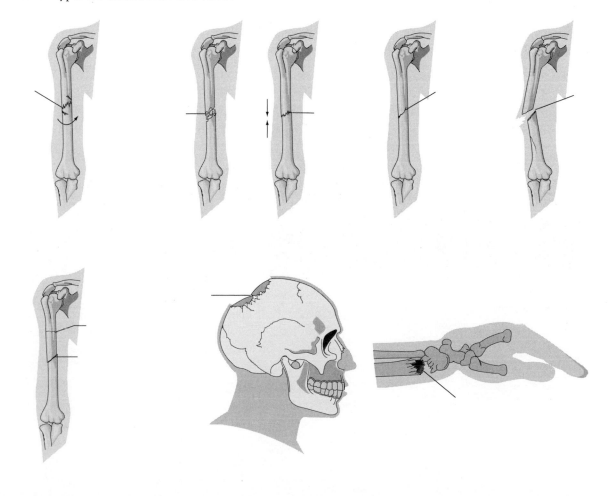

2. Identify the crutch gaits based on the illustrations below.

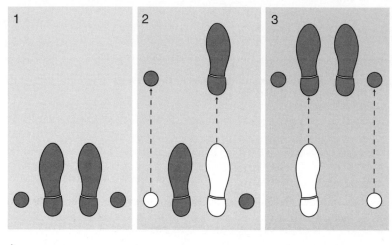

A. _____

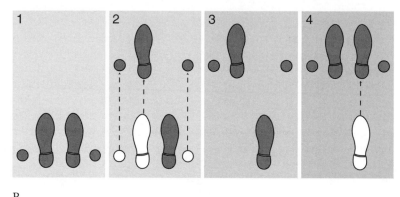

B. _____

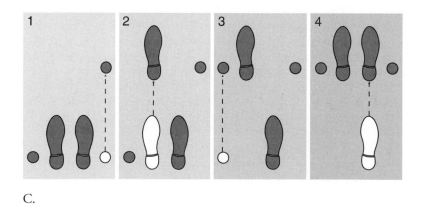

C. _____

FIELD APPLICATION CHALLENGE

Assignment 22-7

Read the following Field Application Challenge and respond to the questions following the scenario.

A patient calls and states that she fell on her left wrist about an hour ago and that the wrist is really swollen. You schedule the patient for an immediate appointment and give the patient some home care instructions to follow prior to being seen. Following an X-ray examination, the physician diagnoses the patient with a sprain to the wrist. Use the matching items to help you answer the questions below.

A. Rest, ice, compression, and elevation

B. Rest, compression, elevation, movement (alternating periods of heat and cold therapy)

C. Immobilize, elevate, and apply ice

____ 1. Which of the above instructions should be given to the patient prior to coming into the office to be seen by the provider?

____ 2. Which of the above instructions should be given to the patient for the first 24 to 48 hours or until all of the swelling is gone?

____ 3. Which of the above instructions may be given to the patient once all of the swelling is diminished?

JOURNALING EXERCISE

Assignment 22-8

What content within this chapter was most meaningful to you? Why? List some examples of how you might apply information contained in this chapter, both during your training and after you enter the health care industry. After reading Davene's mentoring scenario, are you drawn toward working in an orthopedic practice? Why or why not? Do you, or a family member, suffer from orthopedic issues? Explain how you would want to be treated, and give some examples of how you, as a medical assistant, would demonstrate professionalism in this setting.

C H A P T E R **23**

Fundamentals of the Medical Laboratory

VOCABULARY REVIEW
Assignment 23-1: Matching

___ 1. Baseline values

___ 2. Centrifuge

___ 3. Clinical diagnosis

___ 4. Differential diagnosis

___ 5. Profile

___ 6. Reference ranges

___ 7. Asymptomatic

___ 8. External controls

___ 9. Flow sheets

___ 10. Internal controls

A. Testing which is performed when the patient's symptoms are indicative of more than one disease

B. Normal values, expected values, or reference intervals for laboratory results

C. Readings establish a starting point for monitoring a patient's lab results

D. Having no symptoms at all

E. Evaluates the entire testing process, including that the control results are in the expected ranges

F. Group of lab tests related by body system or function

G. An instrument that spins tubes at high speeds to separate the liquid portion of the sample from the cells and other formed elements

H. These evaluate whether or not the test is working as it was designed, that the correct amount of sample was added, that the sample is moving through the test correctly, or whether the instrument is in good working order

I. Identification of a disease or condition from facts obtained through medical history, physical exam, laboratory studies, and radiological studies

J. Found in paper form in the chart, or tracked electronically; contain data collected on patients that can be reviewed and updated each time the patient visits their health care provider

Assignment 23-2: Sentence Completion

Fill in the blanks below with Essential Terms from this chapter.

1. A _____ containing all pertinent information and tests requested, must accompany each specimen.

2. Satellite locations where samples are collected are known as _____.

3. The _____ is the eyepiece of the microscope.

4. A patient who is without symptoms is _____.

5. Examples of _____ include cytologic evaluation (Pap smears), cytogenetic testing, tests in histopathology, and histocompatibility.

6. _____ results usually identify the presence or absence of a substance and are interpreted as positive or negative.

7. _____ (low-complexity) are simple to perform, require a minimum of quality control and documentation, and a minimum of judgment and interpretation.

8. _____ are equipped with either one eyepiece (monocular) or two eyepieces (binocular).

9. Prior to 2012, the CMS stated that only licensed health care professionals had the authority to enter orders into an EHR. However, on August 23, 2012, the CMS issued a final rule on Stage 2 Meaningful Use of the Medicare and Medicaid EHR incentive program stating that credentialed medical assistants also qualify to enter medication orders into the

   _____.

10. _____ procedures are designed to ensure the accuracy and precision of laboratory tests and to discover and eliminate human error.

CHAPTER REVIEW

Assignment 23-3: Abbreviation Review

Write what each of the following abbreviations stands for.

1. CLIA '88: _____

2. COLA: _____

3. DHHS: _____

4. SDS: _____

5. POCT: _____

6. POL: _____

7. PPM: _____

8. QA: _____

9. QC: _____

10. ABR-OE: _____

11. CPOE: _____

12. BUN: _____

13. CEUs: _____

14. SOP: _____

15. ESR: _____

16. PT: _____

Assignment 23-4: Short Answer

1. List at least four reasons for performing laboratory tests.

   _____

   _____

   _____

2. Explain the purpose of the CLIA '88 federal standards and cite the regulation's four sets of rules.

   _____

   _____

   _____

   _____

3. Describe the following laboratory classifications.

   A. Reference lab: _____

   _____

   B. Hospital: _____

   _____

   C. Physician's office laboratory (POL): _____

   _____

   _____

   _____

   D. Point-of-care testing: _____

   _____

   E. Procurement station/satellite lab: _____

   _____

4. Describe the terms quality control and quality assurance.

   A. Quality control: _____

   _____

   _____

   _____

   B. Quality assurance: _____

   _____

5. Hazards in the lab are divided into what three categories?

   _____

CERTIFICATION PRACTICE

Assignment 23-5

Choose the best answer and place the corresponding letter in the blank.

___ 1. Performance of waived tests does not require the laboratory to participate in proficiency testing by outside inspectors or to employ specially trained personnel. The laboratory is required, however, to obtain _____ in order to perform low-complexity tests.

    A. approval by DHHS

    B. CLIA approval

    C. a certificate of waiver

    D. a passing grade on proficiency tests

___ 2. All of the following are CLIA-waived tests, *except:*

    A. HbA1c.

    B. differential count.

    C. hematocrit.

    D. Erythrocyte sedimentation rate.

___ 3. Into which of the following categories does PPM fall?

    A. Low-complexity

    B. Waived

    C. Moderate-complexity

    D. High-complexity

___ 4. Which of the following tests is classified as PPM?

    A. Hemoglobin

    B. Urine sediment examinations

    C. Occult blood testing

    D. Hematocrit

___ 5. Procedures that are designed to ensure the accuracy and precision of laboratory tests are known as:

    A. proficiency testing.

    B. quality assurance.

    C. quality control.

    D. CEUs.

___ 6. You are reading the temperature on the refrigerator where patient samples and test kits are stored. The acceptable range is 35.6–46.4°F, but the thermometer reads 49°F. Which of the following statements is true regarding the impact of the samples and test kits in this refrigerator at that temperature?

    A. None, since there really isn't that much of a difference.

    B. Reagents may need to be discarded.

    C. There may be a bit of an odor, but this shouldn't affect the overall condition.

    D. It will vary depending on the tests that are to be performed.

___ 7. The Occupational Exposure to Hazardous Chemicals in the Laboratory Standard law was designed to:

    A. inform employees of the risks involved while working with exposure to chemicals in the laboratory.

    B. set the standards for the types of chemicals used in a laboratory setting.

    C. establish protocol for documenting test methods.

    D. educate lab personnel regarding the molecular structure of each chemical.

___ 8. Which of the following activities would *not* fall under chemical hazards cautions?

A. Immediately recap bottles containing toxic substances

B. Labeling of all bottles of hazardous chemicals

C. Store flammable or volatile chemicals following manufacturer's guidelines

D. A listing of all the uses for each chemical

___ 9. All of the following items are required information on a laboratory requisition form *except:*

A. clinical diagnosis.

B. specimen source.

C. date and time of collection.

D. an explanation of how the specimen was stored.

___ 10. A patient calls the office demanding to know the results of her laboratory tests that were drawn over a week ago. You notice that they have not been reviewed by the physician. Which of the following statements is correct about what you should tell the patient?

A. If results are normal, it is always okay to inform the patient of the results.

B. Tell the patient that results seem to be normal but that you will have to talk to the physician for confirmation.

C. Read the report to the patient, but inform her that you cannot interpret the results.

D. Inform the patient that the physician has not had an opportunity to review the results but that you will get back in touch with her just as soon as the physician does.

SKILL APPLICATION CHALLENGE

Assignment 23-6: Labeling

Label the parts of the microscope and describe their use in the table below.

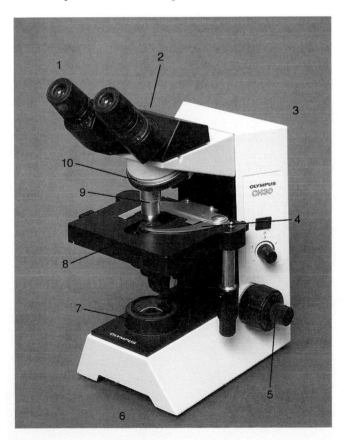

Name of Part	Use
1.	
2.	
3.	
4.	
5.	
6.	
7.	
8.	
9.	
10.	

COMPLETING SPECIAL FORMS

Assignment 23-7: Completing a Lab Requisition

Work Form Necessary: FORM 23-1

Directions: Complete the laboratory requisition form (Work Form 23-1) using the following information. The bill is to be sent directly to the provider so no insurance information is listed for the patient. (Hint: You will not use all of the information that is listed.)

Provider information: Robert Aniso, MD, Welleville Family Physicians, 1010 Carter Drive, Welleville, OH 12345-0987, Dr ID 20A

Patient information: Jane Karnes, 18168 August Avenue, Hometown, OH, 12345-7780, DOB: 05-11-60

Specimen source: Whole blood and serum

Date and time of collection: 05-12-XX, 14:00, patient is fasting

Tests requested: Hemoglobin A1c, and cholesterol

Medications: Lisinopril, Glucophage, Lipitor

Clinical diagnosis: ICD-10 codes E11.65 and E78.0

FIELD APPLICATION CHALLENGE
Assignment 23-8

Read the following Field Application Challenge and respond to the questions following the scenario.

The provider has requested that you obtain a blood sample to be sent to the lab for a blood glucose, cholesterol, and PT/INR. After consulting the lab catalog, you notice that the patient must be fasting for the glucose and cholesterol levels and that serum is the specimen requirement. The PT does not require fasting but the specimen requirement is plasma. You obtain one SST tube and one light-blue top tube. After centrifugation, you pour off the serum and the plasma into tubes that will be sent to the lab. You forgot to label the tubes before pouring off the samples so you do not know which one is serum and which one is plasma.

1. How can you rectify the problem?

_____

_____

2. What could happen if you send the specimens to the lab anyway?

_____

3. How could you prevent this kind of mistake from happening again?

_____

JOURNALING EXERCISE
Assignment 23-9

What content within this chapter was most meaningful to you? Why? As Davene stressed in her mentoring scenario, medical assistants are responsible for assuring that patients comprehend instructions for specific laboratory tests to ensure accuracy. What will you do if you do not understand the test instructions yourself? How will you establish that the patient has a clear understanding of the instructions? How will you handle patients with limited English? Which professionalism keys would be most helpful? Why?

Work Form 23-1

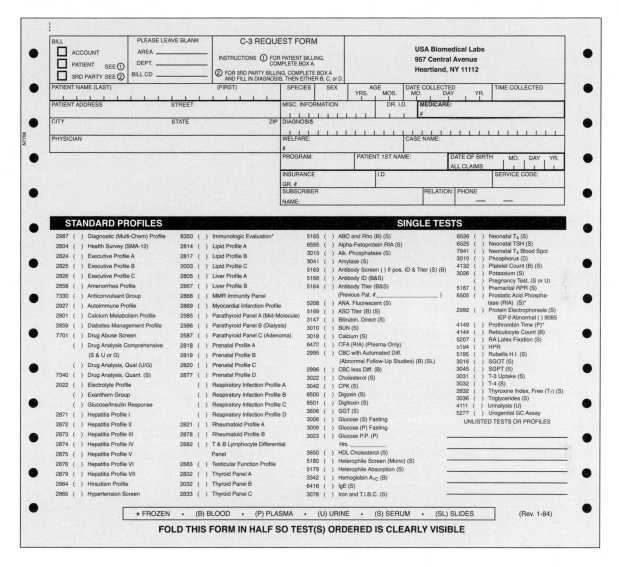

BILL	PLEASE LEAVE BLANK	C-3 REQUEST FORM		USA Biomedical Labs
☐ ACCOUNT	AREA _____	INSTRUCTIONS ① FOR PATIENT BILLING, COMPLETE BOX A.		957 Central Avenue
☐ PATIENT SEE ①	DEPT. _____	② FOR 3RD PARTY BILLING, COMPLETE BOX A		Heartland, NY 11112
☐ 3RD PARTY SEE ②	BILL CD _____	AND FILL IN DIAGNOSIS, THEN EITHER B, C, or D.		

PATIENT NAME (LAST)   (FIRST)   SPECIES   SEX   AGE YRS. MOS.   DATE COLLECTED MO. DAY YR.   TIME COLLECTED

PATIENT ADDRESS   STREET   MISC. INFORMATION   DR. I.D.   MEDICARE: #

CITY   STATE   ZIP   DIAGNOSIS

PHYSICIAN   WELFARE: #   CASE NAME:

PROGRAM: PATIENT 1ST NAME: DATE OF BIRTH ALL CLAIMS   MO. DAY YR.

INSURANCE   I.D.   SERVICE CODE:
GR. #
SUBSCRIBER   RELATION: PHONE
NAME: ___ ___

STANDARD PROFILES

2987 ( ) Diagnostic (Multi-Chem) Profile	8350 ( ) Immunologic Evaluation*
2804 ( ) Health Survey (SMA-12)	2814 ( ) Lipid Profile A
2824 ( ) Executive Profile A	2817 ( ) Lipid Profile B
2825 ( ) Executive Profile B	2003 ( ) Lipid Profile C
2826 ( ) Executive Profile C	2805 ( ) Liver Profile A
2858 ( ) Amenorrhea Profile	2867 ( ) Liver Profile B
7330 ( ) Anticonvulsant Group	2868 ( ) MMR Immunity Panel
2927 ( ) Autoimmune Profile	2869 ( ) Myocardial Infarction Profile
2801 ( ) Calcium Metabolism Profile	2585 ( ) Parathyroid Panel A (Mid-Molecule)
2859 ( ) Diabetes Management Profile	2586 ( ) Parathyroid Panel B (Dialysis)
7701 ( ) Drug Abuse Screen	2587 ( ) Parathyroid Panel C (Adenoma)
( ) Drug Analysis Comprehensive (S & U or G)	2818 ( ) Prenatal Profile A
	2819 ( ) Prenatal Profile B
( ) Drug Analysis, Qual (U/G)	2820 ( ) Prenatal Profile C
7340 ( ) Drug Analysis, Quant. (S)	2877 ( ) Prenatal Profile D
2022 ( ) Electrolyte Profile	( ) Respiratory Infection Profile A
( ) Exanthem Group	( ) Respiratory Infection Profile B
( ) Glucose/Insulin Response	( ) Respiratory Infection Profile C
2871 ( ) Hepatitis Profile I	( ) Respiratory Infection Profile D
2872 ( ) Hepatitis Profile II	2821 ( ) Rheumatoid Profile A
2873 ( ) Hepatitis Profile III	2878 ( ) Rheumatoid Profile B
2874 ( ) Hepatitis Profile IV	2882 ( ) T & B Lymphocyte Differential
2875 ( ) Hepatitis Profile V	Panel
2876 ( ) Hepatitis Profile VI	2883 ( ) Testicular Function Profile
2879 ( ) Hepatitis Profile VII	2832 ( ) Thyroid Panel A
2864 ( ) Hirsutism Profile	2032 ( ) Thyroid Panel B
2865 ( ) Hypertension Screen	2833 ( ) Thyroid Panel C

SINGLE TESTS

5165 ( ) ABO and Rho (B) (S)	6526 ( ) Neonatal T_4 (S)
6555 ( ) Alpha-Fetoprotein RIA (S)	6525 ( ) Neonatal TSH (S)
3015 ( ) Alk. Phosphatase (S)	7941 ( ) Neonatal T_4 Blood Spot
3041 ( ) Amylase (S)	3010 ( ) Phosphorus (S)
5163 ( ) Antibody Screen ( ) If pos. ID & Titer (S) (B)	4132 ( ) Platelet Count (B) (S)
5166 ( ) Antibody ID (B&S)	3026 ( ) Potassium (S)
5164 ( ) Antibody Titer (B&S)	( ) Pregnancy Test, (S or U)
(Previous Pat. #_____)	5187 ( ) Premarital RPR (S)
5208 ( ) ANA. Fluorescent (S)	6505 ( ) Prostatic Acid Phospha-
5169 ( ) ASO Titer (B) (S)	tase (RIA) (S)*
3147 ( ) Bilirubin, Direct (S)	2992 ( ) Protein Electrophoresis (S)
3010 ( ) BUN (S)	IEP if Abnormal ( ) 9085
3018 ( ) Calcium (S)	4149 ( ) Prothrombin Time (P)*
6472 ( ) CEA (RIA) (Plasma Only)	4144 ( ) Reticulocyte Count (B)
2995 ( ) CBC with Automated Diff.	5207 ( ) RA Latex Fixation (S)
(Abnormal Follow-Up Studies) (B) (SL)	5194 ( ) HPR
2996 ( ) CBC less Diff. (B)	5195 ( ) Rubella H.I. (S)
3022 ( ) Cholesterol (S)	3016 ( ) SGOT (S)
3042 ( ) CPK (S)	3045 ( ) SGPT (S)
6500 ( ) Digoxin (S)	3031 ( ) T-3 Uptake (S)
6501 ( ) Digitoxin (S)	3032 ( ) T-4 (S)
3606 ( ) GGT (S)	2832 ( ) Thyroxine Index, Free (T_7) (S)
3006 ( ) Glucose (S) Fasting	3036 ( ) Triglycerides (S)
3009 ( ) Glucose (P) Fasting	4111 ( ) Urinalysis (U)
3023 ( ) Glucose P.P. (P)	5277 ( ) Urogenital GC Assay
Hrs.	UNLISTED TESTS OR PROFILES
3650 ( ) HDL Cholesterol (S)	
5180 ( ) Heterophile Screen (Mono) (S)	_____
5179 ( ) Heterophile Absorption (S)	_____
3342 ( ) Hemoglobin A_{1C} (B)	_____
6416 ( ) IgE (S)	_____
3078 ( ) Iron and T.I.B.C. (S)	_____

★ FROZEN • (B) BLOOD • (P) PLASMA • (U) URINE • (S) SERUM • (SL) SLIDES   (Rev. 1-84)

FOLD THIS FORM IN HALF SO TEST(S) ORDERED IS CLEARLY VISIBLE

N7708

C H A P T E R **24**

Blood Collection Techniques

VOCABULARY REVIEW

Assignment 24-1: Matching

Match the term with its definition and place the corresponding letter in the blank.

____ 1. Aliquot

____ 2. Constrict

____ 3. Lipemia

____ 4. Evacuated tube

____ 5. Hematoma

____ 6. Lancet

____ 7. Gauge

____ 8. Phlebotomy

____ 9. Serum

____ 10. Tourniquet

____ 11. Primary container

____ 12. Venipuncture

____ 13. Plasma

____ 14. Butterfly

____ 15. Integrity

A. Device used to distend veins to assist with venipuncture

B. Liquid portion of the blood that remains after the blood has clotted

C. Piercing a vein with a needle to obtain a blood specimen

D. Small winged needle used for venipuncture

E. Narrowing of a blood vessel

F. Portion of a specimen that is used for testing

G. Sterile disposable sharp-pointed blade used to puncture the skin to collect a blood sample

H. Diameter of the lumen of a needle

I. Guarantees the purity or quality of the specimen

J. Swelling or accumulation of blood due to leakage from a blood vessel during or after venipuncture

K. Abnormal amount of fat in the blood causing the serum or plasma to appear cloudy or milky

L. Collection tube which contains a vacuum that facilitates the collection of blood during venipuncture

M. Original container in which the specimen is collected

N. Puncture of a vein to collect a blood sample

O. Liquid portion of whole blood which comes from a sample which contains an anticoagulant

Assignment 24-2: Sentence Completion

Fill in the blanks below with Essential Terms from this chapter.

1. A gel contained in some separator tubes which forms a barrier between the cellular portion of the specimen and the serum or plasma after centrifugation is _____.

2. _____ is a pooling of blood at the venipuncture site that is caused by leaving the tourniquet in place too long.

3. The medical assistant will _____ the vein to determine its location.

4. A rupturing of the red blood cells during venipuncture is known as _____.

5. The veins used for venipuncture are located in the _____.

6. A _____ is a skin puncture method used to obtain small amounts of blood for testing.

7. An _____ in the vacuum tube can help to preserve the integrity of the specimen.

8. An _____ added to a collection tube prevents the blood from clotting.

9. Each health care facility will have specific professionals (_____) designated to perform phlebotomy.

10. A sufficient amount of specimen must be available for testing. If there is an insufficient amount, the specimen will be referred to as _____ and must be redrawn.

11. Venipuncture is an invasive procedure in which a vein is punctured to obtain a blood sample. It can be performed using any of the following types of equipment: _____ or evacuated tube and holder, syringe, or butterfly and related equipment.

12. The _____ or butterfly set is used to collect blood from small or difficult veins, usually in the hand.

CHAPTER REVIEW

Assignment 24-3: Abbreviation Review

Write what each of the following abbreviations stands for.

1. QNS: _____
2. EDTA: _____
3. CLSI: _____
4. CBC: _____
5. ESR: _____
6. PT: _____
7. aPTT: _____
8. INR: _____
9. SPS: _____
10. SST: _____
11. PPE: _____

12. MCV: _____

13. POCT: _____

14. OSHA: _____

15. BMP: _____

Assignment 24-4: Fill in the Blank

Fill in the blanks below with the appropriate word or phrase.

1. To ensure patient _____ with fasting instructions, the patient should be questioned to determine if fasting instructions were followed.

2. Venipuncture requires special equipment, _____ , and supervision.

3. _____ tourniquets should be used for patients with a latex sensitivity.

4. Color-coding of needles is not _____ and may vary by manufacturer.

5. The range of syringe volumes most commonly used for blood collection is _____ .

6. It is best to have patients _____ if they have a history of fainting (syncope) during a venipuncture.

7. When palpating for a vein, _____ located near the surface will feel hard and cord-like and should not be mistaken for a vein.

8. A _____ is one of the most common complications resulting from a venipuncture, a swelling or bruising resulting from an accumulation of blood at the puncture site.

9. A _____ puncture, also known as a skin or dermal puncture, is the preferred method for blood collection for infants and children under the age of two and for patients with extremely small, fragile veins.

10. When performing a capillary puncture, the _____ (red-topped) should be collected last.

Assignment 24-5: Short Answer

1. List all the equipment needed to perform a venipuncture (vacuum tube method).

   _____

   _____

   _____

2. Explain the purpose of following the correct order of draw.

   _____

   _____

3. CLSI recommends the following order of draw for capillary punctures:

   1. _____

   2. _____

   3. _____

4. In the table below, list the possible remedies for the causes for failed attempts listed:

Causes of Failed Attempt	Possible Remedy
Needle position, bevel against wall of vein	
Needle position, bevel partially inserted	
Needle too deep	
Needle to the side of the vein	
Collapsed vein	
Tube vacuum insufficient	

5. Explain the importance of mixing the blood sample in a tube that contains an additive.

_____

_____

_____

_____

_____

6. List at least five hematoma prevention tips.

A. _____

B. _____

_____

C. _____

D. _____

E. _____

F. _____

G. _____

_____

_____

7. List and describe six criteria for specimen rejection.

A. _____

B. _____

C. _____

D. _____

E. _____

F. _____

CERTIFICATION PRACTICE

Assignment 24-6

Choose the best answer and place the corresponding letter in the blank.

____ 1. You have collected several tubes of blood to be sent to the lab for testing. Which of the following methods applies to the transportation of all of the tubes?

A. Protected from light

B. Placed on ice

C. Placed in a bag, lying down

D. Kept in an upright position

____ 2. All of the following are reasons for a failed venipuncture *except:*

A. the bevel is partially exposed.

B. a collapsed vein.

C. the needle is to the side of the vein.

D. the needle was inserted bevel up.

____ 3. Leaving a tourniquet on the patient's arm for more than one minute can result in:

A. hematoma.

B. reflux.

C. hemoconcentration.

D. reduced specimen volume.

____ 4. Which of the following is the correct level of placement for the tourniquet on the arm?

A. One inch above the puncture site

B. Three to four inches above the elbow

C. Anywhere on the arm as long as it is above the puncture site

D. As close to the axilla as possible

____ 5. After cleansing the venipuncture site, the medical assistant cannot remember where the vein is located and palpates the site again. Which of the following actions should be the next step in performing the venipuncture?

A. Clean the site again following palpation

B. Collect the sample

C. Remove the tourniquet

D. Start over

____ 6. After inspecting both of the patient's arms and applying the tourniquet, you realize that the veins are very small and fragile and very hard to palpate. Which of the following should be your next step?

    A. Inspect the veins of the hand.

    B. Inspect the veins of the wrist.

    C. Ask for help.

    D. Inform the provider that the patient has no veins.

____ 7. Which of the following is an OSHA requirement regarding a blood collection tray?

    A. Should be well-stocked

    B. Should be black in color

    C. Should be red in color or have the biohazard symbol prominently displayed

    D. Should have an ammonia capsule taped on the tray in the event the patient faints

____ 8. You are asked to collect a blood sample from a new patient. All of the following questions should be asked of the patient, *except:*

    A. Have you ever had a reaction to an adhesive bandage?

    B. Are you on aspirin therapy or blood thinners?

    C. Is there any reason I shouldn't draw blood on one side or the other (patient has had a mastectomy, has a shunt or port, and so on)?

    D. Are you afraid of needles?

____ 9. Which of the following techniques would you *not* use when selecting a vein for venipuncture?

    A. Always inspect both arms.

    B. Always select veins in the antecubital regions first, before looking at other sites.

    C. Always select veins in the forearm region first, before looking at other sites.

    D. Always palpate the vein so that you get a grasp of the direction the vein is running.

____ 10. Which of the following is the rationale for wiping away the first drop of blood following a capillary puncture?

    A. Contains electrolytes

    B. Contains skin cells

    C. Diluted with tissue fluid

    D. None of the above

SKILL APPLICATION CHALLENGES

Assignment 24-7: Tube Label Exercise

Complete the tube label below using the following information:

Patient: Carter Leonard

Time collected: 9:30 a.m.

Date collected: 10-10-20XX

Tests ordered: CBC and ESR

You are the phlebotomist

Assignment 24-8: Selecting the Proper Color Tube

Choose the appropriate tube top color that should be collected for the following laboratory tests.

1. CBC: _____

2. Blood glucose: _____

3. Cholesterol level: _____

4. PT/INR: _____

5. Liver Panel: _____

6. Medication level: _____

7. Differential: _____

8. Alcohol level: _____

9. STAT chemistry test: _____

10. ESR: _____

Assignment 24-9: Documentation Exercise

Correctly document the following information in charting format in the progress note below.

Dr. Julieanne Young has ordered the following laboratory tests for patient Julie Vance: CBC, PT, and a basic metabolic panel (BMP). You collect a lavender top tube, a light blue top tube, and a SST tube from the patient's left antecubital space using the vacuum tube method. The tests are sent to ABC Laboratories. The patient complains of pain following the venipuncture. There is no swelling, numbness, or tingling in the area. Dr. Young advises you to tell the patient to put some ice over the site upon returning home. The patient is to call if there are any complications.

COMPLETING SPECIAL FORMS

Assignment 24-10: Outside Specimen Tracking Log

Work Form Necessary: FORM 24-1

Directions: Complete the outside specimen tracking form (Work Form 24-1) using the following information.

10-10-20XX, Dr. Young orders a CBC, PT, and a BMP on Carter Leonard. Enter the correct tube types, your initials, and ABC Laboratories.

FIELD APPLICATION CHALLENGE

Assignment 24-11

Read the following Field Application Challenge and respond to the questions following the scenario.

After processing specimens collected for a CBC and potassium level, you notice that the serum in the red top tube is hemolyzed. The provider needs the results STAT so you send the specimen to the lab for testing. Will the results be accurate? What are the common collection errors that cause hemolysis?

_____

_____

_____

_____

_____

_____

_____

_____

JOURNALING EXERCISE

Assignment 24-12

Reflecting on Davene's mentoring tips, demonstrating professionalism and self-confidence is key to putting your patient at ease. Having a positive attitude and showing compassion will help patients who are nervous get through the procedure. List some examples of how you might apply information contained in this chapter, both during your training and after you enter the health care industry. Think about what you might say to a patient who is fearful of needles. How would you demonstrate professionalism and what would you say to your patient to help put them at ease?

Form 24-1

DOUGLASVILLE MEDICINE ASSOCIATES
5076 BRAND BLVD
DOUGLASVILLE, NY 01234
(123) 456-7890

OUTSIDE LAB SPECIMEN TRACKING LOG								
Date Sent	Patient Name/ ID	Ordering Provider	Tests Ordered	Number and Type of Specimens Sent to Laboratory (Include Tube Colors)	Prepared By	Laboratory	Date Results Received	Results Received By

C H A P T E R **25**

Urinalysis

VOCABULARY REVIEW

Assignment 25-1: Matching

Match the term with its definition and place the corresponding letter in the blank.

_____ 1. Turbid

_____ 2. Urochrome

_____ 3. pH

_____ 4. Hemoglobinuria

_____ 5. Bilirubin

_____ 6. Casts

_____ 7. Refractometer

_____ 8. Renal threshold

_____ 9. Sediment

_____ 10. Ketones

A. Point at which a substance reaches a concentration high enough for it to spill over into the urine

B. Opaque, or unable to see through the urine specimen

C. Structures formed in urine due to the accumulation of protein, cells, and fats in the renal tubules

D. Orange-yellow pigment found in bile which is formed when RBCs are broken down

E. Blood found in urine without the presence of intact red blood cells

F. Instrument used to measure the refractive index of urine, which is directly related to its specific gravity

G. The orange-yellow pigment that gives urine its color

H. Solid material found in urine, after centrifugation, that is examined microscopically

I. Acidity or alkalinity of a urine specimen

J. Normal products of fat metabolism

Assignment 25-2: Sentence Completion

Fill in the blanks below with Essential Terms from this chapter.

1. A _____ is used to perform a chemical urinalysis.

2. A _____ method is used to collect urine that requires no special preparation and in lab-provided sterile container with tight-fitting lids.

3. The _____ is the clear liquid portion of urine that remains after spinning, and is discarded after centrifugation.

4. The amount of dissolved substances found in the urine is measured as its _____.

5. _____ is the presence of blood in the urine with the presence of intact red cells upon microscopic examination.

6. The distal urethra and the urinary meatus usually contain normal flora (nonpathogenic bacteria normally present), which can interfere with test results. For this reason, providers will usually request a _____
_____.

7. A sterile container is always used for _____ specimens.

8. _____ is when red cells have ruptured and hemoglobin has been released into the urine.

9. Odor can become stronger due to bacterial growth and the breakdown of _____ to ammonia.

10. The patient should begin _____ into the toilet, then catch a portion of the stream in a sterile specimen container, and finish _____ (urinating) into the toilet. (*Note:* Same word is used twice.)

CHAPTER REVIEW

Assignment 25-3: Short Answer

1. List changes that will occur in a urine specimen allowed to be unpreserved or unrefrigerated at room temperature.

Clarity: _____

Odor: _____

pH: _____

Glucose: _____

Ketones: _____

Bilirubin: _____

Urobilinogen: _____

Nitrites: _____

RBCs and WBCs: _____

Casts: _____

Bacteria: _____

2. Describe the different collection methods for urine specimens.

Random: _____

_____

_____

_____

Clean-catch midstream: _____

_____

_____

_____

_____

_____

Catheterization: _____

_____

24-hour collection: _____

_____

_____

_____

_____

3. List and describe the three parts of a complete urinalysis, including test methods used in each.

    A. Physical examination: _____

    _____

    _____

    _____

    B. Chemical exam: _____

    _____

    _____

    _____

    C. Microscopic examination: _____

    _____

    _____

    _____

    _____

    _____

    _____

    _____

    _____

    _____

    _____

    _____

    _____

    _____

    _____

4. Describe the proper procedure for preparing a slide for a microscopic urinalysis.

_____

_____

_____

_____

_____

_____

_____

_____

_____

_____

_____

_____

_____

_____

_____

6. Fill in the missing information in the following urine color chart.

Color	Potential Cause
Colorless	
	Normal color
Dark yellow/amber	
	Red cells present in the urine (hematuria) due to kidney stones, UTI, or menstrual contamination. Hemoglobinuria: red cells have ruptured and hemoglobin has been released into the urine
	Bilirubin present; bilirubin converted to biliverdin, such as in liver disease
	Urinary tract infection caused by *Pseudomonas* bacteria; various medications
Brown	
Black	

Assignment 25-4: Abbreviation Review

Write what each of the following abbreviations stands for.

1. C&S: _____

2. RBCs: _____

3. CCMS: _____

4. RTE: _____

5. CLIA: _____

6. SG or SpGr: _____

7. HPF: _____

8. UA: _____

9. LPF: _____

10. U/C: _____

11. PPM: _____

12. UTI: _____

13. QNS: _____

14. WBCs: _____

CERTIFICATION PRACTICE

Assignment 25-5

Choose the best answer and place the corresponding letter in the blank.

____ 1. What percentage of urine is water?

    A. 50%

    B. 75%

    C. 95%

    D. 80%

____ 2. If a patient with diabetes has a positive glucose in their urine, which of the following has occurred?

    A. Patient is not following diet.

    B. Renal threshold has been reached.

    C. Patient is not taking medication properly.

    D. Patient is in acidosis.

____ 3. All of the following pieces of information may be requested to appear on a urine specimen container *except* the:

    A. patient's name.

    B. date and time of collection.

    C. diagnosis.

    D. patient's gender.

____ 4. Which of the following specimen types would be the most concentrated?

    A. Clean-catch

    B. Random

    C. Catheterization

    D. First-morning

____ 5. What is the purpose of a clean-catch midstream urine specimen?

   A. It is the most concentrated.

   B. This method flushes the normal flora from the urethra and urinary meatus before the specimen is collected.

   C. It is the most sterile.

   D. It is the most accurate.

____ 6. A urine specimen collected by catheterization should be placed into which of the following containers?

   A. Sterile container

   B. Urine specimen cup

   C. Any type of container as long as it has been thoroughly cleaned

   D. Centrifuge tube

____ 7. If the provider orders a quantitative test for urine creatinine, which of the following types of specimen should be collected?

   A. First-morning

   B. Clean-catch midstream

   C. 24-hour

   D. Random

____ 8. Which of the following amounts of urine is minimum necessary for testing?

   A. 5 mL

   B. 8 mL

   C. 10 mL

   D. 15 mL

____ 9. Which of the following might a sweet, fruity odor in a urine specimen indicate?

   A. Ingestion of fruit

   B. Contamination

   C. Ketoacidosis

   D. Presence of glucose

____ 10. If a control test does not fall within the acceptable range, which of the following steps should be taken?

   A. Repeat the control test, using a new set of controls and/or new bottle of test strips.

   B. Recheck the expiration date of the reagent strips.

   C. Recheck the expiration date of the control sample.

   D. All of the above

SKILL APPLICATION CHALLENGES

Assignment 25-6: Application Activity

Using the two urinalysis reports on the following pages, identify the abnormal results in the blanks below and state the clinical significance of each abnormal result.

Example A

1. _____
2. _____
3. _____
4. _____
5. _____
6. _____
7. _____
8. _____
9. _____
_____
_____

Example B

1. _____
2. _____
3. _____
4. _____

Example A

URINALYSIS REPORT FORM

PHYSICIAN INFORMATION	PATIENT INFORMATION
DOUGLASVILLE MEDICINE ASSOCIATES **5076 BRAND BLVD.** **DOUGLASVILLE, NY 01234** **(123) 456-7890** Ordering Physician: Dr. C. Leonard Physician ID #345679234	Name: Mr. Joshua Leonard Address: 1234 Main Street City / State / Zip: Mytown, OH 23333 Phone #: 216-888-8888 ID #: 12345678

Date and Time of Collection		Date Results Received
02-24-XX 9:00 a.m.		02-25-XX

Test Ordered	Results	Reference Range
Complete Urinalysis (UA):		
Physical UA:		
Color	Reddish/brown	Straw to Dark Yellow
Clarity/Transparency	Turbid	Clear to Hazy
Chemical UA/Reagent Strip:		
Specific Gravity	1.040	1.005–1.030
pH	8.0	4.5–7.0
Protein	3+ (300)	Negative/trace
Glucose	Negative	Negative
Ketones	Negative	Negative
Blood	2+ (moderate)	Negative
Bilirubin	2+ (moderate)	Negative
Urobilinogen	1	0.1–1.0
Nitrite	Positive	Negative
Leukocytes	2+ (moderate)	Negative
Microscopic UA:		
Hyaline Casts		0–2/LPF
Granular Casts		0/LPF
Cellular Casts	4–6 WBC	0/LPF
WBCs	5–10/HPF	0–5/HPF
RBCs	Too numerous to count (TNTC)	0–2/HPF
Squamous epithelial cells	Few	Few
Transitional epithelial cells		Rare
Bacteria	Moderate	Rare to few
Yeast		Small amount
Crystals:		
Artifacts:		

Example B

URINALYSIS REPORT FORM

PHYSICIAN INFORMATION	PATIENT INFORMATION
DOUGLASVILLE MEDICINE ASSOCIATES **5076 BRAND BLVD.** **DOUGLASVILLE, NY 01234** **(123) 456-7890** Ordering Physician: Dr. Alan Manning Physician ID #345679234	Name: Ms. Kelly Lynn ID #: 456-88-6523

Date and Time of Collection		Date Results Received
02-15-XX 2:00 p.m.		02-19-XX

Test Ordered	Results	Reference Range
Complete Urinalysis (UA):		
Physical UA:		
Color	Dark yellow	Straw to Dark Yellow
Clarity/Transparency	Hazy	Clear to Hazy
Chemical UA/Reagent Strip:		
Specific Gravity	1.025	1.005–1.030
pH	6.0	4.5–7.0
Protein	Trace	Negative/trace
Glucose	1/4 (250)	Negative
Ketones	Moderate	Negative
Blood	Negative	Negative
Bilirubin	Negative	Negative
Urobilinogen	Negative	0.1–1.0
Nitrite	Negative	Negative
Leukocytes	Negative	Negative
Microscopic UA:		
Hyaline Casts	0–1/LPF	0–2/LPF
Granular Casts		0/LPF
Cellular Casts		0/LPF
WBCs	None seen	0–5/HPF
RBCs	None seen	0–2/HPF
Squamous epithelial cells	Moderate	Few
Transitional epithelial cells		Rare
Bacteria		Rare to few
Yeast		Small amount
	Few mucus threads	
Crystals:		
Artifacts:		

Assignment 25-7: Documentation Exercise

Document the physical and chemical lab results from Assignment 25-6, Example B, as though you performed the urinalysis, using correct charting format. Use 02/19/XX as the date and 9:30 a.m. as the time you performed the testing. (The order from Dr. Manning is for a Physical and Chemical UA.)

COMPLETING SPECIAL FORMS

Assignment 25-8: Lab Requisition Form

Work Form Necessary: FORM 25-1

Directions: Complete the lab requisition (Work Form 25-1) with the scenario information given below.

Today's date: 02/15/20XX Time: 2:00 p.m. Patient name: Kelly J. Lynn, Address: 725 Mapleview Ave, Polaris, NY 01658, Telephone number: (123)888-8888, Patient ID # 4523, DOB: 08-12-1984, Sex: female, Fasting: no, Tests ordered: complete UA, Urine Culture, Sample: Urine specimen, and UA Culture Tube, Referring provider: Dr. Alan Manning, Address: Douglasville Medicine Associates, 5076 Brand Blvd., Douglasville, NY 01234, Telephone number: (123) 456-7890, Provider ID#: 345679234. Bill to patient. Patient is a self-pay with no insurance.

Assignment 25-9: Outside Specimen Tracking Log

Work Form Necessary: FORM 25-2

Directions: Enter the following information regarding Kelly Lynn's urine sample and requested tests into the outside lab specimen tracking log (Work Form 25-2). Additional information that you will need is listed below.

Name of lab: ABC Lab

Initials of employee who prepared the specimen: LMV

Initials of employee who received the results: MEH

Date results received: 02/19/20XX

FIELD APPLICATION CHALLENGE

Assignment 25-10

Read the following Field Application Challenge and respond to the questions following the scenario.

A patient being treated for the past 10 days for a UTI has dropped off a urine sample at the office for a recheck. You obtain the sample from the front desk and take it to the lab for a complete urinalysis. You place the sample on the counter and prepare to complete the physical and chemical urinalysis. Another medical assistant calls for your help with obtaining a blood sample from the patient in exam room two. You are then called to the front desk to speak with a patient who has a question about his medication. You room three more patients and return to the lab and realize that it has been over two hours since the patient dropped off the urine specimen. The specimen is quite cloudy and has an abnormal odor. You perform the reagent strip testing. Some tests are abnormal. You prepare the slide for the microscopic exam and notify the provider that it is ready for viewing.

1. Should the results you received be reported as accurate? Why or why not?

   _____

   _____

2. What should you have done with the urine specimen when you received it?

   _____

   _____

   _____

3. What implication could your actions have on the treatment of this patient?

   _____

   _____

   _____

JOURNALING EXERCISE

Assignment 25-11

What content within this chapter was most meaningful to you? Why? Now consider Davene's comment, "*When I asked the group of medical assistants what they could do to ensure the most accurate urine test results, the room became silent. It seems they were so used to performing this 'routine' test that they had forgotten that even the most routine test has specific criteria that should be followed each time testing is performed in order to ensure accuracy.*" How would you avoid becoming complacent when performing routine tests? How will you be vigilant in every detail of each test you perform?

Work Form 25-1

LABORATORY REQUISITION

	PATIENT LAST NAME	FIRST		M.I.	REFERRING PROVIDER		

PROVIDER ID #	PATIENT ID #	BILL: ☐ PHYSICIAN	☐ MEDICAL ☐ MEDICARE	☐ HMO ☐ INSURANCE	☐ CHDP ☐ PATIENT	D.O.B	AGE	SEX

PLEASE COMPLETE INSURANCE BILLING INFORMATION AT BOTTOM

PROVIDER NAME, ADDRESS, AND PHONE NUMBER	PATIENT ADDRESS		PATIENT PHONE NUMBER ( )	DATE COLLECTED	TIME COLLECTED
	CITY	STATE	ZIPCODE	FASTING YES	NO	STAT	CALL RESULT
	PATIENT MEDICARE #	PATIENT MEDICAID #		INFO. BELOW WILL APPEAR ON REPORT

CUSTOM PROFILES & ADDITIONAL TESTS

173 [ ] CHEMISTRY PANEL, COMPLETE BLOOD COUNT (ZPP), LIPID PROFILE, T4

05050 [ ] CHOL, TRIG, HDL CHOL, VLDL CHOL, LDL CHOL, RISK FACTOR

PROFILES

Code	Test		Code	Test	
00011 ☐	SPECIAL COMPREHENSIVE	2 SS,L	03536 ☐	HYPERTHYROID PROFILE	SS
00001 ☐	COMPREHENSIVE HEALTH SURVEY	SS,L	05037 ☐	HYPOTHYROID PROFILE	SS
00002 ☐	GENERAL SURVEY	SS,L	05051 ☐	LIPID PROFILE	SS
00003 ☐	CHEMISTRY PANEL	SS,L	05021 ☐	LIVER PROFILE	SS
CH7 ☐	CHEM 7 PANEL	SS	03359 ☐	LUPUS PROFILE	SS
03280 ☐	ANEMIA PROFILE	SS,L	03959 ☐	MENOPAUSAL PROFILE SS /03960 ☐ POST MENOPAUSAL	SS
06016 ☐	ARTHRITIS PROFILE	SS,L	02280 ☐	OVARIAN FUNCTION PROFILE SS /02281 ☐ TESTICULAR FUNC. PROF.	SS
05725 ☐	COMPREHENSIVE THYROID SURVEY	SS	02808 ☐	PRENATAL PROFILE	L,R
02691 ☐	EPSTEIN BARR PROFILE	SS	05006 ☐	THYROID PROFILE	SS
05010 ☐	ELECTROLYTES	SS	03191 ☐	TORCH PANEL	SS
06826 ☐	HEPATITIS PROFILE	SS	5756 ☐	URINE DRUG SCREEN U / ☐ VENIPUNCTURE	

TESTS

0361 ☐ ABO & Rh TYPE	R,L	0141 ☐ C-REACTIVE PROTEIN	SS	0673 ☐ HEPATITIS B SURFACE ANTIGEN	SS	0237 ☐ PTT	B
0302 ☐ ALKALINE PHOSPHATASE	SS	1341 ☐ DHEA-S	SS	0245 ☐ HEPATITIS C ANTIBODY	SS	0317 ☐ RA FACTOR	SS
0109 ☐ AMYLASE	SS	0119 ☐ DIGOXIN	SS	0257 ☐ IRON	SS	0321 ☐ RUBELLA	SS
0613 ☐ ANA	SS	0224 ☐ DILANTIN	SS	LDL-A ☐ LDL CHOLESTEROL	SS	0331 ☐ RPR	SS
0366 ☐ ANTIBODY SCREEN	R	0835 ☐ ESTRADIOL	SS	0283 ☐ LEAD BLOOD	RB	0335 ☐ SEMEN ANALYSIS	SEMEN
0110 ☐ ASO (STREPTOZYME)	SS	0833 ☐ FERRITIN	SS	0281 ☐ LIPASE	SS	0328 ☐ SEDIMENTATION RATE (ESR)	L
0126 ☐ BILIRUBIN TOTAL	SS	0003 ☐ FOLIC ACID & VITAMIN B12	SS	8225 ☐ LH	SS	0349 ☐ SGOT (AST)	SS
0132 ☐ BUN	SS	0651 ☐ FSH	SS	0247 ☐ MONONUCLEOSIS	SS	0348 ☐ SGPT (ALT)	SS
8726 ☐ CA125	SS	0140 ☐ FTA-ABS	SS	0778 ☐ PHENOBARBITAL	SS	0330 ☐ SICKLE CELL SCREEN	L
0142 ☐ CALCIUM	SS	0210 ☐ GGTP	SS	0307 ☐ POTASSIUM	SS	0354 ☐ T4 (THYROXINE)	SS
0130 ☐ CBC	L	0536 ☐ GLUCOSE, FASTING	GY	0557 ☐ PREGNANCY (SERUM)	SS	1358 ☐ T4 FREE	SS
0388 ☐ CEA-ROCHE	SS	☐ GLUCOSE, ____ HR PP	GY	0308 ☐ PREGNANCY (URINE)	U	8456 ☐ TESTOSTERONE	SS
0152 ☐ CHOLESTEROL	SS	0771 ☐ GLYCOHEMOGLOBIN	L	0359 ☐ PROGESTERONE	SS	0824 ☐ THEOPHYLLINE	SS
0788 ☐ CORTISOL	SS	0534 ☐ H. PYLORI	SS	8041 ☐ PROLACTIN	SS	0360 ☐ TRIGLYCERIDE	SS
0162 ☐ CPK	SS	0823 ☐ HGG QUANTITATIVE	SS	0103 ☐ PROTEIN, TOTAL	SS	0672 ☐ TSH	SS
0445 ☐ CKMB ISOENZYME	SS	1856 ☐ HIV (ANTIBODY)	SS	2000 ☐ PROSTATE SPECIFIC ANTIGEN (PSA)	SS	0373 ☐ URIC ACID	SS
0161 ☐ CREATININE	SS	0558 ☐ HDL CHOLESTEROL	SS	0310 ☐ PT (PROTHROMBIN TIME)	B	0219 ☐ URINALYSIS	U

CYTOPATHOLOGY

☐ PREGNANT ☐ ABORTION ☐ POST-PARTUM ☐ POST-MENOPAUSE

HISTORY _____

PREV. ABNORMAL CYTOL FINDINGS _____

☐ CONTRACEPTIVES   DATE _____
☐ HYSTERECTOMY   ☐ HORMONES   ☐ IUD
☐ COPHORECTOMY   ☐ TOTAL   ☐ SUPRA CX
☐ RADIATION Rx   DATE _____
☐ OTHER _____   ☐ HORMONES Rx   ☐ CHEMO Rx

LMP _____ DATE COLLECTED _____
SOURCE ☐ CERVIX   ☐ ENDOCERVIX   ☐ VAGINA
       ☐ CYTOBRUSH   ☐ OTHER SITE _____

MICROBIOLOGY

THCUL ☐ THROAT	URTHC ☐ URETHRAL	9391 ☐ CHLAMYDIA DNA
EACUL ☐ EAR	VACUL ☐ VAGINAL	9390 ☐ GONORRHEA DNA
EYCUL ☐ EYE	WOCUL ☐ WOUND	9391 ☐ OCCULT BLOOD
GOCUL ☐ GC	ROCUL ☐ CULTURE (Routine)	0293 ☐ OVA & PARASITE
SPCUL ☐ SPUTUM	URCUL ☐ URINE	WTM ☐ WET MOUNT
STCUL ☐ STOOL	GSP ☐ GRAM STAIN	

SOURCE _____   OTHER _____

DIAGNOSIS OR COMMENTS

LAB USE ONLY (DO NOT WRITE BELOW THIS SPACE)

DATE RECEIVED	DATE REPORTED

STATEMENT OF SPECIMEN ADEQUACY

GENERAL CATEGORIZATION

DESCRIPTIVE DIAGNOSIS

HORMONAL EVALUATION

ADDITIONAL COMMENT

CYTOTECHNOLOGIST	PATHOLOGIST

INSURANCE BILLING INFORMATION

PRIMARY INSURED	INSURANCE COMPANY

ADDRESS

POLICY NO. & I.D. NO.	ICD9 CODE

LEGEND

SS	Serum Separator	GY	Grey	B	Blue	U	Urine
R	Red	L	Lavender	RB	Royal Blue	G	Green

Work Form 25-2

DOUGLASVILLE MEDICINE ASSOCIATES
5076 BRAND BLVD
DOUGLASVILLE, NY 01234
(123) 456-7890

				OUTSIDE LAB SPECIMEN TRACKING LOG				
Date Sent	Patient Name/ ID	Ordering Provider	Tests Ordered	Number and Type of Specimens Sent to Laboratory (Include Tube Colors)	Prepared By	Laboratory	Date Results Received	Results Received By

CHAPTER **26**

Hematology and Coagulation Studies

VOCABULARY REVIEW

Assignment 26-1: Matching

Match the term with its definition and place the corresponding letter in the blank.

___ 1. Differential count

___ 2. Complete blood count

___ 3. Erythrocyte sedimentation rate

___ 4. Thrombocyte

___ 5. Normocyte

___ 6. Serum

___ 7. Lymphocyte

___ 8. Hematocrit

___ 9. Monocyte

___ 10. Macrocyte

___ 11. Hemoglobin

___ 12. Microcyte

___ 14. Leukocyte

A. Term used to describe a larger than normal red blood cell

B. Percentage of packed red blood cells in the total volume of blood

C. The largest of all white blood cells; contains no granules in cytoplasm; has a large, irregularly shaped nucleus; may contain holes in the cytoplasm because it is active in phagocytosis

D. Term used to describe a normal sized cell

E. Platelet

F. Liquid portion of the blood after the blood has been allowed to clot; contains no coagulation factors

G. Group of blood tests that includes a hemoglobin, hematocrit, red and white blood counts, differential count, platelet count or estimate, and red blood cell indicies

H. Measurement of how far red cells fall in a given amount of blood in a one-hour time frame

I. Count of 100 white blood cells on a stained blood smear for the purpose of determining the approximate percentage of each type of white blood cell

J. The smallest of all white blood cells; contains no granules in cytoplasm; elevated in viral infections

K. Another name for white blood cell; its main function is to fight infection

L. Iron pigment on the red blood cells that carries oxygen

M. Term used to describe a smaller than normal red blood cell

Assignment 26-2: Misspelled Words

Underline the correctly spelled term.

1. morphology   mourphology   morphologie
2. eaosenophil   eosinophil   eosenophil
3. poickilocytosis   poicilocitosis   poikilocytosis
4. newtrofil   neutrophil   neutraphil
5. erythrocyte   erythracyte   erythrocite
6. hemostasis   homeostasis   hemeostasis
7. anisocitosis   anisositosis   anisocytosis
8. bascophil   basophil   bazophil

CHAPTER REVIEW

Assignment 26-3: Abbreviation Review

Write what each of the following abbreviations stands for.

1. CBC: _____
2. WBC: _____
3. RBC: _____
4. ESR: _____
5. MCV: _____
6. MCH: _____
7. MCHC: _____
8. PT: _____
9. INR: _____
10. aPPT: _____
11. Hgb: _____
12. Hct: _____
13. PPE: _____

Assignment 26-4: Short Answer

1. Describe the process of hematopoesis (or hemopoiesis) and state the different parts of the body in which hematopoesis takes place throughout a person's life.

_____

_____

_____

_____

_____

_____

_____

2. Describe the function of each of the following cellular components.

   Cellular Components   *Function*

   Erythrocytes (RBCs)   _____

                                 _____

                                 _____

                                 _____

                                 _____

   Leukocytes (WBCs)   _____

                                 _____

                                 _____

                                 _____

                                 _____

   Thrombocytes (Platelets)   _____

                                 _____

                                 _____

                                 _____

                                 _____

                                 _____

3. List the normal values for components of the CBC.

   Component   *Normal Value*

   Red blood cell count   Males: _____

                                 Females: _____

                                 Neonates: _____

   White blood cell count   Adults: _____

                                 Neonates: _____

   Thrombocytes (Platelets)   _____

   Hemoglobin   Males: _____

                                 Females: _____

                                 Neonates: _____

   Hematocrit   Males: _____

                                 Females: _____

                                 Neonates: _____

   Differential   Neutrophils: _____

                                 Bands: _____

                                 Eosinophils: _____

                                 Basophils: _____

                                 Lymphocytes: _____

                                 Monocytes: _____

4. Give an explanation of why the hematocrit would be increased in a patient with dehydration.

_____

_____

_____

5. Explain the importance of the information obtained from the red cell indices.

_____

_____

_____

_____

_____

CERTIFICATION PRACTICE

Assignment 26-5

Choose the best answer and place the corresponding letter in the blank.

_____ 1. The following laboratory results have been received on a 79-year-old female. Which of the following results is abnormal?

    A. WBC: 11,500 x 10^9/L

    B. RBC: 3.5 million x 10^{12}/L

    C. Hgb: 10 gm/dL

    D. All of the above

_____ 2. Which of the following is a component of red blood cells that allows for flexible movement through small blood vessels?

    A. Their small diameter

    B. The viscosity of the hemoglobin found on the RBC

    C. Their biconcave shape

    D. Their cellular coating

_____ 3. Without a nucleus, the erythrocyte remains functional in the blood stream for approximately:

    A. 21 days.

    B. 120 days.

    C. 30 days.

    D. 180 days.

_____ 4. If anisocytosis is reported on a differential count, this means that there are variations in the:

    A. hemoglobin content of the red blood cells.

    B. size of the red blood cells.

    C. shape of the red blood cells.

    D. color of the red blood cells.

___ 5. Which of the following is an inherited disorder caused by the presence of abnormal hemoglobin (Hemoglobin S)?

   A. Shistocytosis

   B. Spherocytosis

   C. Sickle cell anemia

   D. Shigellocytosis

___ 6. Which of the following counts within a CBC would help with the diagnosing, evaluating, and treating different types of anemias and bleeding disorders?

   A. RBC count

   B. Hemoglobin

   C. Hematocrit

   D. Red blood cell indices

___ 7. The readings of both tubes for a hematocrit determination must be:

   A. within 2%.

   B. within 1%.

   C. within 3%.

   D. exactly the same.

___ 8. Medical assistants are generally permitted to perform which of the following hematology tests?

   A. Nonautomated ESR

   B. Coagulation tests

   C. Differential

   D. Only A and B are correct

___ 9. If the neutrophil count on a differential is reported as 75%, which of the following conditions would likely be responsible?

   A. Bacterial infection

   B. Viral infection

   C. Polycythemia

   D. All of the above

___ 10. All of the following are true of the ESR *except* the:

   A. test must be timed precisely for one hour.

   B. tube must remain in a vertical position for one hour.

   C. tube rack should be placed on a surface free from vibrations.

   D. tube should be placed in a cool, dark place.

SKILL APPLICATION CHALLENGES

Assignment 26-6: Normal and Abnormal Results

1. Read and record the following ESR result and state whether it is normal or abnormal. The patient is male.

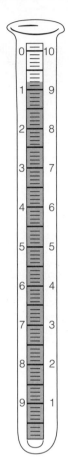

A. The result is: _____

B. This result is normal/abnormal. (Circle one.)

2. Identify the abnormal results from the following lab report and explain their clinical significance in the blanks on the next page.

ABC LABORATORY HEMATOLOGY REPORT FORM

PHYSICIAN INFORMATION		PATIENT INFORMATION	
DOUGLASVILLE MEDICINE ASSOCIATES **5076 BRAND BLVD.** **DOUGLASVILLE, NY 01234** **(123) 456-7890** Ordering Physician: Dr. Carl Veach Physician ID #23658A		Name: Kathleen Beavers ID #: 25698	
Date and Time of Collection		**Date Results Received**	
10-29-XX 8:30 a.m.		10-30-XX	
Test Ordered	**Results**	**Reference Range**	
Complete blood count (CBC):			
White Blood Cell Count	15,000 × 10⁹/L	4,500–11,000 × 10⁹/L	
Red Blood Cell Count	5.0 million × 10¹²/L	M: 4.5–6.0 million/cu mm F: 4.0–5.5/cu mm	
Hemoglobin	10 gm/dL	M: 13–18 gm/dL F: 12–16 gm/dL	
Hematocrit	32%	M: 42–52% F: 36–45%	
MCV	96 fL	80–100 fL	
MCH	30 pG	27–33 pg	
MCHC	34 g/dL	32–37 g/dL	
Platelet Count	300,000 × 10⁹/L	140,000–400,000 × 10⁹/L	
Differential white blood cell count:			
Neutrophilic Bands	6%	0–7%	
Neutrophils	75%	50–65%	
Eosinophils	1%	1–3%	
Basophils	0	0–1%	
Lymphocytes	10%	25–40%	
Monocytes	9%	3–9%	
RBC Morphology:	Hypochromic	Normochromic	
	Microcytic	Normocytic	
Coagulation Studies:			
PT		10–13 seconds	
INR		2.0–3.0 but will vary by laboratory and the patient's condition	

_____

_____

_____

_____

_____

_____

COMPLETING SPECIAL FORMS

Assignment 26-7: Lab Requisition Form

Work Form Necessary: FORM 26-1

Directions: Complete the lab requisition form (Work Form 26-1) with the scenario information given below.

Today's date 10-29-XX, 8:30 a.m., Patient name: Kathleen L. Beavers, Address: 8900 Gracie Blvd., Westerville, NY 01563, Telephone number: 123-469-7449, DOB: 10-29-47, Sex: female, Billing information: The patient should be billed for the lab work (patient does not have any health insurance), Fasting: no, Tests ordered: CBC, Referring provider information: Dr. Carl Veach, Address: Douglasville Medicine Associates, 5076 Brand Blvd., Douglasville, NY 01234, Telephone number: 123-456-7890, Provider ID#: 23658A, Billing information: Dr. Veach, Diagnosis: ICD-10 Code: Z13.2

Assignment 26-8: Outside Specimen Tracking Log

Work Form Necessary: FORM 26-2

Directions: Enter the specimen from the lab requisition in Work Form 26-1 into the lab log (Work Form 26-2). Additional information is included below.

- Type of specimen: One lavender-top tube
- Prepared by: LMV
- Date received: 10-30-XX
- Received by: MEH
- Lab name: ABC Laboratory

FIELD APPLICATION CHALLENGE

Assignment 26-9

Read the following Field Application Challenge and respond to the questions following the scenario.

You are asked to run a hemoglobin and hematocrit on a female patient who suffers from anemia. The hematocrit results are 46% and the hemoglobin is 11 g/dL.

1. Are the test results normal?

_____

2. Do the results correlate with one another? Why or why not?

_____

3. After performing both tests again, you obtain the same results. You check the chart and see that the patient also complains of frequent watery diarrhea over the past two weeks. Could there be a correlation? If so, what?

_____

_____

JOURNALING EXERCISE
Assignment 26-10
What content within this chapter was most meaningful to you? Why? Considering the seriousness of the scenario outlined by Davene, what you would have done if you couldn't get a hold of the patient. Do you think the medical assistant should have been fired? Why or why not? How do the professionalism keys listed apply to this scenario? Which professionalism keys would be most appropriate in this situation?

Work Form 26-1

LABORATORY REQUISITION

PATIENT LAST NAME		FIRST		M.I.	REFERRING PROVIDER

PROVIDER ID #	PATIENT ID #	BILL: ☐ PHYSICIAN	☐ MEDICAL　☐ HMO　☐ CHDP ☐ MEDICARE　☐ INSURANCE　☐ PATIENT PLEASE COMPLETE INSURANCE BILLING INFORMATION AT BOTTOM	D.O.B	AGE	SEX

PROVIDER NAME, ADDRESS, AND PHONE NUMBER	PATIENT ADDRESS		PATIENT PHONE NUMBER ( )	DATE COLLECTED	TIME COLLECTED
	CITY	STATE	ZIP CODE	FASTING YES | NO	STAT | CALL RESULT
	PATIENT MEDICARE #	PATIENT MEDICAID #		INFO. BELOW WILL APPEAR ON REPORT	

CUSTOM PROFILES & ADDITIONAL TESTS

```
173    [ ] CHEMISTRY PANEL, COMPLETE BLOOD COUNT (ZPP), LIPID PROFILE, T4
05050  [ ] CHOL, TRIG, HDL CHOL, VLDL CHOL, LDL CHOL, RISK FACTOR
```

PROFILES

Code	Test		Code	Test	
00011 ☐	SPECIAL COMPREHENSIVE	2 SS,L	03536 ☐	HYPERTHYROID PROFILE	SS
00001 ☐	COMPREHENSIVE HEALTH SURVEY	SS,L	05037 ☐	HYPOTHYROID PROFILE	SS
00002 ☐	GENERAL SURVEY	SS,L	05051 ☐	LIPID PROFILE	SS
00003 ☐	CHEMISTRY PANEL	SS,L	05021 ☐	LIVER PROFILE	SS
CH7 ☐	CHEM 7 PANEL	SS	03359 ☐	LUPUS PROFILE	SS
03280 ☐	ANEMIA PROFILE	SS,L	03959 ☐	MENOPAUSAL PROFILE　SS /03960 ☐ POST MENOPAUSAL	SS
06016 ☐	ARTHRITIS PROFILE	SS,L	02280 ☐	OVARIAN FUNCTION PROFILE　SS /02281 ☐ TESTICULAR FUNC. PROF.	SS
05725 ☐	COMPREHENSIVE THYROID SURVEY	SS	02808 ☐	PRENATAL PROFILE	L,R
02691 ☐	EPSTEIN BARR PROFILE	SS	05006 ☐	THYROID PROFILE	SS
05010 ☐	ELECTROLYTES	SS	03191 ☐	TORCH PANEL	SS
06826 ☐	HEPATITIS PROFILE	SS	5756 ☐	URINE DRUG SCREEN　U / ☐ VENIPUNCTURE	

TESTS

Code	Test		Code	Test		Code	Test	
0361 ☐	ABO & Rh TYPE	R,L	0141 ☐	C-REACTIVE PROTEIN	SS	0673 ☐	HEPATITIS B SURFACE ANTIGEN	SS
0302 ☐	ALKALINE PHOSPHATASE	SS	1341 ☐	DHEA-S	SS	0245 ☐	HEPATITIS C ANTIBODY	SS
0109 ☐	AMYLASE	SS	0119 ☐	DIGOXIN	SS	0257 ☐	IRON	SS
0613 ☐	ANA	SS	0224 ☐	DILANTIN	SS	LDL-A ☐	LDL CHOLESTEROL	SS
0366 ☐	ANTIBODY SCREEN	R	0835 ☐	ESTRADIOL	SS	0283 ☐	LEAD BLOOD	RB
0110 ☐	ASO (STREPTOZYME)	SS	0833 ☐	FERRITIN	SS	0281 ☐	LIPASE	SS
0126 ☐	BILIRUBIN TOTAL	SS	0003 ☐	FOLIC ACID & VITAMIN B12	SS	8225 ☐	LH	SS
0132 ☐	BUN	SS	0651 ☐	FSH	SS	0247 ☐	MONONUCLEOSIS	SS
8726 ☐	CA125	SS	0140 ☐	FTA-ABS	SS	0778 ☐	PHENOBARBITAL	SS
0142 ☐	CALCIUM	SS	0210 ☐	GGTP	SS	0307 ☐	POTASSIUM	SS
0130 ☐	CBC	L	0536 ☐	GLUCOSE, FASTING	GY	0557 ☐	PREGNANCY (SERUM)	SS
0388 ☐	CEA-ROCHE	SS	☐	GLUCOSE, ____ HR PP	GY	0308 ☐	PREGNANCY (URINE)	U
0152 ☐	CHOLESTEROL	SS	0771 ☐	GLYCOHEMOGLOBIN	L	0359 ☐	PROGESTERONE	SS
0788 ☐	CORTISOL	SS	0534 ☐	H. PYLORI	SS	8041 ☐	PROLACTIN	SS
0162 ☐	CPK	SS	0823 ☐	HGG QUANTITATIVE	SS	0103 ☐	PROTEIN, TOTAL	SS
0445 ☐	CKMB ISOENZYME	SS	1856 ☐	HIV (ANTIBODY)	SS	2000 ☐	PROSTATE SPECIFIC ANTIGEN (PSA)	SS
0161 ☐	CREATININE	SS	0558 ☐	HDL CHOLESTEROL	SS	0310 ☐	PT (PROTHROMBIN TIME)	B

Code	Test	
0237 ☐	PTT	B
0317 ☐	RA FACTOR	SS
0321 ☐	RUBELLA	SS
0331 ☐	RPR	SS
0335 ☐	SEMEN ANALYSIS	SEMEN
0328 ☐	SEDIMENTATION RATE (ESR)	L
0349 ☐	SGOT (AST)	SS
0348 ☐	SGPT (ALT)	SS
0330 ☐	SICKLE CELL SCREEN	L
0354 ☐	T4 (THYROXINE)	SS
1358 ☐	T4 FREE	SS
8456 ☐	TESTOSTERONE	SS
0824 ☐	THEOPHYLLINE	SS
0360 ☐	TRIGLYCERIDE	SS
0672 ☐	TSH	SS
0373 ☐	URIC ACID	SS
0219 ☐	URINALYSIS	U

CYTOPATHOLOGY

☐ PREGNANT　☐ ABORTION　☐ POST-PARTUM　☐ POST-MENOPAUSE
HISTORY _____

PREV. ABNORMAL CYTOL FINDINGS _____
☐ CONTRACEPTIVES　　　DATE _____
☐ HYSTERECTOMY　☐ HORMONES　☐ IUD
☐ COPHORECTOMY　☐ TOTAL　☐ SUPRA CX
☐ RADIATION Rx　　　DATE _____
☐ OTHER _____　☐ HORMONES Rx　☐ CHEMO Rx

LMP _____　DATE COLLECTED _____
SOURCE ☐ CERVIX　☐ ENDOCERVIX　☐ VAGINA
　　　　☐ CYTOBRUSH　☐ OTHER SITE _____

MICROBIOLOGY

THCUL ☐ THROAT	URTHC ☐ URETHRAL	9391 ☐ CHLAMYDIA DNA
EACUL ☐ EAR	VACUL ☐ VAGINAL	9390 ☐ GONORRHEA DNA
EYCUL ☐ EYE	WOCUL ☐ WOUND	9391 ☐ OCCULT BLOOD
GOCUL ☐ GC	ROCUL ☐ CULTURE (Routine)	0293 ☐ OVA & PARASITE
SPCUL ☐ SPUTUM	URCUL ☐ URINE	WTM ☐ WET MOUNT
STCUL ☐ STOOL	GSP ☐ GRAM STAIN	
SOURCE _____	OTHER _____	

DIAGNOSIS OR COMMENTS

LAB USE ONLY (DO NOT WRITE BELOW THIS SPACE)

DATE RECEIVED	DATE REPORTED

STATEMENT OF SPECIMEN ADEQUACY

GENERAL CATEGORIZATION

DESCRIPTIVE DIAGNOSIS

HORMONAL EVALUATION

ADDITIONAL COMMENT

CYTOTECHNOLOGIST	PATHOLOGIST

INSURANCE BILLING INFORMATION

PRIMARY INSURED	INSURANCE COMPANY
ADDRESS	
POLICY NO. & I.D. NO.	ICD-10 CODE

LEGEND

SS	Serum Separator	GY	Grey	B	Blue	U	Urine
R	Red	L	Lavender	RB	Royal Blue	G	Green

Work Form 26-2

DOUGLASVILLE MEDICINE ASSOCIATES
5076 BRAND BLVD
DOUGLASVILLE, NY 01234
(123) 456-7890

OUTSIDE LAB SPECIMEN TRACKING LOG								
Date Sent	Patient Name/ID	Ordering Provider	Tests Ordered	Number of and Type of Specimens Sent to Laboratory (Include Tube Colors)	Prepared By	Laboratory	Date Results Received	Results Received By

C H A P T E R **27**

Microbiology

VOCABULARY REVIEW

Assignment 27-1: Matching

Match the term with its definition and place the corresponding letter in the blank.

____ 1 Culture

____ 2. Agar

____ 3. Aerobic

____ 4. Inoculation

____ 5. Opportunistic infection

____ 6. Pathogenic

____ 7. Pathogen

____ 8. Pure culture

____ 9. Sensitivity testing

____ 10. Taxonomy

____ 11. Bacilli

____ 12. Cocci

____ 13. Culture medium

____ 14. Normal flora

____ 15. Microbiology

____ 16. Incubation

____ 17. Fungi

A. Liquid or solid material in which bacteria are grown

B. Class of bacteria that do not require oxygen to grow

C. A group of microbes growing on nutrient-rich media

D. Infection that develops in compromised patients and those taking certain medications such as immunosuppressive drugs

E. Group of microorganisms that includes yeasts and molds

F. Applying a microorganism onto a culture medium

G. Study of microorganisms, especially as they relate to diseases

H. Place a culture in an apparatus that provides optimum conditions for growth and multiplication of microorganisms

I. Disease producing

J. Single-celled microbes that lack a nucleus (the most prevalent of all microorganisms)

K. Disease-causing microorganism

L. Culture that contains only one organism

M. Technique that evaluates which antibiotics will destroy a particular pathogen

N. Classification of living organisms into the proper category using a specific set of laws and principles

O. Microorganisms normally present in different parts of the human body which pose no health threat under ordinary circumstances

P. Organism that lives within, upon, or at the expense of the host

Q. Round-shaped bacteria

____ 18. Parasite

R. Rod-shaped bacteria; may contain spores

____ 19. Gram positive

S. Class of bacteria that requires oxygen to grow

____ 20. Anaerobic

T. Gelatin-like substance that may contain additives and nutrients that will support the growth and multiplication of microorganisms

____ 21. Bacteria

U. Visible growth of microorganisms that appear on a culture medium

____ 22. Colonies

V. Term used to describe bacteria that stain purple during the Gram staining process

Assignment 27-2: Sentence Completion

1. In order to identify which pathogen is causing the patient's condition and which antibiotic will most likely destroy the organism, the provider will order a _____ .

2. Bacteria that cannot retain the dye after being decolorized must be counterstained with a red dye (safranin) to make them visible under the microscope. These bacteria are classed as _____ and appear pink in color.

3. A differential stain is one that produces variable results based on the composition of the bacterial cell wall. A common differential staining method, the _____ , was developed over 100 years ago and is still used today. This method differentiates bacteria based on their color reactions to various stains.

4. Some bacteria retain the purple color after decolorization and are classed as _____ .

5. A _____ is a common cause of infectious diseases in humans. They are responsible for such maladies as influenza (flu), measles, mumps, and the common cold.

CHAPTER REVIEW

Assignment 27-3: Abbreviation Review

Write what each of the following abbreviations stands for.

1. DNA: _____

2. CSF: _____

3. C&S: _____

4. EBV: _____

5. RSV: _____

6. KOH: _____

7. ELISA: _____

8. BC: _____

9. C-Diff: _____

10. CMV: _____

11. Cx: _____

12. O&P: _____

13. STIs: _____

14. UTI: _____

15. POLs: _____

16. CLIA: _____

17. CDC: _____

18. PID: _____

19. HIV: _____

20. HPV: _____

21. HBV: _____

22. HCV: _____

23. EIA: _____

24. VZV: _____

Assignment 27-4: Short Answer

1. Draw examples of each of the following.

Cocci	Bacilli	Spirilla
Diplococci	Bacilli (flagellated)	Spirilla
Streptococci	Diplobacilli	Spirochete
Staphylococci	Streptobacilli	

2. List the different reagents used in the Gram staining process and explain the purpose of each.

_____

_____

_____

_____

3. Describe the three methods used to identify viruses.

A. _____

_____

B. _____

_____

C. _____

_____

4. Explain the purpose of a safety hood when working with molds.

_____

_____

_____

5. List precautions that should be observed to ensure safe handling of microbiology specimens.

A. _____

B. _____

_____

C. _____

D. _____

E. _____

F. _____

6. For the following specimen types, state whether or not normal flora could be present and list two possible pathogens that might be found in each.

Type of Specimen	Normal Flora Present	Types of Pathogens
Urine		
Blood		
Cerebrospinal fluid (CFS)		

Sputum		
Stool		
Wound		
Genital		
Nasal		
Throat		
Eyes		
Ears		

7. Name and describe the three general classifications of growth media contained in culture plates.

    A. _____

    _____

    _____

    _____

    B. _____

    _____

    C. _____

    _____

    _____

    _____

    _____

8. List common diseases caused by the following types of bacteria.

    A. *Escherichia coli*: _____

    B. *Salmonella* species: _____

    C. *Citrobacter*: _____

    D. *Bacillus* species: _____

    E. *Psuedomonas* species: _____

    _____

    F. *Listeria* species: _____

    G. *Helicobacter pylori*: _____

    H. *Bordetella pertussis*: _____

9. List pathogenic conditions caused by the following common viruses.

    A. Rhinovirus: _____

    B. Epstein-Barr virus: _____

    C. Respiratory syncytial virus: _____

    D. Rotavirus: _____

    E. Varicella-zoster virus: _____

    F. Human papillomavirus: _____

CERTIFICATION PRACTICE

Assignment 27-5

Choose the best answer and place the corresponding letter in the blank.

_____ 1. Microorganisms are usually classified using a set of laws and principles known as:

    A. binomial standards.

    B. taxonomy.

    C. microbe classification standards.

    D. prokaryote standards.

_____ 2. Which of the following is reportable to the Public Health Department?

    A. *Salmonella*

    B. *Shigella*

    C. Sexually transmitted infections

    D. All of the above

_____ 3. Bacteria have two names, the first being the genus, the second being the:

    A. species.

    B. class.

    C. family.

    D. group.

_____ 4. All of the following are correct procedures regarding the four-quadrant streaking method except to:

    A. allow plate to come to room temperature before inoculation.

    B. replace the lid immediately after streaking.

    C. not use a plate that has reached its expiration date.

    D. label the bottom of the plate and place in the incubator with the lid facing upward.

_____ 5. A wide clear zone around the colonies on a blood agar plate indicates which of the following?

    A. Alpha hemolysis

    B. Gamma hemolysis

    C. Beta hemolysis

    D. Epi hemolysis

_____ 6. One method of identifying group A beta strep is by performing which type of test?

    A. Methicillin

    B. Bacitracin

    C. Optichin

    D. Zithrocin

_____ 7. A wet mount is valuable when trying to diagnose the cause of which of the following?

    A. STDs

    B. Vaginosis

    C. UTI

    D. URI

___ 8. Which of the following organisms would be suspect in a case of necrotizing fasciitis?

    A. *Streptococcus pneumoniae*

    B. *Streptococcus agalactiae*

    C. *Streptococcus pyogenes*

    D. Beta hemolytic group A strep

___ 9. Which of the following organisms is known to cause wound infections?

    A. *Staphylococcus epidermidis*

    B. *Staphylococcus aureus*

    C. *Proteus* species

    D. *Pseudomonas* species

___ 10. *Salmonella* species can cause all of the following illnesses *except:*

    A. typhoid fever.

    B. urethritis.

    C. food poisoning.

    D. bacteremia.

SKILL APPLICATION CHALLENGES

COMPLETING SPECIAL FORMS

Assignment 27-6: Lab Requisition Form

Work Form Necessary: FORM 27-1

Directions: Complete the lab requisition (Work Form 27-1) with the scenario information given below.
Patient name: Maryn L. Leonard, Address: 6789 Avery Lane, Blondeville, NY 12345, Telephone number: (123) 891-5030, DOB: 05/09/90, Date of collection: 07/24/20XX, Time of collection: 9:00 a.m., Bill the provider for the lab services, Sex: female, Fasting: no, Tests ordered: Throat culture, ICD-10 Code: J02.9, Referring provider: Dr. Carl Daniels, Douglasville Medicine Associates, 5076 Brand Blvd., Douglasville, NY 01234, (123) 456-7890, ID#: 23658B

Assignment 27-7: Outside Specimen Tracking Log

Work Form Necessary: FORM 27-2

Directions: Enter the following information regarding outside specimen tracking into the log (Work Form 27-2). Additional information is included below.

- Type of specimen: Throat swab
- Prepared by: LMV
- Date received: 07/26/20XX
- Received by: MEH
- Lab name: ABC Laboratory

Assignment 27-8: Application Activity

The lab report is back on Maryn Leonard. Read the findings on the following page and state whether or not treatment will be necessary and why you feel that treatment is or is not necessary.

_____

_____

ABC LABORATORY MISCELLANEOUS LABORATORY
TEST REPORT FORM

PHYSICIAN INFORMATION		PATIENT INFORMATION	
DOUGLASVILLE MEDICINE ASSOCIATES 5076 BRAND BLVD. DOUGLASVILLE, NY 01234 (123) 456-7890 **Ordering Physician:** Dr. Carl Daniels **Physician ID** # 23658B		**Name:** Maryn Leonard **Address:** 6789 Avery Lane **City/State/Zip:** Blondeville, NY 12345 **Phone #:** 123-891-5030 **ID #:** 87652364546	
Date and Time of Collection		**Reporting Date**	
07/24/XX 9:00 a.m.		07/26/XX	
Test Ordered	**Results**	**Reference Range**	**Abnormal Results**
Pregnancy Test			
Rapid Strep Test		Negative	
Mono Test		Negative	
Influenza Test		Negative	
H. Pylori		Negative	
Culture Results	**No Growth**	No Growth	
Serology Tests:			
VDRL/RPR		Nonreactive	
HIV		Negative	
CRP		Less than 6 mg/L	
Rheumatoid Factor		Negative	
ASO titer		Negative	

Assignment 27-9: Research Activity

1. Research MRSA (methicillin-resistant *Staphylococcus aureus*) infections and design an informational pamphlet to distribute to patients who might be at-risk for developing this type of infection, such as those using gyms or workout facilities, students using equipment in school gymnasiums, and hospital patients. (*Note: Alternatively, search the patient education tab of the EHR for the topic and print the information related to the subject.*)

2. Search the Internet and obtain information on diseases that were once thought to be eradicated in the United States, such as tuberculosis and whooping cough, but are now making a comeback. (*Note: Alternatively, search the patient education tab of the EHR for the topic and print the information related to the subject.*)

3. Search the Internet for information related to sepsis and septicemia. Write a two-page paper on the subject, including the medical definition of each, signs, symptoms, diagnosis, causes, and treatment. (*Note: Alternatively, search the patient education tab of the EHR for the topic and print the information related to the subject.*)

FIELD APPLICATION CHALLENGE
Assignment 27-10

Read the following Field Application Challenge and respond to the questions following the scenario.
When collecting a wound specimen from a patient, you accidentally touch the swab to the skin at the edge of the wound. The area appears to be infected and the patient appears to be in a lot of pain and asks you to stop swabbing the wound. You don't want to upset the patient any further, so you place the swab in the appropriate transport media to be sent to the lab.

1. What type of transport media should be used for a wound specimen?

   _____

   _____

2. Should you have collected another sample? Why or why not?

   _____

   _____

   _____

   _____

3. What impact could your actions have on this patient's treatment?

   _____

   _____

JOURNALING EXERCISE
Assignment 27-11

The field of medical microbiology includes the study of microscopic organisms such as bacteria, viruses, parasites, and fungi. What content within this chapter was most meaningful to you? Why? List some examples of how information contained in this chapter would apply to your training and after you enter the health care industry. After reviewing the patient visit described by Davene, how do you see yourself handling this or a similar situation? Record how the professionalism keys listed apply to this scenario.

Work Form 27-1

LABORATORY REQUISITION

	PATIENT LAST NAME			FIRST				M.I.	REFERRING PROVIDER		

PROVIDER ID #	PATIENT ID #		BILL: ☐ PHYSICIAN	☐ MEDICAL	☐ HMO	☐ CHDP	D.O.B	AGE	SEX
				☐ MEDICARE	☐ INSURANCE	☐ PATIENT			

PLEASE COMPLETE INSURANCE BILLING INFORMATION AT BOTTOM

PROVIDER NAME, ADDRESS, AND PHONE NUMBER	PATIENT ADDRESS	PATIENT PHONE NUMBER ( )	DATE COLLECTED	TIME COLLECTED
	CITY	STATE	ZIP CODE	FASTING YES NO	STAT	CALL RESULT
	PATIENT MEDICARE #	PATIENT MEDICAID #	INFO. BELOW WILL APPEAR ON REPORT	

CUSTOM PROFILES & ADDITIONAL TESTS

```
173    [ ] CHEMISTRY PANEL, COMPLETE BLOOD COUNT (ZPP), LIPID PROFILE, T4
05050 [ ] CHOL, TRIG, HDL CHOL, VLDL CHOL, LDL CHOL, RISK FACTOR
```

PROFILES

Code	Profile		Code	Profile		
00011	☐ SPECIAL COMPREHENSIVE	2 SS,L	03536	☐ HYPERTHYROID PROFILE		SS
00001	☐ COMPREHENSIVE HEALTH SURVEY	SS,L	05037	☐ HYPOTHYROID PROFILE		SS
00002	☐ GENERAL SURVEY	SS,L	05051	☐ LIPID PROFILE		SS
00003	☐ CHEMISTRY PANEL	SS,L	05021	☐ LIVER PROFILE		SS
CH7	☐ CHEM 7 PANEL	SS	03359	☐ LUPUS PROFILE		SS
03280	☐ ANEMIA PROFILE	SS,L	03959	☐ MENOPAUSAL PROFILE	SS /03960 ☐ POST MENOPAUSAL	SS
06016	☐ ARTHRITIS PROFILE	SS,L	02280	☐ OVARIAN FUNCTION PROFILE	SS /02281 ☐ TESTICULAR FUNC. PROF.	
05725	☐ COMPREHENSIVE THYROID SURVEY	SS	02808	☐ PRENATAL PROFILE		L,R
02691	☐ EPSTEIN BARR PROFILE	SS	05006	☐ THYROID PROFILE		SS
05010	☐ ELECTROLYTES	SS	03191	☐ TORCH PANEL		SS
06826	☐ HEPATITIS PROFILE	SS	5756	☐ URINE DRUG SCREEN	U / ☐ VENIPUNCTURE	

TESTS

0361	☐ ABO & Rh TYPE	R,L	0141	☐ C-REACTIVE PROTEIN	SS	0673	☐ HEPATITIS B SURFACE ANTIGEN	SS	0237	☐ PTT	B
0302	☐ ALKALINE PHOSPHATASE	SS	1341	☐ DHEA-S	SS	0245	☐ HEPATITIS C ANTIBODY	SS	0317	☐ RA FACTOR	SS
0109	☐ AMYLASE	SS	0119	☐ DIGOXIN	SS	0257	☐ IRON	SS	0321	☐ RUBELLA	SS
0613	☐ ANA	SS	0224	☐ DILANTIN	SS	LDL-A	☐ LDL CHOLESTEROL	SS	0331	☐ RPR	SS
0366	☐ ANTIBODY SCREEN	R	0835	☐ ESTRADIOL	SS	0283	☐ LEAD BLOOD	RB	0335	☐ SEMEN ANALYSIS	SEMEN
0110	☐ ASO (STREPTOZYME)	SS	0833	☐ FERRITIN	SS	0281	☐ LIPASE	SS	0328	☐ SEDIMENTATION RATE (ESR)	L
0126	☐ BILIRUBIN TOTAL	SS	0003	☐ FOLIC ACID & VITAMIN B12	SS	8225	☐ LH	SS	0349	☐ SGOT (AST)	SS
0132	☐ BUN	SS	0651	☐ FSH	SS	0247	☐ MONONUCLEOSIS	SS	0348	☐ SGPT (ALT)	SS
8726	☐ CA125	SS	0140	☐ FTA-ABS	SS	0778	☐ PHENOBARBITAL	SS	0330	☐ SICKLE CELL SCREEN	L
0142	☐ CALCIUM	SS	0210	☐ GGTP	SS	0307	☐ POTASSIUM	SS	0354	☐ T4 (THYROXINE)	SS
0130	☐ CBC	L	0536	☐ GLUCOSE, FASTING	GY	0557	☐ PREGNANCY (SERUM)	SS	1358	☐ T4 FREE	SS
0388	☐ CEA-ROCHE	SS		☐ GLUCOSE, ____ HR PP	GY	0308	☐ PREGNANCY (URINE)	U	8456	☐ TESTOSTERONE	SS
0152	☐ CHOLESTEROL	SS	0771	☐ GLYCOHEMOGLOBIN	L	0359	☐ PROGESTERONE	SS	0824	☐ THEOPHYLLINE	SS
0788	☐ CORTISOL	SS	0534	☐ H. PYLORI	SS	8041	☐ PROLACTIN	SS	0360	☐ TRIGLYCERIDE	SS
0162	☐ CPK	SS	0823	☐ HGG QUANTITATIVE	SS	0103	☐ PROTEIN, TOTAL	SS	0672	☐ TSH	SS
0445	☐ CKMB ISOENZYME	SS	1856	☐ HIV (ANTIBODY)	SS	2000	☐ PROSTATE SPECIFIC ANTIGEN (PSA)	SS	0373	☐ URIC ACID	SS
0161	☐ CREATININE	SS	0558	☐ HDL CHOLESTEROL	SS	0310	☐ PT (PROTHROMBIN TIME)	B	0219	☐ URINALYSIS	U

CYTOPATHOLOGY

☐ PREGNANT ☐ ABORTION ☐ POST-PARTUM ☐ POST-MENOPAUSE

HISTORY _____

PREV. ABNORMAL CYTOL FINDINGS _____

☐ CONTRACEPTIVES DATE _____
☐ HYSTERECTOMY ☐ HORMONES ☐ IUD
☐ COPHORECTOMY ☐ TOTAL ☐ SUPRA CX
☐ RADIATION Rx DATE _____
☐ OTHER _____ ☐ HORMONES Rx ☐ CHEMO Rx

LMP _____ DATE COLLECTED _____
SOURCE ☐ CERVIX ☐ ENDOCERVIX ☐ VAGINA
☐ CYTOBRUSH ☐ OTHER SITE

MICROBIOLOGY

THCUL ☐ THROAT	URTHC ☐ URETHRAL	9391 ☐ CHLAMYDIA DNA
EACUL ☐ EAR	VACUL ☐ VAGINAL	9390 ☐ GONORRHEA DNA
EYCUL ☐ EYE	WOCUL ☐ WOUND	9391 ☐ OCCULT BLOOD
GOCUL ☐ GC	ROCUL ☐ CULTURE (Routine)	0293 ☐ OVA & PARASITE
SPCUL ☐ SPUTUM	URCUL ☐ URINE	WTM ☐ WET MOUNT
STCUL ☐ STOOL	GSP ☐ GRAM STAIN	
SOURCE _____	OTHER _____	

DIAGNOSIS OR COMMENTS

LAB USE ONLY (DO NOT WRITE BELOW THIS SPACE)

DATE RECEIVED	DATE REPORTED

STATEMENT OF SPECIMEN ADEQUACY

GENERAL CATEGORIZATION

DESCRIPTIVE DIAGNOSIS

HORMONAL EVALUATION

ADDITIONAL COMMENT

CYTOTECHNOLOGIST	PATHOLOGIST

INSURANCE BILLING INFORMATION

PRIMARY INSURED	INSURANCE COMPANY
ADDRESS	
POLICY NO. & I.D. NO.	ICD-10 CODE

LEGEND

SS	Serum Separator	GY	Grey	B	Blue	U	Urine
R	Red	L	Lavender	RB	Royal Blue	G	Green

Work Form 27-2

DOUGLASVILLE MEDICINE ASSOCIATES
5076 BRAND BLVD
DOUGLASVILLE, NY 01234
(123) 456-7890

OUTSIDE LAB SPECIMEN TRACKING LOG								
Date Sent	Patient Name/ID	Ordering Provider	Tests Ordered	Number of and Type of Specimens Sent to Laboratory (Include Tube Colors)	Prepared By	Laboratory	Date Results Received	Results Received By

C H A P T E R **28**

Clinical Chemistry and CLIA-Waived Testing

VOCABULARY REVIEW

Assignment 28-1: Matching

Match the term with its definition and place the corresponding letter in the blank.

_____ 1. Antiserum

_____ 2. Agglutination

_____ 3. Blood urea nitrogen

_____ 4. Analyte

_____ 5. Homeostasis

_____ 6. Lipoprotein

_____ 7. Triglyceride

_____ 8. Antibody

A. Another type of lipid or fat found in the blood

B. When fats are combined with protein in the blood

C. Serum that contains antibodies to a specific antigen used to perform blood typing

D. Antigen-antibody reaction which involves clumping of cells due to the antibody attaching itself to the antigen

E. Any substance that is being chemically analyzed

F. Kidney function indicator test which measures the amount of nitrogen in the blood

G. Particle produced in response to an antigen for the purpose of neutralizing or destroying that antigen

H. In a healthy body, specific mechanisms monitor and make adjustments to the internal environment to help maintain a constant state of balance

Assignment 28-2: Sentence Completion

Fill in the blanks below with Essential Terms from this chapter.

1. _____ is a waste product of hemoglobin breakdown formed in the liver and excreted in bile.

2. The cholesterol level is divided into _____ ("good" cholesterol) and _____ _____ ("bad" cholesterol).

3. Once your body produces an antibody to a particular _____, you will always have antibodies stored in your bloodstream to fight it.

4. The term for high blood glucose levels is _____ and the term for low blood glucose levels is _____.

5. HDL is the lipoprotein that removes _____ from the body by taking it to the liver, where it is excreted in bile.

6. The presence of the hormone _____, released by the placenta, may be detectable in the patient's sample as early as one to five days after the first missed menstrual cycle.

CHAPTER REVIEW

Assignment 28-3: Abbreviation Review

Write what each of the following abbreviations stands for.

1. HDL: _____

2. LDL: _____

3. BUN: _____

4. hCG: _____

5. OGTT: _____

6. ALT: _____

7. AST: _____

8. LDH: _____

9. GGT: _____

10. ALP: _____

11. CK, CPK: _____

12. TSH: _____

13. HbA1c: _____

14. CRP: _____

15. ALB: _____

16. CEA: _____

17. PSA: _____

18. TP, TPRO: _____

19. UA: _____

20. SST: _____

21. ABG: _____

22. BMP: _____

23. CMP: _____

24. IDDM: _____

25. NIDDM: _____

26. FBS: _____

27. 2HPP: _____

28. RBCs: _____

29. Mg, Mag: _____

30. Ca: _____

31. ABO: _____

32. VDRL: _____

33. RPR: _____

34: RF or RA: _____

35. HDN: _____

36. AMS: _____

37. Na: _____

38. K: _____

39. Cl: _____

40. P: _____

Assignment 28-4: Short Answer

1. List the clinical significance for performing the following tests, along with the normal values for the tests.

Test	Normal Value	Clinical Significance
FBS		
BUN		
HbA1c		
Creatinine		
Total cholesterol		
HDL		
LDL		
Triglycerides		

2. Explain the purpose of a laboratory profile.

_____

_____

_____

3. Explain the importance of proper specimen collection and handling.

_____

_____

_____

_____

4. Explain the purpose of the two-hour postprandial blood glucose level test.

_____

_____

_____

_____

_____

_____

_____

_____

5. List the electrolytes and explain their function in the body.

A. _____

_____

_____

_____

B. _____

_____

_____

C. _____

_____

_____

6. Discuss the role of HbA1c in the management of diabetes.

_____

_____

_____

_____

_____

_____

7. Explain the differences between type 1, type 2, and gestational diabetes.

A. _____

_____

B. _____

_____

_____

_____

C. _____

_____

_____

8. Describe the appearance and causes of icteric, lipemic, and hemolyzed serum.

A. _____

_____

B. _____

_____

C. _____

_____

9. Explain the difference between serum and plasma.

_____

_____

_____

10. Explain the purpose of the chain of custody.

_____

_____

_____

CERTIFICATION PRACTICE

Assignment 28-5

Choose the best answer and place the corresponding letter in the blank.

_____ 1. Which of the following is a screening test for syphilis?

A. HEC

B. SYP

C. STD

D. VDRL

_____ 2. If a patient's blood demonstrates a positive reaction when tested with Anti-B serum, it indicates which of the following blood types?

A. AB

B. B

C. A

D. O

_____ 3. A blood glucose result of 140 mg/dL would indicate which of the following?

A. Hypoglycemia

B. Glycogenemia

C. Impaired glucose tolerance

D. Glycemia

____ 4. When homeostasis is disrupted, the body responds by doing which of the following?

A. It shuts down altogether.

B. It interrupts blood flow.

C. It increases or lowers chemicals that are out of normal range.

D. It retains water.

____ 5. All of the following tests would be included in a hepatic profile, *except:*

A. total and direct bilirubin.

B. ALT.

C. AST.

D. CO_2.

____ 6. Before collecting a specimen for an OGTT, the patient is required to:

A. fast for 10 hours prior to testing.

B. fast for 6 hours prior to testing.

C. eat a high carbohydrate meal.

D. None of the above

____ 7. Which of the following is a tumor marker for colorectal cancer?

A. PSA

B. CEA

C. SST

D. ALP

____ 8. Which of the following is the most common cause of a peptic ulcer?

A. Diet

B. Alcohol consumption

C. Smoking

D. *Helicobacter pylori*

____ 9. Which of the following determines a person's blood type?

A. Antibodies

B. Antigens

C. T-cells

D. B-cells

____ 10. When performing an ABO blood typing, the antigen on the red blood cells reacts with an antibody in the test serum, causing which of the following reactions?

A. Neutralization

B. Specificity

C. Agglutination

D. Autoagglutination

SKILL APPLICATION CHALLENGES

Assignment 28-6: ABO Blood Chart

Fill in the following ABO blood group chart.

ABO Blood Type	Antigen Present on the Red Blood Cells	Antibody Present in the Plasma
Type A		
Type B		
Type AB		
Type O		

COMPLETING SPECIAL FORMS

Assignment 28-7: Lab Requisition Form

Work Form Necessary: FORM 28-1

Directions: Complete the lab requisition (Work Form 28-1) with the scenario information given below. (Hint: All of the information listed may or may not be used.)

Complete the lab requisition with the following information: Patient name: April R. Lindsey, Address: 1234 Lark Lane, Douglasville, NY 01234, Telephone number: 123-456-9087, DOB: 10-12-76, Sex: female, Fasting: yes, Date of visit: 06/26/XX, Time of collection: 8:00 a.m., Tests ordered: Liver and lipid profile. Primary insurance through husband, Dennis Lindsey, Address: Same as patient: ID #: 56987, Payer: Meditel, 9000 Green Ave., Anytown, OH 45229, ICD-10 code: I25.10, Referring provider: Dr. Miguel Gonzales, Address: Douglasville Medicine Associates, 5076 Brand Blvd., Douglasville, NY 01234, Telephone number: 123-456-7890, ID# 298739750023.

Assignment 28-8: Outside Specimen Tracking Log

Work Form Necessary: FORM 28-2

Directions: Enter the information from Assignment 28-7 into the log (Work Form 28-2).

Assignment 28-9: Normal and Abnormal Results

The lab results are back for April Lindsey. Medical assistants cannot diagnose or prescribe; however, knowing the significance of lab results and possible contributing factors for abnormal results will assist you when educating patients in person or over the phone. Record the abnormal results on the lines below, then note the indication(s) as to why particular results may be abnormal and state what may be a likely course of action (plan) by the provider based on the findings.

Abnormal Results

_____

_____

_____

_____

_____

_____

Indications/Plan

_____

_____

_____

_____

_____

_____

_____   _____
_____   _____
_____   _____
_____   _____
_____   _____
_____   _____
_____   _____

CLINICAL CHEMISTRY REPORT FORM

PHYSICIAN INFORMATION	PATIENT INFORMATION
DOUGLASVILLE MEDICINE ASSOCIATES 5076 BRAND BLVD. DOUGLASVILLE, NY 01234 (123) 456-7890 **Physician Name:** Dr. J. Leonard **Physician ID #:** 298739750023	**Name:** April Lindsey **Address:** 1234 Lark Lane **City/State/Zip**: Douglasville, NY 01234 **Phone #:** 123-456-9087 **ID #:** 877387477

Date and Time of Collection	Date Results Received
10/12/XX 9:00 a.m.	10/15/XX

Fasting Sample	Random Sample
Yes __X__	Yes ___

Test Ordered	Results	Reference Range
Profiles/Panels:		
Liver/Hepatic Panel		
Direct Bilirubin	1.0 mg/dL	0.0–0.2 mg/dL
Total Bilirubin	1.4 mg/dL	0.2–1.0 mg/dL
Total Protein	7.8 mg/dL	6.0–8.0 mg/dL
ALT	54 U/L	7–56 U/L
AST	42 U/L	5–40 U/L
LDH	147 mg/dL	Less than 130 mg/dL
GGT	42	M: 9–70 U/L F: 5–45 U/L
ALP	116	30–130 mU/L
Renal Panel		
Sodium (Na)		136–145 mEq/L
Potassium (K)		3.5–5.0 mEq/L
Chloride (Cl)		96–110 mEq/L
BUN/Blood Urea Nitrogen		8–25 mg/dL
Creatinine		0.4–1.5 mg/dL

Uric Acid		M: 3.5–7.2 mg/dL F: 2.6–6.0 mg/dL
Carbon Dioxide/CO_2		22–32 mmol/L
Glucose		70–110 mg/dL
Lipid Panel		
Total Cholesterol	256 mg/dL	Less than 200 mg/dL
HDL	75 mg/dL	M: 37–70 mg/dL F: 40–85 mg/dL
LDL	150 mg/dL	Less than 130 mg/dL
Triglycerides	140 mg/dL	20–180 mg/dL
Thyroid Panel		
	3.0 mU/mL	4.5–13.0 mU/mL
	2.5 mcg/dL	4–11.5 mcg/dL
	6.0 mU/mL	0.3–4.5 mU/mL
Test Ordered	**Results**	**Reference Range**
Cardiac Panel		
LDH		100–225 U/L
CPK		M: 12–70 mcg/L F: 10–55 mcg/L
SGOT		5–40 U/L
Miscellaneous Tests		
Glucose Tests:		
FBS		70–110 mg/dL
2HPP		Less than 140 mg/dL
OGTT:		
1/2 hour		110–170 mg/dL
1 hour		120–170 mg/dL
2 hours		70–120 mg/dL
3 hours		60–120 mg/dL
HgbA1c		4.5–6.5
Albumin		3.0–5.0 gm/dL
Globulin		2.3–3.5 mg/dL
Calcium		8.5–10.5 mg/dL
CEA		Nonsmoker: less than 2.5 ng/mL Smoker: less than 5 ng/mL
PSA		
Amylase		Adults: 25–125 IU/L Adults over 70: 21–160 IU/L
Lipase		Adults: 0–1.5 U/mL
Magnesium (Mg)		1.2–2.4 mEq/L
Phosphorous (P)		2.5–4.5 mg/dL

FIELD APPLICATION CHALLENGE
Assignment 28-10

Read the following Field Application Challenge and respond to the questions following the scenario.
You have been asked to perform a rapid test for infectious mononucleosis on a patient specimen. You obtain the proper specimen and perform the test according to manufacturer's directions. You obtain a negative result and report your result to the provider.

1. What important step was left out?

   _____

2. Can the results be considered accurate? Why or why not?

   _____

   _____

   _____

3. What impact could this have on the patient?

   _____

JOURNALING EXERCISE
Assignment 28-11

After reading this chapter, do you have a better appreciation for your role in laboratory testing and the validity of the results? What content within this chapter was most meaningful to you? Why? Consider Davene's scenario "if a result doesn't come out as expected." What critical thinking measures to would you use to determine possible flaws in testing preparation or performance? Apply the professionalism keys to your journal entries.

Work Form 28-1

LABORATORY REQUISITION

PATIENT LAST NAME		FIRST		M.I.	REFERRING PROVIDER

PROVIDER ID #	PATIENT ID #	BILL: ☐ PHYSICIAN	☐ MEDICAL ☐ HMO ☐ CHDP ☐ MEDICARE ☐ INSURANCE ☐ PATIENT PLEASE COMPLETE INSURANCE BILLING INFORMATION AT BOTTOM	D.O.B	AGE	SEX

PROVIDER NAME, ADDRESS, AND PHONE NUMBER	PATIENT ADDRESS	PATIENT PHONE NUMBER ( )	DATE COLLECTED	TIME COLLECTED
	CITY STATE ZIP CODE		FASTING YES NO	STAT	CALL RESULT
	PATIENT MEDICARE # PATIENT MEDICAID #		INFO. BELOW WILL APPEAR ON REPORT	

CUSTOM PROFILES & ADDITIONAL TESTS

```
173   [ ]  CHEMISTRY PANEL, COMPLETE BLOOD COUNT (ZPP), LIPID PROFILE, T4
05050 [ ]  CHOL, TRIG, HDL CHOL, VLDL CHOL, LDL CHOL, RISK FACTOR
```

PROFILES

00011 ☐ SPECIAL COMPREHENSIVE	2 SS,L	03536 ☐ HYPERTHYROID PROFILE			SS
00001 ☐ COMPREHENSIVE HEALTH SURVEY	SS,L	05037 ☐ HYPOTHYROID PROFILE			SS
00002 ☐ GENERAL SURVEY	SS,L	05051 ☐ LIPID PROFILE			SS
00003 ☐ CHEMISTRY PANEL	SS,L	05021 ☐ LIVER PROFILE			SS
CH7 ☐ CHEM 7 PANEL	SS	03359 ☐ LUPUS PROFILE			SS
03280 ☐ ANEMIA PROFILE	SS,L	03959 ☐ MENOPAUSAL PROFILE	SS /03960 ☐ POST MENOPAUSAL		SS
06016 ☐ ARTHRITIS PROFILE	SS,L	02280 ☐ OVARIAN FUNCTION PROFILE	SS /02281 ☐ TESTICULAR FUNC. PROF.		SS
05725 ☐ COMPREHENSIVE THYROID SURVEY	SS	02808 ☐ PRENATAL PROFILE			L,R
02691 ☐ EPSTEIN BARR PROFILE	SS	05006 ☐ THYROID PROFILE			SS
05010 ☐ ELECTROLYTES	SS	03191 ☐ TORCH PANEL			SS
06826 ☐ HEPATITIS PROFILE	SS	5756 ☐ URINE DRUG SCREEN	U / ☐ VENIPUNCTURE		

TESTS

0361 ☐ ABO & Rh TYPE	R,L	0141 ☐ C-REACTIVE PROTEIN	SS	0673 ☐ HEPATITIS B SURFACE ANTIGEN	SS	0237 ☐ PTT	B
0302 ☐ ALKALINE PHOSPHATASE	SS	1341 ☐ DHEA-S	SS	0245 ☐ HEPATITIS C ANTIBODY	SS	0317 ☐ RA FACTOR	SS
0109 ☐ AMYLASE	SS	0119 ☐ DIGOXIN	SS	0257 ☐ IRON	SS	0321 ☐ RUBELLA	SS
0613 ☐ ANA	SS	0224 ☐ DILANTIN	SS	LDL-A ☐ LDL CHOLESTEROL	SS	0331 ☐ RPR	SS
0366 ☐ ANTIBODY SCREEN	R	0835 ☐ ESTRADIOL	SS	0283 ☐ LEAD BLOOD	RB	0335 ☐ SEMEN ANALYSIS	SEMEN
0110 ☐ ASO (STREPTOZYME)	SS	0833 ☐ FERRITIN	SS	0281 ☐ LIPASE	SS	0328 ☐ SEDIMENTATION RATE (ESR)	L
0126 ☐ BILIRUBIN TOTAL	SS	0003 ☐ FOLIC ACID & VITAMIN B12	SS	8225 ☐ LH	SS	0349 ☐ SGOT (AST)	SS
0132 ☐ BUN	SS	0651 ☐ FSH	SS	0247 ☐ MONONUCLEOSIS	SS	0348 ☐ SGPT (ALT)	SS
8726 ☐ CA125	SS	0140 ☐ FTA-ABS	SS	0778 ☐ PHENOBARBITAL	SS	0330 ☐ SICKLE CELL SCREEN	L
0142 ☐ CALCIUM	SS	0210 ☐ GGTP	SS	0307 ☐ POTASSIUM	SS	0354 ☐ T4 (THYROXINE)	SS
0130 ☐ CBC	L	0536 ☐ GLUCOSE, FASTING	GY	0557 ☐ PREGNANCY (SERUM)	SS	1358 ☐ T4 FREE	SS
0388 ☐ CEA-ROCHE	SS	☐ GLUCOSE, ____ HR PP	GY	0308 ☐ PREGNANCY (URINE)	U	8456 ☐ TESTOSTERONE	SS
0152 ☐ CHOLESTEROL	SS	0771 ☐ GLYCOHEMOGLOBIN	L	0359 ☐ PROGESTERONE	SS	0824 ☐ THEOPHYLLINE	SS
0788 ☐ CORTISOL	SS	0534 ☐ H. PYLORI	SS	8041 ☐ PROLACTIN	SS	0360 ☐ TRIGLYCERIDE	SS
0162 ☐ CPK	SS	0823 ☐ HGG QUANTITATIVE	SS	0103 ☐ PROTEIN, TOTAL	SS	0672 ☐ TSH	SS
0445 ☐ CKMB ISOENZYME	SS	1856 ☐ HIV (ANTIBODY)	SS	2000 ☐ PROSTATE SPECIFIC ANTIGEN (PSA)	SS	0373 ☐ URIC ACID	SS
0161 ☐ CREATININE	SS	0558 ☐ HDL CHOLESTEROL	SS	0310 ☐ PT (PROTHROMBIN TIME)	B	0219 ☐ URINALYSIS	U

CYTOPATHOLOGY

☐ PREGNANT   ☐ ABORTION   ☐ POST-PARTUM   ☐ POST-MENOPAUSE
HISTORY _____

PREV. ABNORMAL CYTOL FINDINGS _____
☐ CONTRACEPTIVES   DATE _____
☐ HYSTERECTOMY   ☐ HORMONES   ☐ IUD
☐ COPHORECTOMY   ☐ TOTAL   ☐ SUPRA CX
☐ RADIATION Rx   DATE _____
☐ OTHER _____   ☐ HORMONES Rx   ☐ CHEMO Rx

LMP _____   DATE COLLECTED _____
SOURCE ☐ CERVIX   ☐ ENDOCERVIX   ☐ VAGINA
☐ CYTOBRUSH   ☐ OTHER SITE _____

MICROBIOLOGY

THCUL ☐ THROAT	URTHC ☐ URETHRAL	9391 ☐ CHLAMYDIA DNA
EACUL ☐ EAR	VACUL ☐ VAGINAL	9390 ☐ GONORRHEA DNA
EYCUL ☐ EYE	WOCUL ☐ WOUND	9391 ☐ OCCULT BLOOD
GOCUL ☐ GC	ROCUL ☐ CULTURE (Routine)	0293 ☐ OVA & PARASITE
SPCUL ☐ SPUTUM	URCUL ☐ URINE	WTM ☐ WET MOUNT
STCUL ☐ STOOL	GSP ☐ GRAM STAIN	
SOURCE _____	OTHER _____	

DIAGNOSIS OR COMMENTS

LAB USE ONLY (DO NOT WRITE BELOW THIS SPACE)

DATE RECEIVED	DATE REPORTED

STATEMENT OF SPECIMEN ADEQUACY

GENERAL CATEGORIZATION

DESCRIPTIVE DIAGNOSIS

HORMONAL EVALUATION

ADDITIONAL COMMENT

CYTOTECHNOLOGIST	PATHOLOGIST

INSURANCE BILLING INFORMATION

PRIMARY INSURED	INSURANCE COMPANY
ADDRESS	
POLICY NO. & I.D. NO.	ICD-10 CODE

LEGEND

SS	Serum Separator	GY	Grey	B	Blue	U	Urine
R	Red	L	Lavender	RB	Royal Blue	G	Green

Work Form 28-2

DOUGLASVILLE MEDICINE ASSOCIATES
5076 BRAND BLVD
DOUGLASVILLE, NY 01234
(123) 456-7890

OUTSIDE LAB SPECIMEN TRACKING LOG								
Date Sent	Patient Name/ID	Ordering Provider	Tests Ordered	Number of and Type of Specimens Sent to Laboratory (Include Tube Colors)	Prepared By	Laboratory	Date Results Received	Results Received By

C H A P T E R **2 9**

Diagnostic Imaging

VOCABULARY REVIEW

Assignment 29-1: Matching

Match the term with its definition and place the corresponding letter in the blank.

_____ 1. Fluoroscopy

_____ 2. Collimator

_____ 3. Angiography

_____ 4. Contrast medium

_____ 5. Radiolucent

_____ 6. Magnetic resonance imaging

_____ 7. Cholangiography

_____ 8. Bucky

_____ 9. Nuclear medicine

_____ 10. Ultrasound

_____ 11. Radiopaque

A. Diagnostic imaging procedure that uses no radiation and produces a high-quality, three-dimensional image that is much clearer than traditional radiographs; the machine uses a powerful magnetic field to produce images of internal organs and soft tissue structure

B. Visualization of the blood vessels to assess blood flow, clots, hemorrhaging, or aneurysm

C. Substance that is either injected or ingested which enhances the internal structures for better visualization

D. Holds a cassette tray in which the Image Receptor is placed; during the radiograph, moves the grid out of the way to prevent it from being visible on the Image Receptor

E. Penetrable by radiographs

F. Diagnostic imaging procedure that does not use radiation but instead bounces high-frequency sound waves to produce an image of an internal body structure, creating a sonogram or picture

G. Branch of medicine that uses radioactive material for the purpose of diagnosing and treating diseases

H. Unable to be penetrated by the radiograph beam (allows visualization of a structure)

I. Visualization of moving body structures in real time, similar to a movie

J. Visualization of the bile ducts for detection of possible stones or lesions

K. Device attached to the radiograph tube that controls the size and shape of the radiograph beam

Assignment 29-2: Sentence Completion

Fill in the blanks below with Essential Terms from this chapter.

1. A(n) _____ is the recorded image produced using X-radiation.

2. The ____ is the component placed below the radiograph table between the table and the image receptor to prevent the radiograph beam from scattering, which helps produce a clearer image.

3. _____ is a procedure that combines upper endoscopy and radiographs to treat problems of the bile and pancreatic ducts.

4. Another name for an X-ray is a(n) _____.

5. The procedure that combines radiograph with a computer analysis of body tissues and organs, performed with or without a contrast medium, and produces cross-sectional images of the body is _____.

6. A(n) _____ is a physician who has received additional training in the use and interpretation of radiological examinations and is usually the medical specialist who oversees a hospital diagnostic imaging department or an outside imaging facility.

7. _____ provides detailed pictures that illustrate disease processes at the cellular or molecular level.

8. The amount of radiation emission is measured in several different ways. The _____ is a measurement of radiation energy per kilogram and is interchangeable with sievert (Sv), as they both are International System of Units (SI).

9. During a radiograph, the radiation that strikes the patient is known as "primary" radiation. _____ is emitted from the patient in all directions, which is considered "secondary" radiation.

10. Substances known as _____, containing radioactive isotopes, are administered to the patient by mouth or by injection.

CHAPTER REVIEW

Assignment 29-3: Abbreviation Review

Write what each of the following abbreviations stands for.

1. AP: _____

2. PA: _____

3. IVP: _____

4. CT: _____

5. MRI: _____

6. KUB: _____

7. ERCP: _____

8. PET: _____

9. GXMO: _____

10. PACS: _____

11. ALARA: _____

12. OSL: _____

13. IVU: _____

14. LGI: _____

15. UGI: _____

16. BE: _____

17. NPO: _____

18. SPECT: _____

19. MRS: _____

20. OTC: _____

Assignment 29-4: Short Answer

1. Explain the advantage of using ultrasound over radiograph during pregnancy.

   _____

2. Define the following patient positions used for radiographs.

   A. AP: _____

      _____

   B. PA: _____

      _____

   C. Lateral: _____

      _____

   D. Oblique: _____

      _____

   E. Erect: _____

   F. Supine: _____

      _____

3. List patient risks associated with radiographs.

   _____

   _____

   _____

4. Explain patient preparation for an IVP and fluoroscopy.

   A. IVP: _____

      _____

   B. Fluoroscopy: _____

      _____

5. List the safety precautions used by health care personnel and patients during radiograph procedures. *The first one has been completed for you.*

Safety Procedures to Protect the Health Care Worker	Safety Procedures to Protect the Patient
Lead apron and gloves should be worn if the radiographer must remain in the room.	Use the smallest amount of radiation possible to achieve the best image.

6. List side effects associated with radiation therapy.

_____

_____

_____

_____

_____

_____

7. List medical assistant duties regarding radiographic procedures.

A. _____

B. _____

C. _____

D. _____

_____

_____

E. _____

_____

F. _____

G. _____

_____

H. _____

I. _____

J. _____

K. _____

L. _____

M. _____

_____

8. List and define the different types of contrast media used to perform radiographs.

A. _____

_____

_____

B. _____

_____

_____

C. _____

_____

_____

CERTIFICATION PRACTICE

Assignment 29-5

Choose the best answer and place the corresponding letter in the blank.

____ 1. Which of the following radiological procedures would require *no* patient preparation?

A. Fluoroscopy

B. IVP

C. Upper GI

D. Radiograph of the hand

____ 2. In which of the following positions would the patient's back be against the film?

A. AP

B. PA

C. Lateral

D. Oblique

___ 3. All of the following are side effects of radiation therapy *except:*

   A. vomiting.

   B. hair loss.

   C. increase in appetite.

   D. nausea.

___ 4. Which of the following radiological procedures provides cross-sectional images of the body?

   A. MRI

   B. CT scan

   C. Bone scan

   D. Both a and b

___ 5. Which of the following controls the size and shape of the radiograph beam?

   A. Grid

   B. Cassette

   C. Bucky

   D. Collimator

___ 6. Which part of the radiograph equipment is designed to prevent scattering of the radiograph beam?

   A. Grid

   B. Processor

   C. Cassette

   D. Bucky

___ 7. In which of the following radiograph positions does the radiograph beam pass from the back to the front?

   A. Lateral

   B. AP

   C. PA

   D. Supine

___ 8. All of the following positions may be used for a radiograph of a fractured ankle *except:*

   A. AP.

   B. lateral.

   C. oblique.

   D. erect.

___ 9. Which of the following imaging procedures never requires film?

   A. CT scan

   B. Bone scan

   C. Digital radiograph

   D. All of the above

___ 10. Which of the following statements is true regarding the radioactive materials used in radiograph procedures?

   A. Radioactive materials must be stored in lead containers.

   B. Radioactive materials should never be handled with bare hands.

   C. Special equipment must be used when handling radioactive materials.

   D. All of the above

SKILL APPLICATION CHALLENGE

Assignment 29-6: Research Activity

Using the Internet to gather information, design a patient information form for one of the following diagnostic imaging procedures:

- MRI
- KUB
- Upper GI
- Cholangiography
- Fluoroscopy
- PET Scan

COMPLETING SPECIAL FORMS

Assignment 29-7: Imaging Request Form

Work Form Necessary: FORM 29-1

Directions: Complete the imaging request form (Work Form 29-1) with the scenario information given below.

Complete the imaging request form with the following information: Patient name: Nancy Tinksy, 5879 Parkside Road, Parkview NY 01652, (123) 259-6632, DOB: 05/22/55, Payer info: Name of insured: Nancy Tinksy, Insurance ID #: 5698AC1, Name of company: Meditel Insurance Company, Address of insurance company: 2345 Long Street, Anytown, OH 43256, (740) 236-9865, Clinical findings: Productive cough × two weeks, (nonsmoker), Referring provider: Dr. Corey Cook, Douglasville Medicine Associates, 5076 Brand Blvd, Douglasville, NY 01234 (123) 456-7890, Radiographs ordered: PA and lateral of the chest to be performed at XYZ Radiology. The provider would like the results transmitted electronically to *ccook@ douglasvillemed.org.*

You contact XYZ Radiology and speak with Kim Grossman. Date of order: 05/19/XX, Date of appointment: 05/19/XX at 3:00 p.m.

Assignment 29-8: Documentation/Charting Exercise

On the following progress note, document that you set the patient up to have a PA and lateral chest X-ray today at 3:00 p.m. at XYZ Radiology and that you spoke with Kim Grossman (date of entry: 05/19/XX, time of entry: 12:45 p.m.) Document that you gave the patient the requisition form (order) to take with her and that the office will call her with the results. Be sure to include an order for the X-ray in your documentation.

FIELD APPLICATION CHALLENGE

Assignment 29-9

Read the following Field Application Challenge and respond to the questions following the scenario.
You are excited because you just received your radiograph certification and are able to take radiographs in your facility. A 27-year-old patient, Claudia Green, has an order from her provider to have a chest radiograph because of a possible broken rib.

1. What is the first question you should ask Claudia?

_____

2. What clothing and other articles should she remove prior to the radiograph?

_____

3. After performing the radiograph, you notice that the patient has a necklace on in the radiograph. Which of the following should you do?

   A. Retake the radiograph.

   B. Check with the provider to see how he wants you to proceed.

   C. Scold the patient for not removing the necklace.

4. How will you make certain that this never occurs again?

_____

_____

JOURNALING EXERCISE

Assignment 29-10

Diagnostic imaging is important for determining the presence of disease or injury. How would you become proficient in educating patients about these procedures? Which professionalism keys would you incorporate into your work in diagnostic imaging?

Work Form 29-1

<table>
<tr><td colspan="3" align="center">

XYZ RADIOLOGY
4598 HIGH STREET
DOUGLASVILLE, NY 01234
(123) 456-9874

</td></tr>
<tr>
<td>

Patient Name:
Address:

Phone #:
DOB:

</td>
<td>

Insured's Name:
Payer Info:

</td>
<td>

Referring Physician Info:

</td>
</tr>
</table>

ULTRASOUND PROCEDURES	X-RAYS/RADIOGRAPHIC PROCEDURES	
Abdomen:	**Abdomen:**	**Upper Extremities**
☐ Complete Abdomen	☐ Plain Film (KUB)	R L AC Joints
☐ Both Abdomen & Pelvic	☐ Acute (2 Views)	R L Clavicle
☐ Other	**Barium Studies:**	R L Digits 1 2 3 4 5
Joint:	☐ BA Swallow	R L Elbow
☐ Shoulder	☐ Upper GI Series	R L Forearm
☐ Knee	☐ GI Small Bowel	R L Hand
☐ Other +Fluid +Mass	☐ BA Enema (Colon)	R L Humerus
Neck:	**Chest:**	R L Scapula
☐ Neck & Thyroid	☐ PA & Lateral	R L Shoulder
Pelvic Female:	☐ Ribs: R L	R L Wrist
☐ Pelvic Routine (Only)	☐ Chest PA	**Lower Extremities**
☐ Transvaginal	☐ Sternum	R L Ankle
☐ Transvaginal & Kidneys	**Head and Neck:**	R L Femur
☐ Obstetrical	☐ Facial	R L Foot
☐ Biophysical	☐ Mandible	R L Hip
Pelvic Male:	☐ Mastoid	R L OS Calcis
☐ Prostate/Bladder	☐ Orbits	R L Toes 1 2 3 4 5
☐ Prostate/Bladder/Kidney	☐ Orbits for MRI	**Spine and Pelvic**
☐ Scrotal	☐ Nasal Bones	☐ Cervical Spine
Vascular Diseases:	☐ Skull	☐ Lumpo-Sacral Spine
☐ Arterial Leg Doppler	☐ Sinuses	☐ Pelvis
☐ Carotid Doppler	☐ Soft Tissue of Neck	☐ Pelvis & Joints
☐ Venous Leg Doppler	☐ TM Joints	☐ Sacrum & Coccyx
☐ Other Doppler		☐ Thoracic Spine

Clinical Data or ICD-10	☐ Email Results: email Address: ☐ Fax Report: Fax #:	
Date of Order:	**Date of Appointment:**	**Time of Appointment:**
Physician's Office Rep:	**XYZ Radiology Rep:**	

CHAPTER **30**

Fundamentals of Pharmacology

VOCABULARY REVIEW

Assignment 30-1: Matching

Match the term with its definition and place the corresponding letter in the blank.

_____ 1. Affinity

_____ 2. Anaphylaxis

_____ 3. Bioavailability

_____ 4. Drug

_____ 5. Drug ceiling

_____ 6. Drug interaction

_____ 7. Efficacy

_____ 8. Pharmacodynamics

_____ 9. Pharmacology

_____ 10. Receptor

_____ 11. Side effect

_____ 12. Therapeutic effect

_____ 13. Therapeutic index

A. Bonding proteins or sites in which a drug attaches; each has a unique structural design

B. Comparing a drug's effectiveness and benefits to its risks

C. Secondary effect in addition to the therapeutic effect

D. Measurement of how tightly a drug attaches or binds to a receptor

E. Advanced systemic reaction; may include bronchial constriction, swelling of the tongue or throat, and an inability to breathe

F. Range between the therapeutic dose of a drug and the dose at which the drug becomes toxic

G. The extent to and the rate at which the drug enters the blood plasma and is made available at the site of action

H. Any substance that produces a change in function of a living organism

I. When one drug diminishes or increases the effects of another drug

J. The study of the effects of drugs on living organisms

K. Maximum dose at which a drug will provide its greatest effect

L. Study of drugs, including their origin, nature, properties, and effects upon living organisms

M. Desired effect that a drug has on the body

Assignment 30-2: Definitions

Define the following terms.

1. Agonists: _____

_____

2. Antagonists: _____

_____

3. Buccal: _____

_____

_____

4. Enteral: _____

5. Parenteral: _____

_____

6. Pharmacokinetics: _____

_____

7. Sublingual: _____

8. Topical: _____

_____

9. Transdermal patches: _____

_____

CHAPTER REVIEW

Assignment 30-3: Abbreviation Review

Write what each of the following abbreviations stands for.

1. OTC: _____
2. FDA: _____
3. APhA: _____
4. DEA: _____
5. CSA: _____
6. USP: _____
7. PDR: _____
8. USP/NF: _____
9. LASA: _____
10. SR: _____
11. GI: _____

12. USAN: _____

13. CPOE: _____

14. PAD: _____

Assignment 30-4: Short Answer

1. List five different sources of drugs.

   A. _____

   B. _____

   C. _____

   D. _____

   E. _____

2. List and describe four processes that affect drug plasma levels.

   A. _____

   _____

   _____

   B. _____

   _____

   _____

   C. _____

   _____

   _____

   D. _____

   _____

   _____

3. List and describe three different names by which a drug may be referred.

   A. _____

   _____

   _____

   _____

   B. _____

   _____

   _____

   _____

   C. _____

   _____

   _____

4. Describe the following terms and which health care professionals can perform the tasks listed.

A. Prescribe: _____

_____

B. Administer: _____

_____

C. Dispense: _____

_____

D. Physicians: _____

_____

E. Nurse practitioners and physician assistants: _____

_____

F. Medical assistants: _____

_____

_____

5. Describe the potential for abuse for each of the five drug schedules, and give an example of a drug for each schedule.

Schedule	*Potential for Abuse*
I (C-I on label)	_____
	_____
	_____
II (C-II on label)	_____
	_____
	_____
	_____
III (C-III on label)	_____
	_____
	_____
	_____
	_____
IV (C-IV on label)	_____
	_____
	_____
V (C-V on label)	_____
	_____
	_____
	_____

6. How often does the DEA require that a full inventory be completed of all controlled substances in the medical office?

   _____

7. How often should inventories be performed in areas in which staff has access?

   _____

8. How long should the controlled substances inventory log be kept?

   _____

9. Define the term prescription and list its parts.

   Prescription: _____

   _____

   Parts of a prescription: _____

   _____

   _____

   _____

   _____

   _____

   _____

   _____

10. List and describe the seven rights of drug administration.

    Right   *Description*

    1. _____   _____

                           _____

                           _____

    2. _____   _____

                           _____

                           _____

                           _____

                           _____

                           _____

    3. _____   _____

                           _____

                           _____

    4. _____   _____

                           _____

                           _____

                           _____

    5. _____   _____

                           _____

6. _____ _____

   _____

   _____

   _____

   _____

   _____

7. _____ _____

   _____

   _____

   _____

   _____

   _____

   _____

   _____

   _____

11. List the two major routes of drug administration and then list and describe all the routes within each major route.

   Route   *Examples*

   _____   _____

   _____   _____

   _____   _____

   _____   _____

   _____   _____

   _____   _____

   _____   _____

   _____   _____

   _____   _____

   _____   _____

   _____   _____

   _____   _____

12. Describe the following forms and list their uses:

   A. DEA Form 224: _____

   _____

   _____

   B. DEA Form 41: _____

   _____

   _____

Assignment 30:5: Fill in the Blank

Fill in the missing components to drug classifications.

Drug Classification	Action	Example
	Prevents or relieves cough	Benylin cough syrup
Miotic	Contracts pupils of the eyes	
Vasodilator		Nitroglycerin
	Relieves mild to moderate fever, pain, and inflammation	Celebrex, Bextra, naproxen, Advil, Motrin
Muscle relaxant	Aids in relaxation of skeletal muscles	
	Reduces nasal congestion and swelling	Sudafed; Afrin
Antiemetic	Counteracts nausea and vomiting	
Laxative		Dulcolax, Metamucil, Miralax
Antimanic		Lithium, Depakene, Depakote, Abilify, Geodon
	Eases breathing by dilating the bronchial tubes	Atrovent, Combivent, albuterol
Cardiac glycoside	Strengthens the heart muscle	
Antihypertensive		Accupril, Altace, enalapril
	Relieves pain	Tylenol, Bayer, Aspro, Dispril (aspirin)
Antiacne	Treats acne	
	Prevents or delays blood clotting	Coumadin, heparin sodium, Lovenox
Antidepressant		Celexa, Effexor XR, Wellbrutrin-SR
Antidiabetic	Helps to lower blood glucose levels	
	Helps to decrease cholesterol or lipid levels	Crestor (rosuvastatin), Lipitor (atorvastatin calcium), Zocor (simvastatin), Zetia (ezetimibe), Niaspan (niacin)

CERTIFICATION PRACTICE
Assignment 30-6

Choose the best answer and place the corresponding letter in the blank.

____ 1. Which of the following drug classifications produces a calming effect?

    A. Sedative

    B. Hypnotic

    C. Tranquilizer

    D. All of the above

____ 2. Drugs may be grouped by the type of action they produce in the body. The application of topical medication to a joint to relieve pain is an example of a:

    A. local action.

    B. remote action.

    C. systemic action.

    D. nerve action.

____ 3. All of the following would be factors that affect drug actions *except:*

    A. body weight.

    B. disease.

    C. blood type.

    D. age.

____ 4. Which of the following is the exclusive name of a drug substance or drug product owned by a company under a trademark law?

    A. Generic name

    B. Trade name

    C. Chemical

    D. Brand name

____ 5. Which of the following is the drug's formula which includes letters and numbers?

    A. Generic name

    B. Trade name

    C. Chemical

    D. Brand name

____ 6. To apply for a DEA number, the provider will need to complete and submit which of the following forms?

    A. DEA Form 222

    B. DEA Form 224

    C. DEA Form 106

    D. DEA Form 41

____ 7. Which of the following sections of the *PDR* provides full-color photographs of the tablets and capsules and is arranged alphabetically by manufacturer?

    A. Section 1 Gray

    B. Section 2 White

    C. Section 3 Blue

    D. Section 4 Gray

___ 8. How long should the patient wait following drug administration?

    A. 10–15 minutes

    B. 15–20 minutes

    C. 20–30 minutes

    D. One hour

___ 9. Which of the following is the minimum number of times a medical assistant should read a label before administering the medication?

    A. Once

    B. Twice

    C. Three times

    D. Four times

___ 10. A medication that is mixed with special binding powder and pressed and molded into a particular shape is called a:

    A. caplet.

    B. capsule.

    C. gel cap.

    D. tablet.

SKILL APPLICATION CHALLENGE

Assignment 30-7: Flash Card Connection

1. Make flash cards for all of the medication abbreviations listed in Appendix A of the textbook.

2. Make flash cards for all of the drug classifications listed in Table 30-1 in this chapter.

COMPLETING SPECIAL FORMS

Assignment 30-8: Prescription Practice

Work Forms Necessary: FORMS 30-1, 30-2, 30-3, and 30-4

Directions: Using the prescription abbreviations in Appendix A of the textbook and the prescription example in the chapter, write prescriptions for the orders given in the following case studies.

Case study information: All of the refills are to be dispensed as written; no generics are to be used. (Note: Remember to write out the quantity.) Use the following patient information for each prescription. The patient's name is Kevin Heller, 5106 Springdale Court, Columbus OH 43227, DOB: 05/07/66, Provider's name, Dr. Paul Timmons.

1. Using Work Form 30-1, write a prescription for Augmentin tablets, 250 mg strength, Dispense amount 30, patient should take one tablet by mouth three times a day for 10 days. No refills are to be given.

2. Using Work Form 30-2, write a prescription for Prilosec tablets, 40 mg strength, Dispense amount 90, patient should take one tablet three times a day before meals. Refill amount three.

3. Using Work Form 30-3, write a prescription for Vicoden ES tablets, Dispense amount 20, patient should take one to two every four to six hours as needed for pain. No refills are to be given. DEA # B2462810

4. Using Work Form 30-4, write a prescription for Procardia capsules, 10 mg strength, Dispense amount 60, patient should take one every morning and one at bedtime. Refill amount one.

Assignment 30-9: Reading Prescriptions

Directions: Using the prescription abbreviations in Appendix A of the textbook and the prescription example in the chapter, rewrite the following prescriptions in lay terms.

1. Rx: Alprazolam 0.25 mg, sig 1 tab tid. Disp #90, 0 refills

_____

_____

2. Rx: Tussionex Susp 5 mg/5 mL, sig 5 mL. q 12 hours prn cough. Disp 50 mL, 0 refills.

_____

_____

3. Rx: Ventolin Inhaler, 90 mcg/actuation, sig 1–2 puffs prn for asthma. Disp 1 inhaler /c 2 refills.

_____

_____

FIELD APPLICATION CHALLENGE

Assignment 30-10

This Field Application Challenge has two parts. In Part A, read the scenario presented and respond to the questions following. In Part B, role play with a partner as instructed below, followed by a documentation exercise.

Part A: Mrs. Peterson has been placed on digoxin 1.5 mg daily due to congestive heart failure (CHF). Digoxin has a narrow therapeutic index and can cause organ toxicity if the blood plasma level exceeds the therapeutic index. The test must be conducted in a very narrow time line (six to eight hours following her last dose). Mrs. Peterson takes her single dose of digoxin at 7:00 a.m. every morning.

1. Based on the above criteria regarding when the blood must be tested and the time that Mrs. Peterson regularly takes her digoxin, what timeline can be used to schedule her testing?

_____

2. Because it may take a while to get the patient back to the drawing station and processed, what time ideally would the patient need to be scheduled by in order to have the blood drawn within the correct timeline?

_____

Part B: Amy from XYZ lab calls the office to state that Mrs. Peterson's digoxin level is 2.8 ng/mL (elevated) and that the provider, Dr. Butcher, will need to be notified right away of the patient's result. You notify the provider and he tells you to call the patient and tell her that she will need to reduce her dose by cutting her 1.5 mg tablets in half for the next seven days. The patient will need to return to the office for another digoxin level on day seven at the new dose. With a lab partner playing the role of Mrs. Peterson, practice calling the patient to give her the provider's instructions. Set the patient up for her next appointment. Remember that the provider wants the patient to be tested on day seven of taking the new dose. (Recall what time of day Mrs. Peterson takes her dose so that you can determine what date and time she will need to be tested.) Chart both the call from the lab and the phone call to the patient on the following progress note. Date both entries as 11/04/XX and use 9:00 a.m. as the time the lab called and 9:30 a.m. as the time you called the patient with the provider's instructions. Be certain to document the instructions given to the patient, the patient's apparent comprehension of the instructions, and the date of the new appointment.

PROGRESS NOTE

Patient Name: _____   DOB: _____

DATE/TIME	PROGRESS NOTES	ALLERGIES

JOURNALING EXERCISE

Assignment 30-11

What content within this chapter was most meaningful to you? Why? After reading Davene's "Professionalism Mentor" feature, has this ever happened to you or a family member? Explain how the professionalism keys apply to the situation described.

Work Form 30-1

Douglasville Medicine Associates
5076 Brand Blvd.
Douglasville, NY 01234
(123)456-7890

Patient Name:

Address:

DOB: Date:

R_X

Disp:

Sig:

Signature:

DEA # _____

☐ **Dispense as Written/Do Not Substitute**

Refills: none 1 2 3 4 5

Work Form 30-2

Douglasville Medicine Associates
5076 Brand Blvd.
Douglasville, NY 01234
(123)456-7890

Patient Name:

Address:

DOB: Date:

R_X

Disp:

Sig:

Signature:

DEA # _____

☐ **Dispense as Written/Do Not Substitute**

Refills: none 1 2 3 4 5

Work Form 30-3

Douglasville Medicine Associates
5076 Brand Blvd.
Douglasville, NY 01234
(123)456-7890

Patient Name:

Address:

DOB: Date:

R_X

Disp:

Sig:

Signature:

DEA # _____

☐ **Dispense as Written/Do Not Substitute**

Refills: none 1 2 3 4 5

Work Form 30-4

Douglasville Medicine Associates
5076 Brand Blvd.
Douglasville, NY 01234
(123)456-7890

Patient Name:

Address:

DOB: Date:

R_X

Disp:

Sig:

Signature:

DEA # _____

☐ **Dispense as Written/Do Not Substitute**

Refills: none 1 2 3 4 5

CHAPTER **31**

Dosage Calculations

VOCABULARY REVIEW

Assignment 31-1: Sentence Completion

Fill in the blanks below with Essential Terms from this chapter.

1. A pharmacist or chemist was formerly known as a(n) _____.

2. The _____ was the original or primary system used for calculating and measuring medication dosages.

3. A(n) _____ is the unit that is used when measuring anything that has mass or weight.

4. A(n) _____ is the fundamental unit for volume and is used when measuring liquids.

5. A(n) _____ is the fundamental unit for length and is used when measuring distance.

6. The _____ is used throughout the world and is the primary system for measuring weight, volume, and length (area).

7. A(n) _____ is a graph that illustrates a relationship between two known values.

8. The medical industry considers the _____ the most accurate method of calculating drug dosages for infants and children up to 12 years of age.

9. The term _____ means to switch from one unit to another.

10. _____ is known as the numbers used to identify the manufacturer, the product, and the size of the container.

Assignment 31-2: Matching I

Match the term with its definition and place the corresponding letter in the blank.

____ 1. Drug dosage

____ 2. Expiration date

____ 3. Generic name

____ 4. Lot control

____ 5. Medication label

____ 6. Prescription

____ 7. Product name

A. An order for a prescribed drug

B. The strength of the drug or amount to be given

C. Gives vital information about the product. Medications normally come with an insert, which has additional information that may be helpful in the administration of the medication.

D. Refers to the trade name or brand name of the medication

E. A drug's official name; can also be a listing of active and nonactive ingredients within the medication

F. Batch number used to track medications in the event that a bulk production of the drug must be recalled due to numerous reports of severe adverse reactions or product contamination

G. Guarantees the effectiveness and safe use of the medication up to the date posted on the drug package or container

CHAPTER REVIEW

Assignment 31-3: Abbreviation Review

Write what each of the following abbreviations stands for.

1. BSA: _____

2. NDC: _____

Assignment 31-4: Matching II

Match the term with its definition and place the corresponding letter in the blank.

____ 1. Centi

____ 2. Milli

____ 3. Micro

____ 4. Kilo

____ 5. Gram

____ 6. Meter

____ 7. Kilogram

____ 8. Milligram

____ 9. Milliliter

____ 10. Centimeter

____ 11. Microgram

____ 12. Millimeter

____ 13. Liter

____ 14. Cubic centimeter

A. One-millionth of a unit

B. One thousand units

C. One-thousandth of a unit

D. One-hundredth of a unit

E. kg

F. g

G. mg

H. cc

I. mm

J. cm

K. m

L. L

M. mL

N. mcg

Assignment 31-5: Short Answer

1. Describe how insulin is measured and what type of syringe is used to administer insulin.

_____

2. List and describe the three different types of human insulin that are available.

   A. _____

   B. _____

   _____

   C. _____

   _____

3. Analogs are insulin medicines that have been altered to help in faster absorption or last longer in the body. Identify, describe, and cite examples.

   A. _____

   _____

   _____

   B. _____

   _____

   _____

   _____

   C. _____

   _____

4. List the important parts of a medication label.

   A. _____

   B. _____

   C. _____

   D. _____

   E. _____

   F. _____

   _____

CERTIFICATION PRACTICE

Assignment 31-6

Choose the best answer and place the corresponding letter in the blank.

____ 1. The patient is to receive 10 mL of Amoxicillin. How many teaspoonfuls should the patient take?

   A. 1.5 teaspoons

   B. 2 teaspoons

   C. 2.5 teaspoons

   D. 3 teaspoons

____ 2. If a physician prescribes 2 tbsp twice a day, how many days will an 8 oz. bottle last?

    A. Two days

    B. Three days

    C. Four days

    D. One week

____ 3. A child weighs 45.9 kg. Convert her weight to pounds (round to the nearest hundredth).

    A. 132.64 lb

    B. 69.58 lb

    C. 87.65 lb

    D. 100.98 lb

____ 4. 2 cups = _____

    A. 8 ounces

    B. 16 tablespoons

    C. 1 quart

    D. 1 pint

____ 5. Dosages of insulin are always measured in which of the following?

    A. Cubic millimeters

    B. Grams

    C. Micromilligrams

    D. Units

____ 6. Which of the following is the unit for length?

    A. Liter

    B. Gram

    C. Meter

    D. Milliliter

____ 7. Which of the following is the unit for volume?

    A. Liter

    B. Gram

    C. Meter

    D. Millimeter

____ 8. Which of the following is the unit for weight or mass?

    A. Liter

    B. Gram

    C. Meter

    D. Kilometer

____ 9. A child weighs 66 pounds and the physician has ordered a daily dose of 30 mg/kg of body weight. The daily dose should divided into three equal doses. Which of the following dosages will be given to the patient per dose?

    A. 300 mg

    B. 600 mg

    C. 900 mg

    D. None of the above

___ 10. The physician orders Amoxicillin 0.05 g. Available is Amoxicillin 150 mg/5 mL. How many milliliters will you give the patient (round to the nearest tenth)?

    A. 1.5 mL

    B. 1.7 mL

    C. 2 mL

    D. 1 mL

SKILL APPLICATION CHALLENGES

Assignment 31-7: Math Review

1. Convert the following measurements. The conversion factor is 1 kg = 2.2 lb (round your answers to the nearest hundredth when applicable).

    A. 38 lb = _____ kg

    B. 14 kg = ____ lb

    C. 67 kg = ____ lb

    D. 45 lb = _____ kg

    E. 113 lb = _____ kg

2. Convert the following units.

    A. 1,000 mcg = ___ mg

    B. 0.6 g = _____ kg

    C. 15.6 L = _____ mL

    D. 8 oz = ___ mL

    E. 1 glass or cup = ___ oz

Assignment 31-8: Dosage Calculations

Calculate the correct number of tablets or capsules to be administered per dose. Tablets are scored. Refer to the prescription abbreviations in Appendix A in the textbook to help you read the orders. Also refer to The Joint Commission's "Do Not Use" list and the ISMP List of Error-Prone Abbreviations, Symbols, and Dose Designations in Appendix B of the textbook. Show your work!

1. Order: 0.5 g of Duricef p.o.r

    Supply: Duricef 500 mg tablets

    Answer: Give the patient _____ of Duricef (500 mg strength)

2. Order: Motrin 600 mg

    Supply: Motrin 300 mg tablets

    Answer: Give the patient _____ of Motrin (300 mg strength)

3. Order: Inderal 15 mg

    Supply: Inderal 10 mg tablets

    Answer: Give the patient _____ of Inderal (10 mg strength)

4. Order: Tylenol 0.5 g

    Supply: Tylenol (acetaminophen) liquid 500 mg in 5 mL

    Answer: Give the patient _____ of Tylenol

Assignment 31-9: Calculations Using Drug Labels

Read the following drug labels and calculate the following medication to be administered per dose. Show your work!

1. Order: Carafate 500 mg

    Answer: Give the patient _____ of Carafate

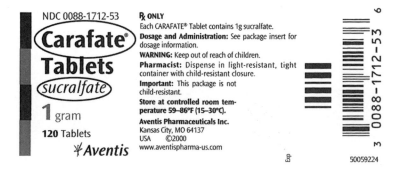

2. Order: 7.5 mg of Terbutaline

   Answer: Give the patient _____ of Terbutaline

USUAL DOSAGE:
See package insert for prescribing information.

Dispense in a tight, light-resistant container as defined in the USP with a child-resistant closure.

Store at 20°-25°C (68°-77°F) [See USP Controlled Room Temperature]. Excursion permitted 15°-30°C (59°-86°F)

Rev. 03/05

N 3 0527-1318-01 5

NDC 0527-1318-01

LANNETT

TERBUTALINE SULFATE TABLETS, USP

2.5 mg

Rx Only

100 TABLETS

Each tablet contains:
Terbutaline, USP ...... 2.5 mg

Inactive Ingredients:
Anhydrous lactose, magnesium stearate, microcrystalline cellulose, povidone, and pregelatinized starch.

Manufactured by:
Lannett Company, Inc.
Philadelphia, PA 19136

Exp. Date:

Lot No.:

3. Order: Promethazine 12.5 mg

   Answer: Give the patient _____ of Promethazine

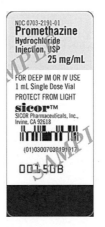

NDC 0703-2191-01
Promethazine
Hydrochloride
Injection, USP
25 mg/mL

FOR DEEP IM OR IV USE
1 mL Single Dose Vial
PROTECT FROM LIGHT

sicor™
SICOR Pharmaceuticals, Inc.,
Irvine, CA 92618

(01)03007032191017

00150B

4. Order: Synthroid 0.3 mg

Answer: Give the patient _____ of Synthroid

NDC 0048-1090-05
NSN 6505-01-153-3338
Code 3P1095

SYNTHROID®

(Levothyroxine Sodium Tablets, USP)

150 mcg   (0.15 mg)

1000 TABLETS

Rx only

BASF Pharma   **knoll®**

See full prescribing information for dosage and administration.

Dispense in a tight, light-resistant container as described in USP.

Store at 25°C (77°F); excursions permitted to 15°-30°C (59°-86°F). [See USP Controlled Room Temperature].

Knoll Pharmaceutical Company
Mount Olive, NJ 07828 USA

7890-03

5. Order: Butorphanol 0.75 mg (round to the nearest hundredth)

Answer: Give the patient _____ of Butorphanol

BUTORPHANOL
TARTRATE INJECTION, USP

2 mg/mL

SINGLE DOSE VIAL
FOR IM OR IV USE
Rx ONLY   **C**ᴵⱽ

1 mL vial

NDC 55390-184-01
USUAL DOSAGE: See package insert.

Store at room temperature, 15° to 30°C (59° to 86°F).

Manufactured for:
Bedford Laboratories™
Bedford, OH 44146

BTP-VB03

6. Order: 4 mg of Inaspine (round to the nearest tenth)

   Answer: Give the patient _____ of Inaspine

   NDC 11098-010-01
   ## INAPSINE®
   (DROPERIDOL)
   INJECTION
   1 mL ampoule
   ## 2.5 mg/mL
   TAYLOR
   PHARMACEUTICALS
   Decatur, IL 62522

   ADPABL   Rev. 7/98

   LOT

   EXP.

7. Order: 50 mg of Amoxil

   Answer: Give the patient _____ of Amoxil

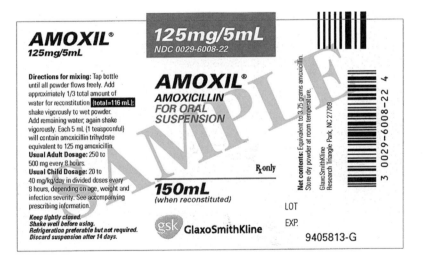

8. Order: 40 mg of Gentamicin

   Answer: Give the patient _____ of Gentamicin

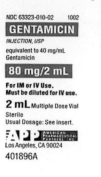

Assignment 31-10: Pediatric Dosage Calculations

1. The 12-year-old patient is to receive 5 mg/kg of Quivadil every eight hours. The patient weighs 132 pounds.

   A. How much of the Quivadil should the patient receive per dose?

       Answer: The patient should receive _____ of the medication per dose

   B. How many total mg should the patient receive of the Quivadil per day? (Show your work.)

       Answer: The patient should receive _____ per day.

2. Referring to the above problem, if the label on the Quivadil bottle reads 250 mg/mL, how many mL should the patient receive per dose?

   Answer: The patient should receive _____ of Quivadil.

3. A two-year-old child has a BSA of 0.5. The adult dose of medication is 25 mg. What dosage should be given to the child? (Round to the nearest whole number.)

   Answer: The child should receive _____ of the medication.

4. A four-year-old child has a BSA of 0.7. The adult dose of medication is 250 mg.

    A. What dosage should be given to the child? (Round your answer to the nearest whole number, but do not round answers until the final step.)

        Answer: The child should receive _____ of the medication

    B. The medication comes available in tablets of 75 mg, 100 mg, 125 mg, and 250 mg. What strength would be the most appropriate strength based on the physician's order?

    C. Why did you select the strength that you did?

    D. Should you check with the physician just to make certain before giving the patient the available dose?

FIELD APPLICATION CHALLENGES

Assignment 31-11

Read the following Field Application Challenges and respond to the questions following each scenario.

1. You just administered an oral medication to a child, and within five minutes the child vomits. Should you re-administer the drug?

2. You are explaining dosage instructions to a 12-year-old patient and her father. You explain that the medication is in capsule form. The father tells you that his daughter (the patient) has a difficult time swallowing any type of pills. What should you do?

JOURNALING EXERCISE

Assignment 31-12

What content within this chapter was most meaningful to you? Why? Reflect on Davene's scenario reminding medical assistants that medication errors can be devastating and once given incorrectly, cannot be undone. What steps would you follow to ensure you are always giving the proper medication to the right patient in the right dose? How will you feel about continuing to learn and attending refresher courses after you have been out of school for a while?

CHAPTER **32**

Administration of Parenteral Medications

VOCABULARY REVIEW

Assignment 32-1: Definitions

Define the following terms.

1. Ampule: _____

2. Aqueous: _____

3. Bolus: _____

4. Cannula: _____

5. Diluent: _____

6. Gauge: _____

7. Occlusion: _____

8. Parenteral: _____

9. Phlebitis: _____

10. Precipitate: _____

11. Taut: _____

12. Vial: _____

_____

Assignment 32-2: Misspelled Words

Underline the correctly spelled term.

1. Aspirate   Asporate   Asipirate
2. Hypudermic   Hyperdermic   Hypodermic
3. Infilration   Infiltrashion   Infiltration
4. Patency   Patoncy   Patiency
5. Thrombisis   Thrombosis   Thormbosis
6. Viscocity   Viscosity   Visocity
7. Wheal   Wheel   Weal
8. Trocarr   Trocar   Trocer

Assignment 32-3: Matching I

Match the term with its definition and place the corresponding letter in the blank.

____ 1. Cartridge unit

____ 2. Cubic centimeter

____ 3. Extravasation

____ 4. Intra-articular

____ 5. Intradermal

____ 6. Intramuscular

____ 7. Luer-Lok

____ 8. Primary drug

____ 9. Secondary drug

____ 10. Subcutaneous

A. The second drug to be drawn up; usually the cloudier medication

B. Within the muscle

C. Threaded end in which the needle can be locked by twisting

D. First drug to be drawn up when combining two drugs into one syringe; often the clearer medication

E. Within a joint

F. Pertaining to under the dermis (or true layer of the skin)

G. Disposable prefilled cartridge of medication that slips into a nondisposable injection device

H. Unit used for the calibration and marking of syringes (no longer used in charting because cc is considered a dangerous abbreviation; mL is used in its place)

I. Medication fluid leaks from the cannula or from the vein into the tissues surrounding the site

J. Pertaining to within the skin

CHAPTER REVIEW

Assignment 32-4: Short Answer

1. List six separate routes used for delivering parenteral medications.

_____

_____

_____

2. List five common parenteral routes by injection and mark those that are routinely performed by the medical assistant with an X.

Performed by Medical Assistant

A. _____   _____

B. _____   _____

C. _____   _____

D. _____   _____

E. _____   _____

(Check your state's Scope of Practice. Many states do not allow medical assistants to perform certain types of administration.)

3. Describe factors that help determine the length of needle, size of the syringe, and the gauge of needle to be used.

A. _____

_____

B. _____

_____

C. _____

_____

4. List several complications that may occur when administering IV therapy.

_____

_____

_____

5. Explain why heparin or insulin injections are not massaged after injection.

_____

_____

6. Based on the latest research, what are the aspiration practices recommended based on the types of medications administered in ambulatory care settings? (*Note: Always check the manufacturer's instructions and with the provider for specifics.*)

• _____

• _____

_____

• _____

7. The purpose of forcing air into the vial is to equalize the pressure within the vial after the medication has been removed.

A. What happens if the proper amount of air is not inserted?

_____

_____

B. What happens when too much air is inserted?

_____

_____

8. What two vaccines should not be given to pregnant patients?

_____

Assignment 32-5: Matching II

Match the type of injection to the description. Answers may be used more than once.

____ 1. Deltoid, ventrogluteal regions, vastus lateralis

____ 2. 10° to 15° angle

____ 3. PPD (tuberculin skin test)

____ 4. 23–25 G

____ 5. Fatty outer portion of the upper arms, the lower abdomen, the middle and lower back, and the thigh region

____ 6. No more than 1 mL per location

____ 7. Needle size 20–23 G, 1–2"

____ 8. 18-20 G for hormones, steroids, penicillin, and certain vitamin preparations

____ 9. 45°; however, a 90°angle may be appropriate for patients with lots of adipose tissue or when using a shorter needle

____ 10. Thicker or oil-based medications; typically a 18-20 G needle

____ 11. 26–27 G

____ 12. Aspirate, except for immunizations

____ 13. ½- to ⅝-inch

____ 14. A longer needle and a steeper angle of 90 degrees

____ 15. ⅜- to ⅝-inch

____ 16. No more than 3 mL

A. Intradermal injection

B. Subcutaneous injection

C. Intramuscular injection

D. Intravenous injection

CERTIFICATION PRACTICE

Assignment 32-6

Choose the best answer and place the corresponding letter in the blank.

____ 1. What type of diluent is typically used to reconstitute powdered medications?

A. Sterile peroxide

B. Sterile alcohol

C. Sterile saline

D. Sterile chloride

____ 2. All of the following are types of medication that are single-dose and available in prefilled cartridges *except:*

    A. Penicillin G benzathine.

    B. Phenergan.

    C. DepoProvera.

    D. Albuterol.

____ 3. At what angle should an intradermal injection be given?

    A. 5-degree

    B. 10- to 15-degree

    C. 45-degree

    D. 90-degree

____ 4. All of the following would be sites for subcutaneous injection *except:*

    A. inner forearm.

    B. upper arm.

    C. lower abdomen.

    D. thigh region.

____ 5. The dorsogluteal site was previously used to administer medications; however, this site is no longer recommended because of the danger of nicking what nerve?

    A. Ulnar

    B. Sciatic

    C. Femoral

    D. Popiliteal

____ 6. All of the following would be common medications given subcutaneously *except:*

    A. MMR.

    B. polio (IPV).

    C. allergy injections.

    D. allergy extracts for testing.

____ 7. Which of the following routes would you use for allergy testing extracts and PPD extract?

    A. Intradermal

    B. Subcutaneous

    C. IM

    D. Z-track

____ 8. Which of the following routes would you use if the medication may cause irritation or discoloration to superficial layers of tissue or to the skin?

    A. Intradermal

    B. Subcutaneous

    C. IM

    D. Z-track

____ 9. Which of the following routes should be used for the MMR vaccine?

    A. Intradermal

    B. Subcutaneous

    C. IM

    D. Z-track

____ 10. Which of the following routes should be used for PPD or tuberculin skin testing?

    A. Intradermal

    B. Subcutaneous

    C. IM

    D. Z-track

SKILLS APPLICATION CHALLENGES
Assignment 32-7: Labeling

1. Label the parts of this syringe.

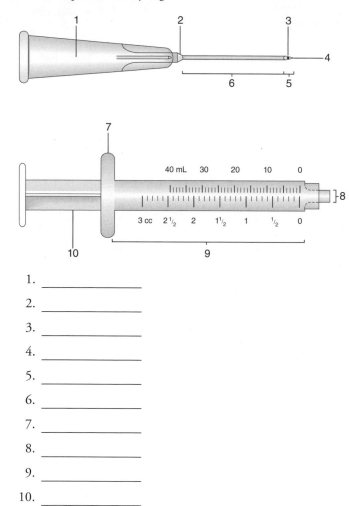

1. _____

2. _____

3. _____

4. _____

5. _____

6. _____

7. _____

8. _____

9. _____

10. _____

2. Label the angles of injections and list the type of injection that matches each angle (i.e., intradermal, subcutaneous, IM) in these pictures.

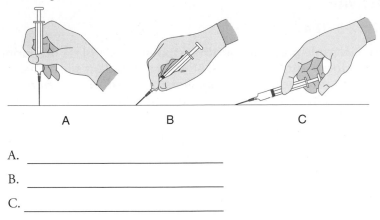

A.   _____

B.   _____

C.   _____

Assignment 32-8: Syringe Review

Illustrate the amount of medication that should be drawn up in each syringe by coloring the amount of medication requested with a colored pencil, marker, or crayon.

A. 2.4 mL

B. 16 U

C. 0.5 mL

D. 3.2 mL

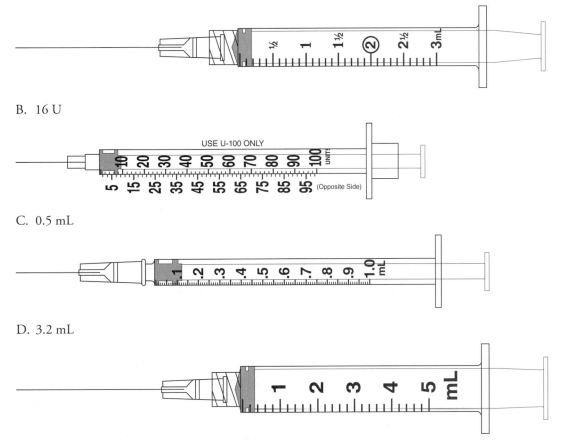

COMPLETING SPECIAL FORMS

Assignment 32-9: Immunization Activity

Work Forms Necessary: FORMS 32-1, 32-2, 32-3, 32-4

Directions: This assignment has two parts. First, role play with another student to simulate preparing a patient to receive an immunization. Second, document the immunization in the patient's progress note and the immunization log. (*Note: You wouldn't ordinarily need to document manufacturer, lot number, and expiration information on both the progress note and log, but for practice purposes, document this information on both forms.*)

A. With one of your fellow students, role play as medical assistant and patient using Work Form 32-1 (a VIS form). The patient's name is Lori Wise. Once you have finished going over the form with the patient, have the patient sign the consent form (Work Form 32-2). Use 07/18/XX as today's date. Sign your name as the witness, followed by SMA. Now, go to the CDC Website (www.cdc.gov) and search for "VIS" and print the most recent version of the influenza (flu) vaccine VIS form. Give this form, along with Work Form 32-2, to your instructor when you turn in this workbook assignment.

B. Using the information below, document that you gave the patient an influenza vaccine on the progress note (Work Form 32-3) and in the vaccination log (Work Form 32-4).

- Today's date: 07/18/XX
- Time: 10:55 a.m.
- Patient's name: Lori Wise
- Amount given: 0.5 mL
- Location: Right deltoid
- Route: IM
- Ordering provider: Dr. Pella
- Manufacturer's name: Glaxo-Smith
- Lot number: 39838
- Expiration date: 02/21/XX
- Medical assistant: Your Name
- Postinjection observation: No reactions
- Vaccination consent form signed and patient signed a consent form

FIELD APPLICATION CHALLENGE

Assignment 32-10

Read the following Field Application Challenge scenario and respond to the questions following.

You work for a busy family practice and are in charge of ordering all of the medications. Unlike most medications, the influenza vaccine has to be ordered early in the year (usually during the months of February and March). If you forget to order the vaccine during those months, when the seasonal flu activity begins (as early as October and continuing to occur as late as May) the office may be unable to obtain the vaccine, leaving patients scrambling to find other places to get their vaccines.

1. Based on this scenario, what can you do to make certain that this same scenario doesn't occur in your office?

_____

_____

_____

2. Flu vaccines are water-soluble and the amount that is given to each patient is 0.5 mL. These vaccines are to be given intramuscularly. What site would be best for adults? What site would be best for children under the age of five?

_____

_____

3. When giving an injection in the deltoid, which arm is the best arm to use and why?

_____

_____

4. Based on the location of the injection, the viscosity of the medication, and the population of patients receiving the vaccine, what gauges and lengths of needles should you have on hand during flu vaccine season?

_____

_____

_____

_____

_____

5. Explain why it is important to ask patients about drug allergies each time they come into your office?

_____

_____

6. What other allergies should you screen patients for before administering an influenza injection? *(Hint: This information can be found in the VIS form obtained in Workbook Assignment 32-8.)*

_____

JOURNALING EXERCISE

Assignment 32-11

What content within this chapter was most meaningful to you? Why? Are you confident that you know, understand, and can follow the seven rights of medication administration? How will you apply the professionalism keys to medication administration and the seven rights? Write a pledge to yourself to always be vigilant when giving medications. Read your pledge often; it will help you to always make the right call.

Work Form 32-1

VACCINE INFORMATION STATEMENT

Influenza (Flu) Vaccine (Inactivated or Recombinant): *What you need to know*

> Many Vaccine Information Statements are available in Spanish and other languages. See www.immunize.org/vis
>
> Hojas de información sobre vacunas están disponibles en español y en muchos otros idiomas. Visite www.immunize.org/vis

1 Why get vaccinated?

Influenza ("flu") is a contagious disease that spreads around the United States every year, usually between October and May.

Flu is caused by influenza viruses, and is spread mainly by coughing, sneezing, and close contact.

Anyone can get flu. Flu strikes suddenly and can last several days. Symptoms vary by age, but can include:
- fever/chills
- sore throat
- muscle aches
- fatigue
- cough
- headache
- runny or stuffy nose

Flu can also lead to pneumonia and blood infections, and cause diarrhea and seizures in children. If you have a medical condition, such as heart or lung disease, flu can make it worse.

Flu is more dangerous for some people. Infants and young children, people 65 years of age and older, pregnant women, and people with certain health conditions or a weakened immune system are at greatest risk.

Each year **thousands of people in the United States die from flu**, and many more are hospitalized.

Flu vaccine can:
- keep you from getting flu,
- make flu less severe if you do get it, and
- keep you from spreading flu to your family and other people.

2 Inactivated and recombinant flu vaccines

A dose of flu vaccine is recommended every flu season. Children 6 months through 8 years of age may need two doses during the same flu season. Everyone else needs only one dose each flu season.

Some inactivated flu vaccines contain a very small amount of a mercury-based preservative called thimerosal. Studies have not shown thimerosal in vaccines to be harmful, but flu vaccines that do not contain thimerosal are available.

There is no live flu virus in flu shots. **They cannot cause the flu.**

There are many flu viruses, and they are always changing. Each year a new flu vaccine is made to protect against three or four viruses that are likely to cause disease in the upcoming flu season. But even when the vaccine doesn't exactly match these viruses, it may still provide some protection.

Flu vaccine cannot prevent:
- flu that is caused by a virus not covered by the vaccine, or
- illnesses that look like flu but are not.

It takes about 2 weeks for protection to develop after vaccination, and protection lasts through the flu season.

3 Some people should not get this vaccine

Tell the person who is giving you the vaccine:
- **If you have any severe, life-threatening allergies.** If you ever had a life-threatening allergic reaction after a dose of flu vaccine, or have a severe allergy to any part of this vaccine, you may be advised not to get vaccinated. Most, but not all, types of flu vaccine contain a small amount of egg protein.

- **If you ever had Guillain-Barré Syndrome (also called GBS).** Some people with a history of GBS should not get this vaccine. This should be discussed with your doctor.

- **If you are not feeling well.** It is usually okay to get flu vaccine when you have a mild illness, but you might be asked to come back when you feel better.

U.S. Department of Health and Human Services Centers for Disease Control and Prevention

Work Form 32-1 (*Cont'd*)

4 | Risks of a vaccine reaction

With any medicine, including vaccines, there is a chance of reactions. These are usually mild and go away on their own, but serious reactions are also possible.

Most people who get a flu shot do not have any problems with it.

Minor problems following a flu shot include:
- soreness, redness, or swelling where the shot was given
- hoarseness
- sore, red or itchy eyes
- cough
- fever
- aches
- headache
- itching
- fatigue

If these problems occur, they usually begin soon after the shot and last 1 or 2 days.

More serious problems following a flu shot can include the following:
- There may be a small increased risk of Guillain-Barré Syndrome (GBS) after inactivated flu vaccine. This risk has been estimated at 1 or 2 additional cases per million people vaccinated. This is much lower than the risk of severe complications from flu, which can be prevented by flu vaccine.
- Young children who get the flu shot along with pneumococcal vaccine (PCV13) and/or DTaP vaccine at the same time might be slightly more likely to have a seizure caused by fever. Ask your doctor for more information. Tell your doctor if a child who is getting flu vaccine has ever had a seizure.

Problems that could happen after any injected vaccine:
- People sometimes faint after a medical procedure, including vaccination. Sitting or lying down for about 15 minutes can help prevent fainting, and injuries caused by a fall. Tell your doctor if you feel dizzy, or have vision changes or ringing in the ears.
- Some people get severe pain in the shoulder and have difficulty moving the arm where a shot was given. This happens very rarely.
- Any medication can cause a severe allergic reaction. Such reactions from a vaccine are very rare, estimated at about 1 in a million doses, and would happen within a few minutes to a few hours after the vaccination.

As with any medicine, there is a very remote chance of a vaccine causing a serious injury or death.

The safety of vaccines is always being monitored. For more information, visit: **www.cdc.gov/vaccinesafety/**

5 | What if there is a serious reaction?

What should I look for?
- Look for anything that concerns you, such as signs of a severe allergic reaction, very high fever, or unusual behavior.

Signs of a severe allergic reaction can include hives, swelling of the face and throat, difficulty breathing, a fast heartbeat, dizziness, and weakness. These would start a few minutes to a few hours after the vaccination.

What should I do?
- If you think it is a severe allergic reaction or other emergency that can't wait, call 9-1-1 and get the person to the nearest hospital. Otherwise, call your doctor.
- Reactions should be reported to the Vaccine Adverse Event Reporting System (VAERS). Your doctor should file this report, or you can do it yourself through the VAERS web site at **www.vaers.hhs.gov**, or by calling **1-800-822-7967**.

VAERS does not give medical advice.

6 | The National Vaccine Injury Compensation Program

The National Vaccine Injury Compensation Program (VICP) is a federal program that was created to compensate people who may have been injured by certain vaccines.

Persons who believe they may have been injured by a vaccine can learn about the program and about filing a claim by calling **1-800-338-2382** or visiting the VICP website at **www.hrsa.gov/vaccinecompensation**. There is a time limit to file a claim for compensation.

7 | How can I learn more?

- Ask your health care provider. He or she can give you the vaccine package insert or suggest other sources of information.
- Call your local or state health department.
- Contact the Centers for Disease Control and Prevention (CDC):
  - Call **1-800-232-4636** (**1-800-CDC-INFO**) or
  - Visit CDC's website at **www.cdc.gov/flu**

Vaccine Information Statement

Inactivated Influenza Vaccine

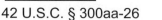
08/07/2015

42 U.S.C. § 300aa-26

Office Use Only

Courtesy of Department of Health and Human Services, Centers for Disease Control and Prevention

Work Form 32-2

DOUGLASVILLE MEDICINE ASSOCIATES
5076 BRAND BLVD
DOUGLASVILLE, NY 01234
(123) 456-7890

IMMUNIZATION CONSENT FORM

I have read the Vaccination Information Statements(s) regarding the following immunizations listed below and am aware of the adverse reactions associated with the vaccine(s). I have had an opportunity to ask questions regarding the possible adverse reactions and benefits of each immunization. I believe that the benefits outweigh the risks and I assume full responsibility for any reactions that may occur.

1. _____   2. _____

3. _____   4. _____

I am requesting that the immunization (s) be given to me or the person listed below for whom I am the legal guardian.

_____   _____
Signature/Legal Guardian   Today's Date

_____   _____
Print Name   Witness

Work Form 32-3

Work Form 32-4

DOUGLASVILLE MEDICINE ASSOCIATES
5076 BRAND BLVD
DOUGLASVILLE, NY 01234
(123) 456-7890

FLU VACCINE LOG								
Today's Date	Patient's Name	Ordering Physician	Amt Given	Manufacturer's Name	Lot Number	Exp. Date	MA	Time
07/18/20XX	Gunter, Thomas	Little	0.5 mL	Glaxo-Smith	39838	02/21/20XX	NS	10:45 am

C H A P T E R **3 3**

Responding to Medical Office Emergencies

VOCABULARY REVIEW

Assignment 33-1: Definitions

Define the following terms.

1. Embolus: _____

2. Diaphoresis: _____

3. Syncope: _____

4. Thrombus: _____

5. Heat stroke: _____

   _____

6. Heat exhaustion: _____

7. Ischemia: _____

Assignment 33-2: Matching

Match the term with its definition and place the corresponding letter in the blank.

____ 1. Abrasions

____ 2. Acute abdomen

____ 3. Anaphylaxis

____ 4. Algorithm

____ 5. Asthma

____ 6. Automated external defibrillator

____ 7. Cardiopulmonary resuscitation

A. Injury in which the brain is jarred

B. Chronic lung disease which causes the bronchial tubes to constrict and block the flow of air to and from the lungs

C. Drugs or electrical shock are used to restore normal contractions to the heart

D. Superficial scrapes that may be very painful

E. Cart that stocks all of the medications and supplies used in an emergency

F. Sudden or abrupt onset of intense abdominal pain

G. Life-threatening condition in which patient's blood sugar is dangerously high

____ 8. Cerebrovascular accident (CVA)   H. A procedure to restore heart and lung function

____ 9. Diabetic ketoacidosis   I. Outlines a detailed sequence of actions to perform in order to accomplish a task

____ 10. Concussion   J. Another term for heart attack

____ 11. Crash cart   K. Another term for stroke or brain attack, referring to a blockage or bleeding within the blood vessels of the brain

____ 12. Defibrillation   L. Severe allergic reaction to an allergen usually in the form of food, medication, a chemical, or an insect sting or bite

____ 13. Diabetic coma   M. A serious complication of diabetes that occurs when the body produces high levels of blood acids called ketones, and develops when the body is unable to produce enough insulin

____ 14. Myocardial infarction   N. Automated unit that defibrillates the heart

____ 15. Frostbite   O. Another term for mini-stroke

____ 16. Hypothermia   P. Process in which patient's symptoms are ranked in terms of importance or priority

____ 17. Transient ischemic attack (TIA)   Q. Sudden attack that result from a malfunction of the brain; the two types are petite mal and grand mal

____ 18. Orthostatic hypotension   R. Life-threatening condition in which the patient's blood sugar drops to a dangerously low level, causing the patient to go into shock

____ 19. Triage   S. A potentially fatal condition that can be brought on by disease, injury, decrease in circulation, and/or fluid loss

____ 20. Ventricular fibrillation   T. Injury to the brain caused by trauma

____ 21. Seizure   U. Cramping that occurs from a combination of factors, including elevated temperature, loss of fluids, and a loss of salt from the body; usually confined to the abdomen and legs

____ 22. Traumatic brain injury   V. Local injury of skin due to freezing or subfreezing conditions

____ 23. Insulin shock   W. Uncontrollable bleeding

____ 24. Shock   X. Blood pressure that drops upon standing

____ 25. Hemorrhaging   Y. Occurs when the ventricles of the heart beats in a disorganized, rapid manner; one of the most common rhythms that occurs in adjust victims of sudden cardia arrest

____ 26. Heat cramp   Z. A condition that occurs when body temperature falls below 95°F (35°C)

CHAPTER REVIEW

Assignment 33-3: Abbreviation Review

Write what each of the following abbreviations stands for.

1. PPE: _____

2. TIA: _____

3. CVA: _____

4. AED: _____

5. CPR: _____

_____ 6. Blood gently oozes

_____ 7. Blood spurts

_____ 8. Is not life-threatening

_____ 9. May cause great blood loss

CERTIFICATION PRACTICE

Assignment 33-7

Choose the best answer and place the corresponding letter in the blank.

____ 1. Which of the following drugs would *not* likely to be found on an emergency cart?

    A. Epinephrine

    B. Imitrex

    C. Lidocaine

    D. Dopamine

____ 2. In order to have the best chance of a full recover, clot-busting drugs such as _____ should be administered within three hours from the onset of stroke symptoms.

    A. aspirin

    B. lovinox

    C. warfarin

    D. tissue plasminogen activator

____ 3. If a victim has a pacemaker, in which of the following locations should the rescuer place AED electrode pads?

    A. No change in placement

    B. 3 inches from the pacemaker

    C. 2 inches from the pacemaker

    D. 1 inch from the pacemaker

____ 4. All of the following symptoms are true for a patient experiencing hypoglycemia (insulin shock) *except:*

    A. skin is red, hot, and dry.

    B. poor coordination.

    C. headache.

    D. confusion and disorientation.

____ 5. Another term for heart attack is:

    A. ischemic attack.

    B. myocardial infarction.

    C. ventricular fibrillation.

    D. angina.

____ 6. Poisons can enter the body through which of the following routes?

    A. Inhalation

    B. Ingestion/Injection

    C. Absorption

    D. All of the above

___ 7. A severe, potentially life-threatening allergic reaction is called _____ shock.

    A. neurogenic

    B. cardiogenic

    C. psychogenic

    D. anaphylactic

___ 8. Which of the following is the first step used to control external bleeding?

    A. Elevation

    B. Pressure points

    C. Direct pressure

    D. Tourniquet

___ 9. Treatment of nosebleed includes all of the following *except:*

    A. tilt head slightly forward.

    B. pinching the nostrils.

    C. cold compress.

    D. having the patient lie down.

___ 10. Which of the following is common for an arterial bleed?

    A. Bright red blood that spurts

    B. Dark red blood that flows steadily

    C. Dark red blood that oozes

    D. Bright red blood that oozes

SKILL APPLICATION CHALLENGE

Assignment 33-8: Case Study

You are working for an urgent care center. Three patients arrive all about the same time. Patient 1 received an eye injury while at work. A tiny piece of wood flew in her eye, and she is unable to keep her eye open. Patient 2 has had severe stomach flu-like symptoms for the past two days and may be dehydrated, and Patient 3 is experiencing chest pain. In what order should these patients be seen? Why? What steps will you take for each patient to get them ready for the provider?

Patient	*Priority (1, 2, 3)*	*Steps Taken to Prepare the Patient for the Provider*
Patient 1	_____	_____
		_____
		_____
		_____
		_____
		_____
		_____
		_____
		_____

Patient 2   _____   _____

_____

_____

_____

_____

_____

_____

Patient 3   _____   _____

_____

_____

_____

_____

_____

_____

_____

_____

Assignment 33-9: Research Activity

Animal bite reporting requirements vary by state and local jurisdiction. Medical assistants should refer to the health department for the state, county, or city they work in to become familiar with reporting requirements. For example, Section 11.03 of the New York City Health Code requires that all animal bites be reported within 24 hours of the event. On their website is a form to be completed and submitted online. Medical assistants should follow state, local, and office policy in regards to reporting animal bites. Go to your local health department website and determine if there is a reporting requirement for animal bites. Then go to the New York City website www.nyc.gov and type "report an animal bite" in the search box. There you will find Form VPHS 55 – EGP which is a form that can be completed online. (*Note:* **Do NOT submit a report**, *just view and/ or print the report for class discussion.*) How do the NYC reporting requirements compare to your local health department?

FIELD APPLICATION CHALLENGES

Assignment 33-10

Read the following Field Application Challenges and respond to the questions following each scenario.

1. You just administered an allergy injection and within a matter of minutes, the patient collapses on the floor.

    A. What could be wrong with the patient?

    _____

    B. What steps should you take in order to assist the patient?

    _____

    _____

    _____

    _____

_____

_____

_____

2. A middle-aged man walks into your office, collapses onto the floor, and begins to shake uncontrollably. Coworkers state that the patient has a history of epilepsy. As you approach him, you see that he is breathing. His eyes are open but he does not respond when you call him by name.

A. What could be wrong with the patient?

_____

B. What measures should you take to help the patient?

_____

_____

_____

_____

_____

_____

3. A father calls in to state that his two-year-old daughter has gotten into the medicine cabinet and has chewed up and swallowed three Xanax tablets.

A. What question should the medical assistant ask the father?

_____

B. If the daughter is unconscious or not breathing, what should be the medical assistant's course of action?

_____

_____

_____

_____

_____

C. If the daughter is both conscious and breathing, what instructions should you give to the father?

_____

_____

_____

JOURNALING EXERCISE

Assignment 33-11

What content within this chapter was most meaningful to you? Why? After reading about the emergency office scenario outlined in Davene's mentor feature, how would you react in an emergency situation and what professionalism keys would you use and why? Apply this to any of the following potential emergency situations: (1) Patient having a cardiac emergency, (2) Patient going into anaphylactic shock, or (3) Patient with a superficial gunshot wound to the shoulder.

2

Competency Checklists

Name _____   Date _____   Score _____

COMPETENCY CHECKLIST

PROCEDURE 1-1   Locate a State's Legal Scope of Practice for Medical Assistants

Task: To locate a state's legal scope of practice for medical assistants

Condition: Using a computer with Internet access, a paper and pen, or a computer with word processing or spreadsheet capabilities, use the following steps and locate a state's legal scope of practice for medical assistants and write a brief summary.

Standards: The student will have 15 minutes to complete the procedure and will need to score an 85% or above to pass the competency. Automatic failure results if any essential steps are omitted or performed incorrectly.

STEPS START TIME: END TIME:	Points Possible	First Attempt	Second Attempt	Third Attempt
1. Using a computer, access the Internet to locate the legal scope of practice for your state, as noted in Step 2.	10			
2. Access the AAMA website (www.aama-ntl.org). Search under "State Scope of Practice Laws." Locate the state where you are located (e.g., Ohio).	10			
3. Using the information obtained in Step 2, click on the Scope of Practice link for your state. Review the information and then access the additional links (if available), for example, Frequently Asked Questions and Laws and Regulations.	10			
4. Using paper and pen (or computer with a word processing program) prepare a written summary of the scope of practice, what you learned from the website and how you would apply it to your medical assisting duties. Cite your sources.	10			
Points Earned / Points Possible:	___ / 40			

Points possible reflect importance of step in meeting the task: Important = (5) Essential = (10). Determine score by dividing points earned by total points possible, and multiplying results by 100.

EVALUATION

Evaluator Signature: _____   Date: _____

Evaluator Comments:

Key Competencies		
ABHES	MA.A.1.4.f(1)	Define scope of practice for the medical assistant within the state that the medical assistant is employed
	MA.A.1.11.b	Demonstrate professional behavior
CAAHEP	X.C.1	Differentiate between scope of practice and standards of care for medical assistants
	X.P.1	Locate a state's legal scope of practice for medical assistants

Name _____ Date _____ Score _____

COMPETENCY CHECKLIST

PROCEDURE 1-2   Apply the Patients' Bill of Rights as it Relates to Choice of Treatment, Consent for Treatment, and Refusal of Treatment

Task: To explain both the practice's expectations for patients as well as what legal and ethical rights the patient can expect, and to apply the Patients' Bill of Rights as it relates to choice of treatment, consent for treatment, and refusal of treatment

Condition: Gather documents (printed policy information, patient education material, etc.), patient's chart (or computer with EHR access), and paper and pen. In a role-play activity, have students pair up. In a quiet room free from distraction, explain the practice expectations for patients and what legal and ethical rights the patient can expect by following the steps listed below.

Standards: The student will have 15 minutes to complete the procedure and will need to score an 85% or above to pass the competency. Automatic failure results if any essential steps are omitted or performed incorrectly.

Sample Procedure Scenario

A new patient to the practice has not been to a primary care doctor in more than five years. She has not taken medication as prescribed. The patient states that she recently went to an orthopedic doctor for carpal tunnel syndrome and needs clearance from her primary care provider (PCP) before surgery.

STEPS START TIME: END TIME:	Points Possible	First Attempt	Second Attempt	Third Attempt
1. Identify the patient.	10			
2. Invite the patient into a room free of distractions and demonstrate sensitivity to patient's privacy by closing the door to maintain and protect the patient's privacy and integrity of the medical record.	10			
3. ***Displaying professionalism through verbal communication***, introduce yourself, identify your role in the practice, and tell the patient what to expect from the conversation, using language the patient can understand and making the patient feel at ease. Display tact, diplomacy, and respect for the patient. Be courteous and treat the patient with dignity.	10			
4. Explain both the practice's expectations for patients as well as what legal and ethical rights the patient can expect.	10			
5. Apply the Patients' Bill of Rights as it relates to choice of treatment, consent for treatment, and refusal of treatment.	10			
6. Provide pre-printed information and policies, preferably in the patient's native language (or with verification through a translator followed by documentation of patient's response to explanations).	10			
7. ***Demonstrating empathy***, provide the patient with an opportunity to ask questions. Individualize the conversation and discussion based on the patient's needs and reason for visit. Analyze communications, providing appropriate responses and feedback.	10			
8. Refer questions to appropriate others for further explanation or clarification.	10			
9. Document time, date, patient response, and any materials provided in the patient record.	10			
Points Earned / Points Possible:	___ / 90			

Points possible reflect importance of step in meeting the task: Important = (5) Essential = (10). Determine score by dividing points earned by total points possible, and multiplying results by 100.

Name _____ Date _____ Score _____

EVALUATION

Evaluator Signature: _____ Date: _____

Evaluator Comments:

Key Competencies		
ABHES	MA.A.1.8.f	Display professionalism through written and verbal communications
	MA.A.1.11.b	Demonstrate professional behavior
CAAHEP	V.C.14	Relate the following behaviors to professional communication: (a) assertive, (b) aggressive, and (c) passive
	V.A.1.a	Demonstrate empathy
	X.C.4	Summarize the Patient Bill of Rights
	X.P.4	Apply the Patient's Bill of Rights as it relates to: (a) choice of treatment, (b) consent for treatment, and (c) refusal of treatment
	X.A.1	Demonstrate sensitivity to patient rights

Name _____ Date _____ Score _____

COMPETENCY CHECKLIST

PROCEDURE 3-1   Create and Organize a Patient's Medical Record

Task: To prepare an accurate and complete patient chart to submit to the provider for final review.

Condition: Using a chart or folder, patient records, privacy forms, and tabs, create an accurate and complete paper patient chart to submit to the provider for final review (if you have access to an EHR, create a patient's medical record).

Standards: The student will have two hours to complete the procedure and will need to score an 85% or above to pass the competency. Automatic failure results if any essential steps are omitted or performed incorrectly.

STEPS START TIME: END TIME:	Points Possible	First Attempt	Second Attempt	Third Attempt
1. Prepare chart or folder for patient (electronic or paper). Verify accurate spelling of name. Include demographics, insurance information, privacy forms, and emergency contact information.	10			
2. Retrieve and compile available reports and information. Verify that all records are for the correct patient before including in the record.	10			
3. Sort and organize records by type: operative notes, progress notes from various providers, laboratory reports, radiology, medication flow sheets, immunization records, and so on.	10			
4. Verify accuracy and completeness and submit to provider for final review.	10			
Points Earned / Points Possible:	___ / 40			

Points possible reflect importance of step in meeting the task: Important = (5) Essential = (10). Determine score by dividing points earned by total points possible, and multiplying results by 100.

EVALUATION

Evaluator Signature: _____ Date: _____

Evaluator Comments:

Key Competencies		
ABHES	MA.A.1.8.a	Gather and process documents
	MA.A.1.8.f	Display professionalism through written and verbal communications
CAAHEP	VI.C.4	Define types of information contained in the patient's medical record
	VI.C.5	Identify methods of organizing the patient's medical record based on: (a) problem-oriented medical record (POMR), and (b) source-oriented medical record (SOMR)
	VI.P.3	Create a patient's medical record
	VI.P.4	Organize a patient's medical record

Name _____ Date _____ Score _____

COMPETENCY CHECKLIST

PROCEDURE 4-1   Documenting the Administration of a Medication

Task: To document the administration of a medication.

Condition: The student will document the information from the sample scenario below in an EHR or on a progress note and medication log supplied by the instructor.

Standards: The student will have five minutes to complete the documentation and will need to score an 85% or above to pass the competency. Automatic failure results if any essential steps are omitted or performed incorrectly.

Sample Procedure Scenario

Use the following information to document the administration of a flu vaccine:

Order: Fluzone (0.5 mL); **Route:** IM; **Location:** R. Deltoid; **VIS:** (03-2018); **Ordering Provider**: Dr. Patel; Patient tolerated well. **Manufacturer:** SANOF PASTEUR; **Lot #**: 569874BD; **Expiration Date:** 04-20XX

STEPS START TIME: END TIME:	Points Possible	First Attempt	Second Attempt	Third Attempt
1. Assemble required information for medication entries such as medication labels and provider orders.	10			
2. Record the date and time of administration.	10			
3. Record the full name of the medication.	10			
4. Record the strength of the medication.	10			
5. Record the route of administration.	10			
6. Record the site of administration.	10			
7. Record the name of physician that ordered the medication.	10			
8. Record any problems during or following administration and actions taken.	10			
9. Record any consent forms signed.	10			
10. Record educational material distributed.	10			
11. Record information in the medication log (if applicable).	10			
12. Record documentation identifier.	10			
13. Document accurately in the patient's chart and make certain there are no spelling errors. Only use standard medical abbreviations that do not appear on the Joint Commission's "Do Not Use List."	10			
Points Earned / Points Possible:	___ / 130			

Points possible reflect importance of step in meeting the task: Important = (5) Essential = (10). Determine score by dividing points earned by total points possible, and multiplying results by 100.

Name _____ Date _____ Score _____

EVALUATION
Evaluator Signature: _____ Date: _____

Evaluator Comments:

DOCUMENTATION
Instructor Note: Retain work products with competency checklist.
Work Products, Procedure 4-1a (Progress Note) and 4-1b (Medication Log). Procedure forms can be downloaded from the student companion website.

Key Competencies		
ABHES	MA.A.1.4.a	Follow documentation guidelines
CAAHEP	I.P.4.f	Verify the rules of medication administration: right documentation
	X.P.3	Document patient care accurately in the medical record

Name _____ Date _____ Score _____

COMPETENCY CHECKLIST

PROCEDURE 4-2   Documenting a Phone Call from a Patient

Task: To document a call from the patient.

Condition: The student will document the call described in the sample scenario below in the patient's chart/EHR, referencing a telephone screening or triage manual provided by the instructor.

Standards: The student will have 10 minutes to complete the documentation and will need to score an 85% or above to pass the competency. Automatic failure results if any essential steps are omitted or performed incorrectly.

STEPS START TIME: END TIME:	Points Possible	First Attempt	Second Attempt	Third Attempt
1. Assemble patient's chart, black pen (if applicable), and telephone screening manual.	10			
2. Document the date and time of the telephone call.	10			
3. Document the general complaint and to whom you are speaking, if not the patient. (Check privacy statement to see if you have permission to discuss patient information with caller.) If not, you will need to speak directly with patient.	10			
4. Open screening manual and document responses to the screening questions listed in the protocol or telephone screening manual.	10			
5. *Incorporate critical thinking skills when performing patient assessment.*	10			
6. Document instructions given to the patient and list where the instructions came from.	10			
7. Document the patient's comprehension of the instructions and the patient's intentions in following the instructions.	10			
8. Record document identifier.	10			
9. Document accurately in the medical record. There should be no spelling errors and you should only use standard medical abbreviations that are not on the Joint Commission's "Do Not Use" List.	10			
Points Earned / Points Possible:	___ / 90			

Points possible reflect importance of step in meeting the task: Important = (5) Essential = (10). Determine score by dividing points earned by total points possible, and multiplying results by 100.

Name _____ Date _____ Score _____

EVALUATION

Evaluator Signature: _____ Date: _____

Evaluator Comments:

DOCUMENTATION

Instructor Note: Retain work products with competency checklist.
Work Product, Procedure 4-2 (Progress Note). Procedure forms can be downloaded from the student companion website.

Key Competencies		
ABHES	MA.A.1.4.a	Follow documentation guidelines
CAAHEP	I.P.3	Perform patient screening using established protocols
	I.A.1	Incorporate critical thinking skills when performing patient assessment
	V.P.6	Demonstrate professional telephone techniques
	X.P.3	Document patient care accurately in the medical record

Name _____ Date _____ Score _____

COMPETENCY CHECKLIST

PROCEDURE 5-1   Conduct a Patient Screening

Task: To accurately complete a patient screening while promoting good therapeutic communications.

Condition: Given a patient chart, history form (or EHR), blank progress note, pen, and a classmate on whom to perform the history, the student will conduct and record a comprehensive patient history while promoting good therapeutic communication.

Standards: The student will have 20 minutes to complete the procedure and will need to score an 85% or above to pass the competency. Automatic failure results if any essential steps are omitted or performed incorrectly.

STEPS START TIME: END TIME:	Points Possible	First Attempt	Second Attempt	Third Attempt
1. Wash hands and prepare the interview area. The interview area should be private, comfortable, and free of distractions.	10			
2. Once the patient has been escorted to the examination room, identify yourself, list your title, and identify the patient using two different identifiers. Ask the patient if she has a certain preference for the way she wants to be addressed throughout the remainder of the interview and future visits.	10			
3. Obtain a height and weight and vital signs on the patient.	10			
4. Update the patient's medication list. Include the name of the medication, the strength, the route if other than oral, and how often the patient takes the medication.	10			
5. Update the patient's allergy history.	10			
6. Obtain the patient's chief complaint and a brief history of the present illness if office protocol.	10			
7. Explain the rationale for gathering the history and inform the patient that everything that is shared during the interview will remain confidential, ***demonstrating empathy***.	10			
8. If the patient completed the form prior to the visit, review all information and check for possible omissions or incomplete responses, ***incorporating critical thinking skills when performing patient assessment***. If the medical assistant is completing the entire form, address all questions on the form, ***demonstrating active listening***.	10			
9. Properly develop all "Yes" responses in the past medical history section. List the exact name of the disease or condition, duration or onset of the disease, treatment, current status, and date of resolve if applicable.	10			
10. Properly expand on all "Yes" responses listed in the family and social history sections.	10			
11. Make certain that all hospitalizations and surgeries are listed on the medical history form.	10			
12. Answer depression screening questions that can be completed by someone other than the provider.	10			
13. Update the patient's preventive care information.	10			
14. Use feedback techniques to obtain patient information including reflection, restatement, and clarification.	10			

Name _____ Date _____ Score _____

15. ***Demonstrate empathy, active listening, and professional nonverbal communication throughout the screening.***	5				
16. Monitor the patient's nonverbal communication throughout the screening.	5				
17. Once the form is completed, summarize the information with the patient.	10				
18. Ask the patient if she would like any additional information added to the history form.	10				
19. Thank the patient for his or her assistance during the interview process.	5				
20. Instruct the patient how to disrobe prior to the exam. Give patient a timeline when the provider will be in and properly exit the room.	10				
21. Report relevant information concisely and accurately to the provider.	10				
22. ***Demonstrate the principles of self-boundaries*** by staying within the boundaries of medical assisting throughout the screening.	10				
Points Earned / Points Possible:	___ / 205				

Points possible reflect importance of step in meeting the task: Important = (5) Essential = (10). Determine score by dividing points earned by total points possible, and multiplying results by 100.

EVALUATION

Evaluator Signature: _____ Date: _____

Evaluator Comments:

DOCUMENTATION

Instructor Note: Retain work products with competency checklist.
Work Products, Procedure 5-1a (Progress Note) and 5-1b (Patient History Form). Procedure forms can be downloaded from the student companion website.

Key Competencies		
ABHES	MA.A.1.4.a	Follow documentation guidelines
	MA.A.1.8.f	Display professionalism through written and verbal communications
	MA.A.1.9.b	Obtain vital signs, obtain patient history, and formulate chief complaint
	MA.A.1.9.c	Assist provider with general/physical examination
	MA.A.1.11.b	Demonstrate professional behavior
CAAHEP	I.P.1	Measure and record: (a) blood pressure, (b) temperature, (c) pulse, (d) respirations, (e) height, (f) weight, and (i) pulse oximetry
	I.P.3	Perform patient screening using established protocols
	I.A.1	Incorporate critical thinking skills when performing patient assessment
	V.C.2	Identify types of nonverbal communication
	V.C.3	Recognize barriers to communication
	V.C.4	Identify techniques for overcoming communication barriers
	V.C.5	Recognize the elements of oral communication using a sender-receiver process
	V.P.1	Use feedback techniques to obtain patient information including: (a) reflection, (b) restatement, and (c) clarification
	V.P.11	Report relevant information concisely and accurately
	V.A.1	Demonstrate (a) empathy, (b) active listening, and (c) nonverbal communication
	V.A.2	Demonstrate the principles of self-boundaries
	V.A.4	Explain to a patient the rationale for performance of a procedure
	X.P.3	Document patient care accurately in the medical record

Name _____ Date _____ Score _____

COMPETENCY CHECKLIST

PROCEDURE 6-1   Effectively Communicate with Patients from Different Cultures

Task: To effectively communicate with patients from different cultures.

Condition: Given a patient's chart/EHR, pen, necessary brochures, any supplies or equipment necessary for the screening, a classmate to play the part of the culturally diverse patient, and another classmate to play the role of the interpreter, the student will interview the patient, following the steps listed below.

Standards: The student will have 15 minutes to complete the procedure and will need to score an 85% or above to pass the competency. Automatic failure results if any essential steps are omitted or performed incorrectly.

STEPS START TIME: END TIME:	Points Possible	First Attempt	Second Attempt	Third Attempt
1. Prepare interview area. The interview area should be private, comfortable, and free of distractions. The furniture should be set up to accommodate the patient and anyone who may be with the patient, including an interpreter. The medical assistant's chair should be set up at least 4 to 6 feet (although up to 12 feet is acceptable in certain settings) directly across from the patient and interpreter if present.	10			
2. Identify yourself, list your title, and identify the patient. If you are uncertain how to properly pronounce the patient's name, ask the patient for the proper pronunciation. Write the phonetic spelling somewhere in the chart.	10			
3. If you are not the same gender as the patient, ask the patient if she would prefer to have a medical assistant of the same gender, ***demonstrating respect for individual diversity***.	10			
4. Ask the patient to introduce any family members who are present.	5			
5. Ask the patient a little bit about her family or career.	10			
6. If the patient has limited English proficiency and a professional interpreter is not present, give the patient written materials that explain the patient's right to a professional interpreter in his or her native language.	10			
7. If the patient states that a family member will be performing the interpreting, explain to the family member the importance of accurate interpreting. If an interpreter is required, contact the agency (or qualified interpreter). Wait until the interpreter is available before proceeding with questioning.	10			
8. Ask the patient to explain the goals for today's visit.	10			
9. Speak clearly and avoid using any slang or medical jargon. Talk directly to the patient even if an interpreter is present. Avoid using many gestures as some common gestures may be considered offensive in some cultures.	10			
10. Have the patient repeat back any instructions to ensure that the patient understands the information.	10			
11. Direct and demonstrate which clothes need to be removed and explain why. Provide the patient with items such as gowns, sheets, or drapes to help ensure modesty.	10			
12. Thank the patient and family members for their cooperation and let them know that the provider will be in shortly.	5			
13. Document the visit and record and explain any paperwork that was given to the patient, as well as if an interpreter was present.	10			
Points Earned / Points Possible:	__ / 120			

Points possible reflect importance of step in meeting the task: Important = (5) Essential = (10). Determine score by dividing points earned by total points possible, and multiplying results by 100.

Name _____ Date _____ Score _____

EVALUATION

Evaluator Signature: _____ Date: _____

Evaluator Comments:

DOCUMENTATION

Instructor Note: Retain work products with competency checklist.

Work Product, Procedure 6-1 (Progress Note). Procedure forms can be downloaded from the student companion website.

Key Competencies		
ABHES	MA.A.1.5.e	Analyze the effect of hereditary, cultural, and environmental influences on behavior
	MA.A.1.8.f	Display professionalism through written and verbal communications
CAAHEP	V.C.3	Recognize barriers to communication
	V.C.4	Identify techniques for overcoming communication barriers
	V.P.5	Coach patients appropriately considering: (a) cultural diversity, and (c) communication barriers
	V.A.3	Demonstrate respect for individual diversity including: (a) gender, (b) race, (c) religion, (d) age, (e) economic status, and (f) appearance
	X.A.1	Demonstrate sensitivity to patient rights

Name _____ Date _____ Score _____

COMPETENCY CHECKLIST

PROCEDURE 6-2   Effectively Communicate with Sight Impaired or Visually Impaired Patients

Task: To assist a patient that is visually impaired by using effective communication techniques.

Condition: Gather the patient's chart/EHR, supplies, and equipment necessary for the screening. Have a classmate play the part of a blind patient. The student will simulate assisting a blind patient during an office visit, by acting as a sighted guide.

Standards: The student will have 20 minutes to complete the procedure and will need to score an 85% or above to pass the competency. Automatic failure results if any essential steps are omitted or performed incorrectly.

STEPS START TIME: END TIME:	Points Possible	First Attempt	Second Attempt	Third Attempt
1. Prepare the patient's room by clearing anything that could cause the patient to trip or fall. Also prepare the walkway from the reception room to the examination room to make certain that it is free of any obstacles.	10			
2. When you go into the reception room, gently call out the patient's name and tell her that you are ready to assist her back to the room. ***Demonstrating the principles of self-boundaries***, do not shake the patient's hand unless the patient extends her hand first.	5			
3. Identify yourself and state your title.	10			
4. If the patient has a guide dog, do not touch or talk to the guide dog while the harness is on. Have the patient and the dog follow you back to the room.	10			
5. If the patient does not have a guide dog, ask the patient if she would like to have sighted guide assistance.	10			
6. If the patient wants sighted guide assistance, ask the patient which side she prefers to be assisted on.	10			
7. Position yourself on the side that the patient indicates and allow the patient to grasp your arm, usually just above the elbow.	10			
8. Walk with your arm down to the side about a half step in front of the patient toward the inside of the patient.	10			
9. Warn the patient about the surroundings and any obstacles, such as a doorway, an elevator, or a staircase.	10			
10. Approach seating in a forward motion. Describe the type of seating that the patient will be placed in, such as a low sofa, upright chair, or an armchair.	10			
11. Walk the patient to the front of the chair, allowing her knees to just gently touch the front of the cushion or seat.	10			
12. Place the patient's hand on the arm of the chair and allow the patient to finish seating herself.	10			
13. Interview the patient in the way that you would any other patient.	5			
14. Lay out all gowns and drapes beside the patient. Let her know their exact location before leaving. Ask the patient if she needs any assistance getting dressed.	10			
15. When performing procedures, alert the patient to every step before you perform it, ***showing awareness of the patient's concerns related to the procedure being performed.***	10			
16. Notify the patient that you are leaving and tell the patient that the provider will knock before entering.	10			
Points Earned / Points Possible:	___ / 150			

Points possible reflect importance of step in meeting the task: Important = (5) Essential = (10). Determine score by dividing points earned by total points possible, and multiplying results by 100.

Name _____ Date _____ Score _____

EVALUATION

Evaluator Signature: _____ Date: _____

Evaluator Comments:

Key Competencies		
ABHES	MA.A.1.5.e	Analyze the effect of hereditary, cultural, and environmental influences on behavior
	MA.A.1.8.f	Display professionalism through written and verbal communications
CAAHEP	I.A.2	Incorporate critical thinking skills when performing patient care
	I.A.3	Show awareness of a patient's concerns related to the procedure being performed
	V.C.3	Recognize barriers to communication
	V.C.4	Identify techniques for overcoming communication barriers
	V.P.5.c	Coach patients appropriately considering communication barriers
	V.A.2	Demonstrate the principles of self-boundaries
	V.A.3	Demonstrate respect for individual diversity including: (a) gender, (b) race, (c) religion, (d) age, (e) economic status, and (f) appearance
	X.A.1	Demonstrate sensitivity to patient rights

Name _____ Date _____ Score _____

COMPETENCY CHECKLIST

PROCEDURE 6-3   Effectively Communicate with Hearing Impaired or Deaf Patients When an Interpreter is Present

Task: To effectively communicate with a deaf patient when an interpreter is present.

Condition: Given a patient's chart/EHR, pen, equipment and supplies necessary for the screening, a classmate to play the part of a deaf patient, and a classmate to play the role of the interpreter, the student will effectively communicate with a deaf patient with the aid of an interpreter, following the steps listed below.

Standards: The student will have 20 minutes to complete the procedure and will need to score an 85% or above to pass the competency. Automatic failure results if any essential steps are omitted or performed incorrectly.

STEPS START TIME: END TIME:	Points Possible	First Attempt	Second Attempt	Third Attempt
1. Set the chairs up in a triangular pattern. The patient's chair should be centered and directly across from both the medical assistant and interpreter.	10			
2. Ask the interpreter to introduce herself.	10			
3. Look directly at the patient during the communication encounter, not at the interpreter. Keep in mind, however, that the patient will be focusing on the interpreter.	10			
4. Talk at a normal rate of speed.	10			
5. Ask the patient to repeat back any instructions.	10			
6. Give the patient written instructions to take home.	5			
7. Thank both the patient and interpreter for their participation. If the patient indicates that she really liked this interpreter, make a note of it in the patient's chart.	5			
8. Document the encounter and state that the interpreter was present.	10			
Points Earned / Points Possible:	___ / 70			

Points possible reflect importance of step in meeting the task: Important = (5) Essential = (10). Determine score by dividing points earned by total points possible, and multiplying results by 100.

Name _____ Date _____ Score _____

EVALUATION

Evaluator Signature: _____ Date: _____

Evaluator Comments:

DOCUMENTATION

Instructor Note: Retain work products with competency checklist.
Work Product, Procedure 6-3 (Progress Note). Procedure forms can be downloaded from the student companion website.

Key Competencies		
ABHES	MA.A.1.5.e	Analyze the effect of hereditary, cultural, and environmental influences on behavior
	MA.A.1.8.f	Display professionalism through written and verbal communications
CAAHEP	I.A.2	Incorporate critical thinking skills when performing patient care
	V.C.3	Recognize barriers to communication
	V.C.4	Identify techniques for overcoming communication barriers
	V.P.5.c	Coach patients appropriately considering communication barriers
	V.A.3	Demonstrate respect for individual diversity including: (a) gender, (b) race, (c) religion, (d) age, (e) economic status, and (f) appearance
	X.A.1	Demonstrate sensitivity to patient rights

Name _____ Date _____ Score _____

COMPETENCY CHECKLIST

PROCEDURE 6-4   Effectively Communicate with a Hearing Impaired or Deaf Patient Who Speech Reads

Task: To effectively communicate with a hearing impaired or deaf patient who speech reads.

Condition: Given a patient chart/EHR, pen, any supplies or equipment needed for the screening, and a classmate to play the part of the hearing impaired patient, the student will provide effective communication for a hearing impaired patient who can read lips by following the steps listed below.

Standards: The student will have 20 minutes to complete the procedure and will need to score an 85% or above to pass the competency. Automatic failure results if any essential steps are omitted or performed incorrectly.

STEPS START TIME: END TIME:	Points Possible	First Attempt	Second Attempt	Third Attempt
1. Prepare the interview area. Choose a quiet room that is well lit and glare free. Lighting should point toward your face.	10			
2. Position yourself directly across from the patient at the same level as the patient.	10			
3. Speak at a normal rate of speed. Do not turn your head away when speaking to the patient.	5			
4. Use gestures, hand cues, and written materials to assist in the communication process.	5			
5. When the patient doesn't understand a statement that you have made, try rephrasing it instead of repeating it.	10			
6. Have the patient communicate back to you any instructions that you have given. This may be through gestures, speaking, or writing.	10			
Points Earned / Points Possible:	___ / 50			

Points possible reflect importance of step in meeting the task: Important = (5) Essential = (10). Determine score by dividing points earned by total points possible, and multiplying results by 100.

Name _____ Date _____ Score _____

EVALUATION
Evaluator Signature: _____ Date: _____

Evaluator Comments:

Key Competencies		
ABHES	MA.A.1.4.f	Comply with federal, state, and local health laws and regulations as they relate to healthcare settings
CAAHEP	I.A.2	Incorporate critical thinking skills when performing patient care
	V.C.3	Recognize barriers to communication
	V.C.4	Identify techniques for overcoming communication barriers
	V.A.3	Demonstrate respect for individual diversity including: (a) gender, (b) race, (c) religion, (d) age, (e) economic status, and (f) appearance
	X.A.1	Demonstrate sensitivity to patient rights

Name _____ Date _____ Score _____

COMPETENCY CHECKLIST

PROCEDURE 7-1   Coach Patients Regarding Office Policies, Health Maintenance, Disease Management, and Disease Prevention

Task: To provide a successful health coaching session regarding office policies by collecting the appropriate learning materials and obtaining the names and numbers of resources that can assist with compliance.

Condition: Given a patient's chart/EHR, health topic to research prior to the session, equipment and supplies as listed in the procedure, and a classmate to play the part of the patient, the student will provide a health coaching session following the steps listed below.

Standards: The student will have 20 minutes to complete the procedure and will need to score an 85% or above to pass the competency. Automatic failure results if any essential steps are omitted or performed incorrectly.

Sample Procedure Scenario

Office Policies: Provide a coaching session for a new patient to the practice. Review information about the financial policy of the practice (copay due at time of visit, any amounts due after insurance has paid, the policy for charging patients for missed or late canceled appointments, and so on); privacy practices (review the notice of privacy practices (NPP) and gather signatures as required) and confidential communication preferences (CCP); review the means of communications (give patient information regarding the practice website and patient portal); and coach regarding expectations and compliance (keeping scheduled appointments, taking medications as prescribed, communicating health concerns openly with provider and staff, and so on).

Health maintenance and disease prevention: Coach on topic of weight management.

Managing current disease: Coach on diabetes management.

STEPS START TIME: END TIME:	Points Possible	First Attempt	Second Attempt	Third Attempt
1. Read and clarify the order from the provider.	10			
2. Collect the learning tools necessary for the session.	10			
3. Collect phone numbers or email addresses of community resources, if applicable.	10			
4. Review the information and ask the provider questions if unclear about certain aspects of the material.	10			
5. Set up the room so that everyone in the session has a seat and can see each other. Make certain that the room is free from distractions and has plenty of electrical outlets for necessary equipment.	10			
6. Identify the patient using two identifiers. Identify any family members or friends who have accompanied the patient.	10			
7. Identify yourself and state your title.	10			
8. List the purpose of the session.	10			

Name _____ Date _____ Score _____

9. Find out the patient's preferred learning style and set goals to determine what the patient and family members want to accomplish from the session.
 	
If educating patients on office policies:
  a. Go over policies regarding missed appointments, copays, and the privacy policy.
  b. Have patient sign privacy statement and establish who can have access to their information.
  c. Go over the patient bill of rights and the patient's responsibilities as a patient.
  d. Instruct patient how to use the patient portal and set up the patient's account if time permits.
 	
If educating the patient on health maintenance and disease prevention:
  a. Review patient's status on preventive testing and immunizations.
  b. Work on a plan for catching the patient up on these items.
  c. Discuss other health care goals with patient including BMI and nutrition goals.
  d. Provide patient with a copy of the goals.
 	
If educating the patient on managing current disease:
  a. Go over educational materials detailing the disease.
  b. Train the patient how to use any monitoring devices and how to properly administer his medications.
	10			

10. Present the information in a clear manner, checking with the patient and family members along the way to make certain that they have a clear understanding of what is being presented.	10			
11. Summarize the information at the end of the session.	10			
12. Have the patient repeat the information. If a demonstration was incorporated into the session, have the patient demonstrate the procedure back to you.	10			
13. Praise the patient for acknowledgment of the material.	10			
14. If applicable, give the patient learning pamphlets, information sheets, prescriptions, and supplies, and provide a list of resources that can assist the patient with any special needs.	5			
15. Give the patient your card or a piece of paper with your name and office phone number. Encourage the patient to call you with any questions.	10			
16. Dismiss the patient and document the session.	10			
Points Earned / Points Possible:	___ / 155			

Points possible reflect importance of step in meeting the task: Important = (5) Essential = (10). Determine score by dividing points earned by total points possible, and multiplying results by 100.

Name _____ Date _____ Score _____

EVALUATION

Evaluator Signature: _____ Date: _____

Evaluator Comments:

DOCUMENTATION

Instructor Note: Retain work products with competency checklist.

Work Product, Procedure 7-1 (Progress Note). Procedure forms can be downloaded from the student companion website.

Key Competencies		
ABHES	MA.A.1.4.a	Follow documentation guidelines
	MA.A.1.5.c	Intervene on behalf of the patient regarding issues/concerns that may arise, i.e., insurance policy information, medical bills, physician/provider orders, etc.
	MA.A.1.9.i	Identify community resources and Complementary and Alternative Medicine practices (CAM)
	MA.A.1.11.b	Demonstrate professional behavior
CAAHEP	V.P.4	Coach patients regarding: (a) office policies, (b) health maintenance, (c) disease prevention, and (d) treatment plan
	V.P.5	Coach patients appropriately considering: (a) cultural diversity, (b) developmental life stage, and (c) communication barriers
	V.P.10	Facilitate referrals to community resources in the role of a patient navigator
	V.P.11	Report relevant information concisely and accurately
	V.A.2	Demonstrate the principles of self-boundaries
	V.A.3	Demonstrate respect for individual diversity including: (a) gender, (b) race, (c) religion, (d) age, (e) economic status, and (f) appearance
	V.A.4	Explain to a patient the rationale for performance of a procedure
	X.P.3	Document patient care accurately in the medical record

Name _____ Date _____ Score _____

COMPETENCY CHECKLIST

PROCEDURE 7-2   Develop a Current List of Community Resources Related to Patients' Health Care Needs

Task: Use research tools and techniques to create a list of community resources related to patients' health care needs.

Condition: Given a topic to research and equipment and supplies as listed in the procedure, develop a current list of community resources related to patients' health care needs following the steps listed below.

Standards: The student will have 30 minutes to complete the procedure and will need to score an 85% or above to pass the competency. Automatic failure results if any essential steps are omitted or performed incorrectly.

Sample Procedure Scenario

A patient is being seen who requires various senior services (for example, housing, transportation, activities, and Alzheimer's support group). Develop a current list of community resources related to the patient's health care needs.

STEPS START TIME: END TIME:	Points Possible	First Attempt	Second Attempt	Third Attempt
1. Assemble required items (telephone, telephone directory, hospital directory, pen, paper, and computer with Internet access).	10			
2. Using the telephone directory and Internet, research the community resources available in your area, create a list of available health care resources, and identify the services provided by each.	10			
3. Verify the information with a follow-up telephone call to the community resource for most current information to be documented.	10			
4. Create a list in a spreadsheet format (using Microsoft Excel or Word, for instance). In the spreadsheet, identify the communication resource(s), services provided, and contact information.	10			
5. Print the resource document.	10			
Points Earned / Points Possible:	___ / 50			

Points possible reflect importance of step in meeting the task: Important = (5) Essential = (10). Determine score by dividing points earned by total points possible, and multiplying results by 100.

Name _____ Date _____ Score _____

EVALUATION
Evaluator Signature: _____ Date: _____

Evaluator Comments:

DOCUMENTATION
Instructor Note: Retain work products with competency checklist.
Work Product, Procedure 7-2 (List of community resources created by student)

Key Competencies		
ABHES	MA.A.1.5.b(3)	List organizations/support groups that can assist patients and family members of patients experiencing terminal illness
	MA.A.1.9.i	Identify community resources and Complementary and Alternative Medicine practices (CAM)
CAAHEP	V.P.9	Develop a current list of community resources related to patients' healthcare needs

Name _____ Date _____ Score _____

COMPETENCY CHECKLIST

PROCEDURE 7-3   Facilitate Referrals to Community Resources in the Role of a Patient Navigator

Task: Use research tools and techniques to facilitate referrals to community resources as a patient navigator.

Condition: Given a patient, patient's chart/EHR, physician/provider order, equipment and supplies as listed in the procedure, and a classmate to play the part of the patient, the student will facilitate referrals to community resources in the role of a patient navigator.

Standards: The student will have 20 minutes to complete the procedure and will need to score an 85% or above to pass the competency. Automatic failure results if any essential steps are omitted or performed incorrectly.

Sample Procedure Scenario

A patient is being seen who requires various senior services (for example, housing, transportation, activities, and Alzheimer's support group). Facilitate referrals to community resources in the role of a patient navigator.

STEPS START TIME: END TIME:	Points Possible	First Attempt	Second Attempt	Third Attempt
1. Assemble required items (telephone, telephone directory, pen, paper, computer with Internet access, patient's chart, or computer with EHR program).	10			
2. Using the telephone book, Internet, and current list of community resources created in Procedure 7-2, facilitate referral in the role of a patient navigator (coaching the patient during the referral process). ***Demonstrate respect for individual diversity***.	10			
3. Verify the information with the patient while in the exam room (or on the telephone). Then place a follow-up telephone call to the patient (or caller) following HIPAA guidelines within 48 hours, ***demonstrating empathy and active listening skills***.	10			
4. Print the referral information and document in the patient's chart.	10			
5. Give the patient your card or a piece of paper with your name and office phone number. Encourage the patient to call you with any questions.	10			
6. Dismiss the patient and document the session.	10			
Points Earned / Points Possible:	___ / 60			

Points possible reflect importance of step in meeting the task: Important = (5) Essential = (10). Determine score by dividing points earned by total points possible, and multiplying results by 100.

Name _____ Date _____ Score _____

EVALUATION

Evaluator Signature: _____ Date: _____

Evaluator Comments:

DOCUMENTATION

Instructor Note: Retain work products with competency checklist.
Work Product, Procedure 7-3 (Progress Note). Procedure forms can be downloaded from the student companion website.

Key Competencies		
ABHES	MA.A.1.4.a	Follow documentation guidelines
	MA.A.1.5.c	Intervene on behalf of the patient regarding issues/concerns that may arise, i.e., insurance policy information, medical bills, physician/provider orders, etc.
	MA.A.1.9.i	Identify community resources and Complementary and Alternative Medicine practices (CAM)
CAAHEP	V.P.10	Facilitate referrals to community resources in the role of a patient navigator
	V.P.11	Report relevant information concisely and accurately
	V.A.1	Demonstrate: (a) empathy, and (b) active listening
	V.A.2	Demonstrate the principles of self-boundaries
	V.A.3	Demonstrate respect for individual diversity including: (a) gender, (b) race, (c) religion, (d) age, (e) economic status, and (f) appearance
	V.A.4	Explain to a patient the rationale for performance of a procedure
	X.P.3	Document patient care accurately in the medical record

Name _____ Date _____ Score _____

COMPETENCY CHECKLIST

PROCEDURE 8-1   Perform Medically Aseptic Handwashing

Task: To perform medically aseptic handwashing.

Condition: Given the equipment and supplies as listed in the procedure, the student will perform the task, adhering to the standards listed below.

Standards: The student will have five minutes to complete the procedure and will need to score an 85% or above to pass the competency. Automatic failure results if any essential steps are omitted or performed incorrectly.

STEPS START TIME: END TIME:	Points Possible	First Attempt	Second Attempt	Third Attempt
1. Remove all jewelry on hands and wrists.	5			
2. Stand at the sink, but do not touch the sink with hands or clothing.	10			
3. Turn on the faucet, and adjust the water temperature.	10			
4. Wet the hands, wrists, and forearms and apply soap; using a circular motion and friction, scrub the backs and palms of hands, wrists, and forearms, interlace fingers and thumbs and rub back and forth to clean surfaces in-between; keep the hands pointing down during the entire washing process.	10			
5. Clean the nails and cuticles with a cuticle stick or soft brush.	10			
6. Rinse the hands and wrists well with the hands pointed downward and not touching the sink.	10			
7. Repeat if this is the first handwashing of the day or when the hands are contaminated with blood or OPIM. ***Recognize the implications for failure to comply with CDC regulations in the health care setting***.	10			
8. Blot the hands, wrists, and forearms dry with a paper towel, and discard the towel. Turn the faucet off with a clean paper towel.	10			
9. Apply lotion.	5			
Points Earned / Points Possible:	___ / 80			

Points possible reflect importance of step in meeting the task: Important = (5) Essential = (10). Determine score by dividing points earned by total points possible, and multiplying results by 100.

Name _____ Date _____ Score _____

EVALUATION

Evaluator Signature: _____ Date: _____

Evaluator Comments:

Key Competencies		
ABHES	MA.A.1.9.a	Practice standard precautions and perform disinfection/sterilization techniques
CAAHEP	III.P.3	Perform handwashing
	III.A.1	Recognize the implications for failure to comply with Center for Disease Control (CDC) regulations in healthcare settings

Name _____ Date _____ Score _____

COMPETENCY CHECKLIST

PROCEDURE 8-2   Perform an Alcohol-Based Hand Rub

Task: To clean hands by using an alcohol-based hand rub.

Condition: Given the equipment and supplies as listed in the procedure, the student will perform the task, adhering to the steps below.

Standards: The student will have three minutes to complete the procedure and will need to score an 85% or above to pass the competency. Automatic failure results if any essential steps are omitted or performed incorrectly.

STEPS START TIME: END TIME:	Points Possible	First Attempt	Second Attempt	Third Attempt
1. Inspect the hands for any visible soil or contamination. If present, the hands must be washed first.	10			
2. Remove all jewelry on hands and wrists.	5			
3. Apply the recommended amount of alcohol-based hand sanitizer.	10			
4. Smooth the hand rub over all surfaces of the hand.	10			
5. Rub the hands together (approximately 15 to 30 seconds) until dry.	10			
Points Earned / Points Possible:	___ / 45			

Points possible reflect importance of step in meeting the task: Important = (5) Essential = (10). Determine score by dividing points earned by total points possible, and multiplying results by 100.

Name _____ Date _____ Score _____

EVALUATION
Evaluator Signature: _____ Date: _____

Evaluator Comment:

Key Competencies		
ABHES	MA.A.1.9.a	Practice standard precautions and perform disinfection/sterilization techniques
CAAHEP	III.P.3	Perform handwashing

Name _____ Date _____ Score _____

COMPETENCY CHECKLIST

PROCEDURE 8-3   Remove Contaminated Gloves

Task: To properly remove contaminated gloves without contaminating hands or other areas.

Condition: Given the equipment and supplies as listed in the procedure, the student will perform the task, adhering to the standards listed below.

Standards: The student will have five minutes to complete the procedure and will need to score an 85% or above to pass the competency. Automatic failure results if any essential steps are omitted or performed incorrectly.

STEPS START TIME: END TIME:	Points Possible	First Attempt	Second Attempt	Third Attempt
1. With the hands pointed downward and away from the body, grab the palm of the right glove with the left hand.	10			
2. Turn the right glove inside out, drop it into the left gloved hand, and crumple it into a ball in the left hand.	10			
3. Form a fist with the left hand, containing the right glove, invert the fist, and insert two fingers of the ungloved hand between the wrist and under the cuff of the back of the contaminated left glove.	10			
4. Turn the left glove inside out over the fist containing the crumpled other glove.	10			
5. Dispose of the contaminated gloves by dropping them into a biohazard waste container (preferably controlled with a step-on lid opening pedal). ***Recognize the implications for failure to comply with CDC regulations in health care settings.***	10			
6. Wash hands.	5			
Points Earned / Points Possible:	___ / 55			

Points possible reflect importance of step in meeting the task: Important = (5) Essential = (10). Determine score by dividing points earned by total points possible, and multiplying results by 100.

Name _____ Date _____ Score _____

EVALUATION

Evaluator Signature: _____ Date: _____

Evaluator Comments:

Key Competencies		
ABHES	MA.A.1.9.a	Practice standard precautions and perform disinfection/sterilization techniques
	MA.A.1.10.c	Dispose of biohazardous materials
CAAHEP	III.P.10.b	Demonstrate proper disposal of biohazardous materials: regulated wastes
	III.A.1	Recognize the implications for failure to comply with Center for Disease Control (CDC) regulations in healthcare settings

Name _____   Date _____   Score _____

COMPETENCY CHECKLIST

PROCEDURE 8-4   Select, Apply, Remove, and Dispose of Appropriate PPE Following Universal or Standard Precautions

Task: To select the appropriate PPE and dispose of contaminated items based on individual procedure or infectious event.

Condition: Given the equipment and supplies as listed in the procedure, the student will demonstrate the proper steps for applying, removing, and disposing of appropriate PPE, adhering to the steps listed below.

Standards: The student will have 15 minutes to complete the procedure and will need to score an 85% or above to pass the competency. Automatic failure results if any essential steps are omitted or performed incorrectly.

STEPS START TIME: END TIME:	Points Possible	First Attempt	Second Attempt	Third Attempt
1. If a procedure is ordered, review the provider's orders and the organization's protocol for applying PPE and procedures for the proper disposal of infectious wastes. If involved in an infectious event, follow protocol for handling such events.	10			
2. Pull the appropriate PPE, cleaning supplies, or spill kit based on the procedure or infectious event.	10			
3. Remove jewelry, lab coat, or any other items that may become contaminated if exposed to bodily fluids.	10			
4. Wash hands, apply gown, and tie securely.	10			
5. Apply shoe and hair covers, if applicable.	10			
6. Apply mask, if applicable.	10			
7. Apply safety glasses, if applicable.	10			
8. Apply gloves and pull over the cuff of gown to ensure that no skin is exposed.	10			
9. Enter exposure area, perform procedure, or clean up infectious wastes following the organization's protocol.	10			
10. Dispose of wastes into the proper receptacles and transport contaminated instruments and equipment to proper area for cleaning, disinfection, or sterilization.	10			
11. Remove contaminated gloves and place in biohazard bag.	10			
12. Remove goggles or face shield and place in biohazard container, if contaminated. (If these items cannot be removed without contaminating hands, apply gloves before removal.)	10			
13. Remove gown or apron/coverall. Untie the ties and peel the gown away from your neck and shoulder, then turn gown inside out, and roll into a ball. If disposable, place in the biohazard container. If cloth, put in a proper laundry receptacle.	10			
14. Remove shoe and/or hair covers and dispose of in proper trash receptacle.	10			
15. Remove mask and place in proper trash receptacle.	10			
16. Wash hands and put away cleaning supplies.	10			
Points Earned / Points Possible:	__ / 160			

Points possible reflect importance of step in meeting the task: Important = (5) Essential = (10). Determine score by dividing points earned by total points possible, and multiplying results by 100.

Name _____ Date _____ Score _____

EVALUATION

Evaluator Signature: _____ Date: _____

Evaluator Comments:

Key Competencies		
ABHES	MA.A.1.9.a	Practice standard precautions and perform disinfection/sterilization techniques
	MA.A.1.9.c	Dispose of biohazardous materials
CAAHEP	III.P.2	Select appropriate barrier/personal protective equipment (PPE)
	III.P.10.b	Demonstrate proper disposal of biohazardous material: regulated wastes

Name _____   Date _____   Score _____

COMPETENCY CHECKLIST
PROCEDURE 9-1   Sanitization and Lubrication of Instruments

Task: To sanitize and lubricate instruments.

Condition: Given the equipment and supplies as listed in the procedure, the student will demonstrate the procedure for sanitizing and lubricating instruments, adhering to the steps listed below.

Standards: The student will have 10 minutes to complete the procedure and will need to score an 85% or above to pass the competency. Automatic failure results if any essential steps are omitted or performed incorrectly.

STEPS START TIME: END TIME:	Points Possible	First Attempt	Second Attempt	Third Attempt
1. Wash your hands and apply utility gloves.	10			
2. Place pre-soaked instruments into basin filled with a solution of warm water and surgical soap.	10			
3. Thoroughly scrub each part of the instruments. Pay close attention to parts of the instruments that contain crevices, teeth, and serrations.	10			
4. Thoroughly rinse each instrument in distilled water or an approved rinsing solution.	10			
5. Place each instrument on a waterproof drape until all instruments have been thoroughly sanitized and rinsed.	10			
6. Dry each instrument with a muslin cloth or comparable material.	10			
7. Inspect each instrument for any defects. Remove any instruments that are damaged.	10			
8. (Optional) Lubricate each instrument, especially on box locks and moving parts.	5			
9. Dry the lubricated instruments according to the instructions found on the lubricant label.	10			
10. Clean the area using an approved disinfectant.	10			
11. Remove utility gloves, hang them upside down (by the finger tips) to dry and wash hands.	5			
Points Earned / Points Possible:	__ / 105			

Points possible reflect importance of step in meeting the task: Important = (5) Essential = (10). Determine score by dividing points earned by total points possible, and multiplying results by 100.

Name _____ Date _____ Score _____

EVALUATION

Evaluator Signature: _____ Date: _____

Evaluator Comments:

Key Competencies		
ABHES	MA.A.1.9.a	Practice standard precautions and perform disinfection/sterilization techniques
CAAHEP	III.P.3	Perform handwashing
	III.P.5	Perform sterilization procedures

Name _____ Date _____ Score _____

COMPETENCY CHECKLIST
PROCEDURE 9-2   Chemical Disinfection of Instruments

Task: To cleanse and disinfect instruments.

Condition: Given the equipment and supplies as listed in the procedure, the student will demonstrate the procedure for disinfecting surgical instruments, adhering to the steps listed below.

Standards: Timing will vary on this competency according to submersion times on the disinfecting bottle. The instructor will set the time limit for this competency. The student will need to score an 85% or above to pass the competency. Automatic failure results if any essential steps are omitted or performed incorrectly.

STEPS START TIME: END TIME:	Points Possible	First Attempt	Second Attempt	Third Attempt
1. Choose a room that is well ventilated and clean. Use a fume hood if available.	10			
2. Check the expiration date of the chemical, its mixing formula and instructions for use, as well as its cautionary information (see SDS).	10			
3. Wash your hands, gather the supplies, and apply PPE.	10			
4. Prepare and pour the solution into an acceptable disinfecting immersion container following the manufacturer's instructions and check the solution with a chemical indicator to confirm it meets the MEC.	10			
5. Directly on the chemical container, record the date that the container was opened and activated along with your initials.	10			
6. Place the instrument to be disinfected into the disinfecting tray until the instrument is completely submerged in the disinfecting solution. Apply the lid securely on the basin.	10			
7. Set the timer according to the manufacturer's instructions.	10			
8. When the timer goes off, lift the tray out of the disinfecting solution and rinse the item according to manufacturer's instructions.	10			
9. Dry the instrument with a clean cloth.	10			
10. Clean the area and replace items.	10			
11. Remove PPE and wash your hands.	10			
Points Earned / Points Possible:	__ / 110			

Points possible reflect importance of step in meeting the task: Important = (5) Essential = (10). Determine score by dividing points earned by total points possible, and multiplying results by 100.

Name _____ Date _____ Score _____

EVALUATION

Evaluator Signature: _____ Date: _____

Evaluator Comments:

DOCUMENTATION

Instructor Note: Retain work products with competency checklist.
Work Product, Procedure 9-2 (Instrument Disinfection Log). Procedure forms can be downloaded from the student companion website.

Key Competencies		
ABHES	MA.A.1.9.a	Practice standard precautions and perform disinfection/sterilization techniques
CAAHEP	III.P.2	Select appropriate barrier/personal protective equipment (PPE)
	III.P.3	Perform handwashing
	III.P.5	Perform sterilization procedures

Name _____ Date _____ Score _____

COMPETENCY CHECKLIST

PROCEDURE 9-3   Wrapping Items for Sterilization in an Autoclave

Task: To wrap instruments for sterilization in an autoclave.

Condition: Given the equipment and supplies as listed in the procedure, the student will demonstrate the procedure for wrapping surgical instruments for sterilization in an autoclave, adhering to the steps listed below.

Standards: The student will have 15 minutes to complete the procedure and will need to score an 85% or above to pass the competency. Automatic failure results if any essential steps are omitted or performed incorrectly.

STEPS START TIME: END TIME:	Points Possible	First Attempt	Second Attempt	Third Attempt
1. Gather the supplies, wash hands, and put on gloves.	10			
2. Check the integrity of the wrapping materials for any flaws.	10			
3. Check the expiration date on the sterilization indicators.	10			
4. Place the items on a clean, dry, flat surface.	10			
Wrapping in Paper or Muslin:				
5. Place one of the sheets of paper or muslin cloth facing diagonally so that they resemble a diamond.	10			
6. Place the sanitized instrument in the center of the paper slightly below the center line. Slightly open instruments with hinges and shield any sharp tips with a piece of gauze. Place a sterilization indicator beside the instrument.	10			
7. Take the bottom edge of the paper that is facing you and fold it upward. Fold the top edge of the diagonal back toward you so that there is a flap.	10			
8. Fold the right side corner of the wrap toward the center. Fold the tip back toward the right side so that there is a flap.	10			
9. Repeat step 8 for the other side. The item should be snuggly encased, but not tight enough to puncture through the wrap.	10			
10. Fold the pack upward from the bottom edge until the article is completely covered, folding the last tip back on itself.	10			
11. Place the wrapped item onto the center of a second piece of autoclave paper. Repeat steps 7 through 9.	10			
12. The last flap is not folded back on itself, but instead is secured with autoclave tape.	10			
13. Label the pack with the name(s) of the items inside, the date, and your first initial and full last name or initials.	10			
Items in Peel-Apart Pouches:				
14. Label the peel-apart pouch with the name(s) of the items inside, the date, and your first initial and full last name or initials.	10			
15. Place instruments in the envelope (handle first).	10			
16. Pull the backing off of the adhesive strip and bend the adhesive flap downward so that it completely seals the envelope. Apply autoclave tape to the edge of the flap if there are any wrinkles or bumps.	10			
Points Earned / Points Possible:	__ / 160			

Points possible reflect importance of step in meeting the task: Important = (5) Essential = (10). Determine score by dividing points earned by total points possible, and multiplying results by 100.

Name _____ Date _____ Score _____

EVALUATION

Evaluator Signature: _____ Date: _____

Evaluator Comments:

Key Competencies		
ABHES	MA.A.1.9.a	Practice standard precautions and perform disinfection/sterilization techniques
CAAHEP	III.P.3	Perform handwashing
	III.P.4	Prepare items for autoclaving
	III.P.5	Perform sterilization procedures

Name _____ Date _____ Score _____

COMPETENCY CHECKLIST
PROCEDURE 9-4   Operate an Autoclave

Task: To properly operate the autoclave to assure complete sterilization of the items in the pack.

Condition: Given the equipment and supplies as listed in the procedure, the student will demonstrate the procedure for sterilizing wrapped instruments in a fully automated autoclave, adhering to the steps listed below.

Standards: The student will have 1 hour to complete the procedure and will need to score an 85% or above to pass the competency. Automatic failure results if any essential steps are omitted or performed incorrectly.

STEPS START TIME: END TIME:	Points Possible	First Attempt	Second Attempt	Third Attempt
1. Wash your hands, apply gloves, and gather the supplies.	10			
2. Arrange the packs on the autoclave trays vertically and separated by at least an inch. Jars should be placed on their sides with their lids removed.	10			
3. Check the water level in the autoclave reservoir and add distilled water to the fill-line if needed.	10			
4. Place loaded trays into the autoclave. Make any necessary adjustments to accommodate the proper positioning of the instruments on each tray.	10			
5. Close and latch the door according to manufacturer's instructions.	10			
6. Select the correct parameters for the type of load you are running.	10			
7. Once the load has gone through the complete sterilization cycle the door will automatically vent. Do not open until venting is complete. Once venting is complete, use an oven mitt or pot holder and remove packs from trays.	10			
8. When the items are cool, examine them for tears, holes, or damages of any kind. Make sure the labels are readable and that the stripes on the indicator tape has darkened.	10			
9. Store the items in a clean, closed environment such as a drawer or a cupboard.	10			
Points Earned / Points Possible:	__ / 90			

Points possible reflect importance of step in meeting the task: Important = (5) Essential = (10). Determine score by dividing points earned by total points possible, and multiplying results by 100.

Name _____ Date _____ Score _____

EVALUATION

Evaluator Signature: _____ Date: _____

Evaluator Comments:

DOCUMENTATION

Instructor Note: Retain work products with competency checklist.

Work Product, Procedure 9-4 (Sterilization Log). Procedure forms can be downloaded from the student companion website.

Key Competencies		
ABHES	MA.A.1.9.a	Practice standard precautions and perform disinfection/sterilization techniques
CAAHEP	III.P.3	Perform handwashing
	III.P.4	Prepare items for autoclaving
	III.P.5	Perform sterilization procedures

Name _____ Date _____ Score _____

COMPETENCY CHECKLIST
PROCEDURE 9-5   Apply Skin Closures

Task: To apply sterile skin closures.

Condition: Given the equipment and supplies as listed in the procedure, the student will demonstrate the proper steps for applying sterile skin closures, adhering to the steps listed below.

Standards: The student will have 15 minutes to complete the procedure and will need to score an 85% or above to pass the competency. Automatic failure results if any essential steps are omitted or performed incorrectly.

STEPS START TIME: END TIME:	Points Possible	First Attempt	Second Attempt	Third Attempt
1. Wash your hands and gather the supplies.	10			
2. Identify the patient using two identifiers, identify yourself. *Explain the rationale for performance of the procedure. Show awareness of the patient's concerns related to the procedure being performed.*	10			
3. Inspect the wound and select the size of adhesive strips that best matches the patient's wound.	10			
4. Position the patient so he is comfortable and position the tray for easy access.	5			
5. Clean the tray and apply items to the tray. Avoid contaminating any of the supplies. Supplies include: • 1 pack of skin antiseptic swabs • 1 package of sterile adhesive strips Open all items in a sterile fashion so that they are completely open for easy access.	10			
6. Wash your hands and apply clean gloves.	10			
7. Clean the patient's skin so that the cleansing extends at least 2 to 3 inches (5 to 7 cm) around the wound using sterile antiseptic swabs.	10			
8. Allow the area to completely dry.	10			
9. Remove the card to which the skin closures are attached using sterile technique. Bend the card at the perforated edge and gently remove the tab. Grasp the skin closure with gloved hands or forceps, lifting straight up. Touch only the edges of the strips.	10			
10. If applying single strips, line the first strip up with the center of the wound. Firmly press one end of the strip on either side of the wound to secure it in place.	10			
11. Gently pull the strip while lining up both edges of the wound so that they come together. (You may need to use the other hand to help oppose the wound edges.)	10			
12. Once the skin is lined up evenly on both sides, pull the tape to the opposite side while pressing down firmly on the skin.	10			
13. Apply the next strip approximately ⅛ inch from the first strip on either side of the first strip.	10			
14. Perform the same step on the opposite side of the wound.	10			

Name _____ Date _____ Score _____

15. Continue this process until the wound is completely closed.	10			
16. If needed, apply one closure approximately ½ inch away from the strip's edges, running parallel to the wound on both sides of the strips.	5			
17. Make certain that there is good approximation of the wound margins.	10			
18. Apply dressing if necessary.	10			
19. Remove gloves and wash your hands.	10			
20. Give the patient home care instructions. (Instruct patient not to pull the strips off, but to let them fall off on their own. The patient may, however, cut the edges as they curl up.)	10			
21. Place trash in trash receptacle.	10			
22. Document the procedure in the patient's chart.	10			
Points Earned / Points Possible:	__ / 210			

Points possible reflect importance of step in meeting the task: Important = (5) Essential = (10). Determine score by dividing points earned by total points possible, and multiplying results by 100.

EVALUATION

Evaluator Signature: _____ Date: _____

Evaluator Comments:

DOCUMENTATION

Instructor Note: Retain work product with competency checklist.
Work Product, Procedure 9-5 (Progress Note). Procedure forms can be downloaded from the student companion website.

Key Competencies			
ABHES	MA.A.1.4.a	Follow documentation guidelines	
	MA.A.1.9.e	Perform specialty procedures including but not limited to minor surgery, cardiac, respiratory, OB-GYN, neurological, gastroenterology	
CAAHEP	I.A.3	Show awareness of a patient's concerns related to the procedure being performed	
	III.P.3	Perform handwashing	
	III.P.8	Perform wound care	
	V.A.4	Explain to a patient the rationale for performance of a procedure	
	X.P.3	Document patient care accurately in the medical record	

Name _____ Date _____ Score _____

COMPETENCY CHECKLIST
PROCEDURE 9-6 Suture or Staple Removal

Task:	To remove sutures and staples.
Condition:	Given the equipment and supplies as listed in the procedure, the student will demonstrate the proper steps for removing sutures or staples, adhering to the steps listed below.
Standards:	The student will have 15 minutes to complete the procedure and will need to score an 85% or above to pass the competency. Automatic failure results if any essential steps are omitted or performed incorrectly.

STEPS START TIME: END TIME:	Points Possible	First Attempt	Second Attempt	Third Attempt
1. Identify the patient using two identifiers.	10			
2. Identify yourself and *explain the rationale for performance of the procedure. Show awareness of the patient's concerns related to the procedure being performed*.	10			
3. Ask if the patient took all of the antibiotic and whether all other home care instructions were followed. *Incorporate critical thinking skills when performing patient care*.	10			
4. Examine the outside of the patient's bandage and make a mental note.	10			
5. Wash your hands and apply examination gloves.	10			
6. Remove the dressing and observe both the inside of the dressing and the wound area for any signs of infection (make a mental note).	10			
7. Discard the dressing into the biohazard container, remove gloves, and wash your hands.	10			
8. Have the provider observe the wound before starting the procedure.	10			
9. Once the provider okays the procedure, open supplies including suture removal kit.	10			
10. If sutures are adhered to the bandage, irrigate dressing with sterile water or saline and dry.	10			
11. Cleanse area with a skin antiseptic.	10			
12. If removing sutures, grasp one side of the first knot with the thumb forceps and gently tug upward on the end of the knot. Using the other hand, work the suture scissors under the knot as close to the skin as possible and cut the suture. Pull the knot toward the wound, making certain that no part of the suture that was on the outside goes through the inside of the wound.	10			
13. If removing staples, gently grasp the staple with the remover and squeeze the handle of the staple remover until the staple is pinched up and out.	10			
14. Continue to remove the sutures or staples until all have been removed.	10			
15. Make sure that the wound still has good approximation and that there is no gapping of the skin (notify the provider if there are any concerns).	10			
16. Apply antiseptic ointment only if ordered and dress the wound according to the provider's instructions.	10			
17. Remove gloves and wash your hands.	10			
18. Give the patient any home care instructions and dismiss.	10			

Name _____ Date _____ Score _____

19. Clean the area and dispose of related items in the biohazardous trash receptacle.	10			
20. Document the procedure.	10			
Points Earned / Points Possible:	__ / 200			

Points possible reflect importance of step in meeting the task: Important = (5) Essential = (10). Determine score by dividing points earned by total points possible, and multiplying results by 100.

EVALUATION

Evaluator Signature: _____ Date: _____

Evaluator Comments:

DOCUMENTATION

Instructor Note: Retain work products with competency checklist.
Work Product, Procedure 9-6 (Progress Note). Procedure forms can be downloaded from the student companion website.

Key Competencies		
ABHES	MA.A.1.4.a	Follow documentation guidelines
	MA.A.1.9.e	Perform specialty procedures including but not limited to minor surgery, cardiac, respiratory, OB-GYN, neurological, gastroenterology
	MA.A.1.10.c	Dispose of biohazardous materials
CAAHEP	I.A.2	Incorporate critical thinking skills when performing patient care
	I.A.3	Show awareness of a patient's concerns related to the procedure being performed
	III.P.3	Perform handwashing
	III.P.8	Perform wound care
	III.P.10.b	Demonstrate proper disposal of biohazardous material: regulated wastes
	V.A.4	Explain to a patient the rationale for performance of a procedure
	X.P.3	Document patient care accurately in the medical record

Name _____ Date _____ Score _____

COMPETENCY CHECKLIST

PROCEDURE 10-1   Perform a Surgical Handwash and Apply Surgical Gloves

Task: To perform a surgical handwash and apply surgical gloves.

Condition: Given the equipment and supplies as listed in the procedure, the student will demonstrate the proper steps for performing a surgical handwash and applying sterile gloves, adhering to the steps listed below.

Standards: The student will have 15 minutes to complete the procedure and will need to score an 85% or above to pass the competency. Automatic failure results if any essential steps are omitted or performed incorrectly.

STEPS START TIME: END TIME:	Points Possible	First Attempt	Second Attempt	Third Attempt
1. Peel apart a sterile towel without contaminating it and lay the towel on a flat, clean surface close to the area where the handwash is to take place.	10			
2. Place gloves beside the sterile towel and remove them from the outer wrapper. Unfold the pack so that it lies flat. Carefully open each flap of the inner wrapper to expose the gloves without contaminating them. (The gloves should be positioned so that the cuffs are facing you, and the thumbs are pointing outward.)	10			
3. Open the sterile scrub pack containing the impregnated scrub brush and nail cleaner. Do not remove them yet. Place them in the sink area.	10			
4. Remove all rings and watches and place them in your pockets. Turn on the water using the automatic sensor or foot or knee control and adjust the temperature (should be warm, not hot).	10			
5. Rinse your hands under the water, keeping the hands and fingers pointed upward and the arms well above the waist.	10			
6. Using just the nail stick and water, clean under each nail. Drop the nail stick in the sink and rinse hands.	10			
7. Completely wet your hands, wrists, and forearms up to the elbow, keeping hands and fingers pointed in an upward position and well above the waist.	10			
8. Obtain the impregnated brush and start the scrub on the palm of the hand and move to the base of the thumb using a circular pattern. Do not go over a section that has already been scrubbed, or you will contaminate it.	10			
9. Next, move to the fingers. Scrub each surface of each finger using several vertical strokes from the base of each finger to the nail (there are a total of four surfaces for each finger). Be certain to scrub the skin between the thumb and index finger as well.	10			
10. Once the fingers are completely scrubbed, turn the hand over and scrub the posterior portion of the hand extending to below the wrists using a circular pattern.	10			
11. Next, scrub the forearm using a circular pattern from the wrists to slightly above the elbow. Make certain to scrub all four surfaces.	10			
12. Rinse both the arm that was just scrubbed and the opposite arm with arms well above the waist and fingers pointed upward. Water should run from the finger tips down the arms and over the elbow. Do not touch any part of the sink while washing or rinsing.	10			
13. Wash the opposite side using the same steps as the first side. Drop the scrub brush in the sink and rinse thoroughly. The entire length of the scrub will vary between two and six minutes.	10			

Name _____ Date _____ Score _____

14. Turn off the water using the foot, knee, or sensor control when applicable.	10			
15. Pick up the towel in your dominant hand by holding onto the corners. The towel should be several inches away from your body. Using just one side of the towel, start at the fingertips on your nondominant hand and pat dry all the way up to the elbow, making sure that you dry all four surfaces simultaneously. Remember to keep the arms and hands above the waist with fingers pointed upward.	10			
16. Repeat the same procedure on your dominant hand using the opposite side of the sterile towel.	10			
17. Once the hands are completely dried, walk to the clean, dry surface where the gloves are laying.	10			
18. Pick up the first glove by the inside cuff using your nondominant hand. Lift the glove up and away from the flat surface to avoid dangling the glove across a nonsterile surface. Slide the glove in an upward motion, over the hand.	10			
19. Pick up the second glove with your dominant hand by slipping the four fingers from the gloved hand underneath the cuff of the second glove. Make certain that the thumb is facing outward. Slide the glove onto the hand without contaminating either glove.	10			
20. Leaving your fingers under the cuff, unfold the cuff so that it slides down over the wrist. Do not allow the gloved thumb from the opposite hand to touch the inside of the cuff. Repeat the same procedure for the first glove.	10			
21. Examine both gloves for any tears or problems.	10			
Points Earned / Points Possible:	__ / 210			

Points possible reflect importance of step in meeting the task: Important = (5) Essential = (10). Determine score by dividing points earned by total points possible, and multiplying results by 100.

EVALUATION

Evaluator Signature: _____ Date: _____

Evaluator Comments:

Key Competencies		
ABHES	MA.A.1.9.a	Practice standard precautions and perform disinfection/sterilization techniques
CAAHEP	III.P.2	Select appropriate barrier/personal protective equipment (PPE)
	III.P.3	Perform handwashing

Name _____ Date _____ Score _____

COMPETENCY CHECKLIST
PROCEDURE 10-2   Prepare the Patient's Skin for the Surgical Procedure Using a One-Step Scrub

Task: To prepare the patient's skin for the surgical procedure using a one-step scrub.

Condition: Given the equipment and supplies as listed in the procedure, the student will demonstrate the proper steps for performing a surgical scrub on the patient's skin using a one-step scrub, adhering to the steps listed below. (This type of scrub is only used if the patient was sent home with special soaps and instructions for cleansing the skin prior to procedure.)

Standards: The student will have 15 minutes to complete the procedure and will need to score an 85% or above to pass the competency. Automatic failure results if any essential steps are omitted or performed incorrectly.

STEPS START TIME: END TIME:	Points Possible	First Attempt	Second Attempt	Third Attempt
1. Wash your hands and gather the supplies.	10			
2. Identify the patient using two identifiers. Verify that the patient followed the site cleansing instructions.	10			
3. Identify yourself and **explain the rationale for the performance of the procedure, showing awareness of the patient's concerns related to the procedure being performed**.	10			
4. Expose the surgical site and drape the patient for modesty if necessary. Some facilities ask the patient to mark the area where the surgery is to take place with an "X" before prepping the skin.	10			
5. Position the patient for comfort and place absorbent drapes under the area to be cleansed, if applicable.	10			
6. Adjust the light so that it illuminates the surgical site. Inspect the skin for any gross contamination. If any gross contamination is visible, the skin will have to be thoroughly cleansed before applying the antiseptic cleanser.	10			
7. Remove absorbent drape and apply sterile drape under the surgical site. Open the skin-prep kit without contaminating the swab or the sponge applicator.	10			
8. Wash your hands and apply sterile gloves.	10			
9. Remove the swab or sponge, touching only the applicator or handle.	10			
10. Apply the antiseptic scrub by painting concentric circles over the site.	10			
11. Scrub normally lasts anywhere from 30 seconds to two minutes, which equates to about three separate applications with three separate applicators. Follow the physician's orders.	10			
12. If the physician orders the area to be shaved, pull skin taut and shave in the direction that the hair grows. Remember that shaving is not recommended unless absolutely necessary!	10			
13. Re-cleanse the skin according to office policy.	10			
14. Apply fenestrated drape according to the physician's preference.	10			
15. Instruct the patient to keep hands below the drapes (when applicable).	10			
Points Earned / Points Possible:	__ / 150			

Points possible reflect importance of step in meeting the task: Important = (5) Essential = (10). Determine score by dividing points earned by total points possible, and multiplying results by 100.

Name _____   Date _____   Score _____

EVALUATION

Evaluator Signature: _____   Date: _____

Evaluator Comments:

Key Competencies			
ABHES	MA.A.1.9.a	Practice standard precautions and perform disinfection/sterilization techniques	
	MA.A.1.9e	Perform specialty procedures included but not limited to minor surgery, cardiac, respiratory, OB-GYN, neurological, gastroenterology	
CAAHEP	III.P.3	Perform handwashing	
	III.P.5	Perform sterilization procedures	

Name _____ Date _____ Score _____

COMPETENCY CHECKLIST
PROCEDURE 10-3   Disinfect a Surgical Tray and Place a Sterile Barrier on the Tray

Task: To disinfect a surgical tray and place a sterile barrier on the tray.

Condition: Given the equipment and supplies as listed in the procedure, and a student to play the part of the patient, the student will demonstrate the proper steps for disinfecting a surgical tray and placing a sterile barrier on the tray, adhering to the steps listed below.

Standards: The student will have 10 minutes to complete the procedure and will need to score an 85% or above to pass the competency. Automatic failure results if any essential steps are omitted or performed incorrectly.

STEPS START TIME: END TIME:	Points Possible	First Attempt	Second Attempt	Third Attempt
1. Wash your hands.	10			
2. Adjust the Mayo stand so that it is right about waist level.	10			
3. Pick up the 4 × 4s saturated with disinfectant (but not dripping) by only touching the top side of the 4 × 4s. Clean the tray using the bottom side of the 4 x 4s using a circular motion, starting from the center and working toward the periphery, until the whole tray is completely covered.	10			
4. Allow the tray to air dry.	10			
5. Select an appropriate sterile barrier and place it on a clean, dry, flat surface.	10			
6. Peel back the top flap of the pack, completely exposing the drape. Make certain that the pack is positioned so that the cut corners are facing you.	10			
7. Using your thumb and forefinger, gently pull up one of the top corner edges of the drape without touching any other part of the drape. Lift the drape well above the counter surface and away from you.	10			
8. Grab the opposing corner so that both corners are now being held along the top edge of the drape. Keep the drape well above your waist and several inches away from your body.	10			
9. Pull the drape over the Mayo stand so that the part of the drape that was facing you is lying against the surface of the tray and the part that was facing away from you is now facing upward on the tray.	10			
Points Earned / Points Possible:	__ / 90			

Points possible reflect importance of step in meeting the task: Important = (5) Essential = (10). Determine score by dividing points earned by total points possible, and multiplying results by 100.

Name _____ Date _____ Score _____

EVALUATION

Evaluator Signature: _____ Date: _____

Evaluator Comments:

Key Competencies		
ABHES	MA.A.1.9.a	Practice standard precautions and perform disinfection/sterilization techniques
CAAHEP	III.P.3	Perform handwashing
	III.P.5	Perform sterilization procedures
	III.P.6	Prepare a sterile field

Name _____ Date _____ Score _____

COMPETENCY CHECKLIST
PROCEDURE 10-4   Open Sterile Items and Place Them on the Sterile Field

Task: To open sterile items and place them on the sterile field.

Condition: Given the equipment and supplies as listed in the procedure, the student will demonstrate the proper steps for opening sterile items and placing them on a sterile field, adhering to the steps listed below.

Standards: The student will have 15 minutes to complete the procedure and will need to score an 85% or above to pass the competency. Automatic failure results if any essential steps are omitted or performed incorrectly.

STEPS START TIME: END TIME:	Points Possible	First Attempt	Second Attempt	Third Attempt
Opening a Sterile Pack and Transferring Items to the Sterile Field Using Sterile Transfer Forceps				
1. Wash your hands.	10			
2. Place a sterilized pack of transfer forceps on the side table.	10			
3. Place the unopened sterilized instrument on the side table, examine the autoclave tape, and make certain that the stripes turned the appropriate color. Check the expiration date and the quality of the wrapper to make certain that the wrap has not been compromised.				
4. Remove the tape from the packet and place it on the side table. Position the pack so that the flap that was taped is facing you.	5			
5. Using only your thumb and index finger, grasp the tip of the folded flap that was covered with tape and pull it away from you.	10			
6. Using only your right thumb and index finger, grasp the tip of the folded-back flap on the right side and pull it all the way to the right.	10			
7. Using only your left thumb and index finger, grasp the tip of the folded-back flap on the left side and pull it all the way to the left.	10			
8. Using only your dominant thumb and index finger, grasp the tip of the last folded-back flap and pull it toward you without touching anything on the inside of the wrap. The entire instrument should be exposed for easy retrieval later. Check the sterilization indicator in the pack to make certain it turned the appropriate color; if not, remove the pack and get a new one.	10			
9. Move to the packet containing the sterile transfer forceps. Open the sterile transfer forceps the same way you opened the first pack.	10			
10. Once the pack is opened, grasp only the handles of the sterile transfer forceps by placing your thumb in one ring and your index finger in the other ring. Do not touch any other part of the instrument. Lift the transfer forceps straight up, keeping the tips facing downward but well above the height of the side table.	10			
11. Move the transfer forceps to the instrument that needs to be transferred to the sterile field. Once you are positioned in front of the sterile instrument, lower the transfer forceps to the sterile instrument and securely grasp the instrument. Lift the instrument well above the height of the side table and approach the sterile tray. Standing a few inches away from the field, gently lower the sterile instrument onto the tray. Do not allow your hand to drop below the level of the handle.	10			

Name _____ Date _____ Score _____

12. Once the instrument has been fully transferred to its appropriate place on the tray, pull the sterile transfer forceps up and away from the field and set them back down on the side table.	10			
Opening a Peel-Apart Pack				
1. Inspect the package and make certain that the integrity of the wrap has not been altered. Check the control strip to make certain that it turned the correct color. Check the expiration date to make certain that the pack is not expired.	10			
2. Position yourself so that you are in front of the tray but several inches away from the field.	10			
3. Grasp both the top edges of the peel-apart pack and carefully peel them apart by rolling the wrap downward on both sides.	10			
4. Once the wrap has been peeled to the point that the item can be transferred to the field, turn your hands inward and push the pack forward so that the item is just slightly over the field. The hands should be well above the field. Gently drop the item onto the field.	10			
Points Earned / Points Possible:	__ / 155			

Points possible reflect importance of step in meeting the task: Important = (5) Essential = (10). Determine score by dividing points earned by total points possible, and multiplying results by 100.

EVALUATION

Evaluator Signature: _____ Date: _____

Evaluator Comments:

Key Competencies		
ABHES	MA.A.1.9.a	Practice standard precautions and perform disinfection/sterilization techniques
CAAHEP	III.P.3	Perform handwashing
	III.P.5	Perform sterilization procedures
	III.P.6	Prepare a sterile field

Name _____ Date _____ Score _____

COMPETENCY CHECKLIST
PROCEDURE 10-5   Set Up a Complete Sterile Tray and Pour a Sterile Solution

Task: To set up a complete sterile tray and pour a sterile solution.

Condition: Given the equipment and supplies as listed in the procedure, the student will demonstrate the proper steps for setting up a sterile tray and pouring sterile solutions, adhering to the steps listed below.

Standards: The student will have 15 minutes to complete the procedure and will need to score an 85% or above to pass the competency. Automatic failure results if any essential steps are omitted or performed incorrectly.

STEPS START TIME: END TIME:	Points Possible	First Attempt	Second Attempt	Third Attempt
1. Perform an aseptic handwash using antibacterial soap and water.	10			
2. Gather the supplies and place them on the side table.	10			
3. Properly position the Mayo stand so that it is at your waist level.	10			
4. Clean the Mayo stand with 4 × 4s that have been saturated with a disinfectant (but not dripping), cleaning in a concentric circular motion.	10			
5. Allow the stand to air dry.	5			
6. Check the instrument pack and make certain that the integrity of the pack has not been compromised.	10			
7. Check the tape on the outside of the pack to make certain that the stripes turned the correct color and that the pack has not reached its expiration date.	10			
8. Pull the tape off of the pack and place it on the side table.	5			
9. Place the sterile pack on the center of the Mayo stand so that the flap that was taped is facing you.	10			
10. Using only your thumb and index finger, grasp the tip of the folded flap that was covered with tape and pull it away from you.	10			
11. Using only your right thumb and index finger, grasp the tip of the folded-back flap on the right side and pull it all the way to the right.	10			
12. Using only your left thumb and index finger, grasp the tip of the folded-back flap on the left side and pull it all the way to the left.	10			
13. Using only your dominant thumb and index finger, grasp the tip of the last folded-back flap and pull it toward you without touching anything on the inside of the wrap.	10			
14. Repeat steps 10 through 13 for the second layer of wrap. (The inner wrap will become your sterile drape.)	10			
15. Move to the side table without turning your back on the field.	10			
16. Open the pack of sterile gloves and remove them from the wrapper.	10			
17. Open the inner wrapper without contaminating the gloves.	10			
18. Wash your hands with alcohol-based hand sanitizer following the directions on the bottle.	10			
19. Apply surgical gloves—remember to hold your hands above the waist.	10			
20. Approach the field facing forward and stand 12 inches away from the field. Remove the items from the inside of the tray and place them on the sterile field in a logical sequence. Place the basins for the sterile solution on one corner of the stand facing upward.	10			

Name _____ Date _____ Score _____

21. Once the field has been totally arranged, remove the sterilization indicator from the inside of the tray and make certain that it is the proper color.	10			
22. Place the tray that held the instruments onto the side table. Do not turn your body away from the sterile tray as you place the instrument tray on the side table.	10			
23. Remove gloves and wash your hands with alcohol-based sanitizer.	10			
24. Pick up the brand new bottle of iodine and read the label. Make certain that you have the correct solution. Check the label to confirm that the solution has not passed its expiration date.	10			
25. Pick up the bottle of iodine, palming the label.	10			
26. Remove the cap and place it to the side so that the lid is facing upward. Remove the protective seal and place it on the side table.	10			
27. Move to the tray and approach the corner on which the basins are sitting.	10			
28. Pour the iodine into the container labeled as iodine, pouring 2 to 6 inches above the field. Be careful not to allow the solution to splash. Fill to the desired level.	10			
29. Repeat steps 24 through 28 with a new bottle of sterile saline, pouring into the container labeled as saline.	10			
30. If the solutions are not used in their entirety, replace the caps and follow the facility's policy for storing the solutions. Keep in mind that these solutions should not be used for any future surgical procedures.	5			
Points Earned / Points Possible:	__ / 285			

Points possible reflect importance of step in meeting the task: Important = (5) Essential = (10). Determine score by dividing points earned by total points possible, and multiplying results by 100.

EVALUATION

Evaluator Signature: _____ Date: _____

Evaluator Comments:

Key Competencies		
ABHES	MA.A.1.9.a	Practice standard precautions and perform disinfection/sterilization techniques
CAAHEP	I.A.3	Perform handwashing
	III.P.5	Perform sterilization procedures
	III.P.6	Prepare a sterile field

Name _____ Date _____ Score _____

COMPETENCY CHECKLIST
PROCEDURE 10-6   Apply Surgical Attire

Task: To apply surgical attire.

Condition: Given the equipment and supplies as listed in the procedure, and a student to play the part of the second medical assistant, the student will demonstrate the proper steps for applying surgical attire, adhering to the steps listed below.

Standards: The student will have 15 minutes to complete the procedure and will need to score an 85% or above to pass the competency. Automatic failure results if any essential steps are omitted or performed incorrectly.

STEPS START TIME: END TIME:	Points Possible	First Attempt	Second Attempt	Third Attempt
1. Gather the supplies.	10			
2. Remove all rings and watches and perform an aseptic handwash. Do not replace rings or watches following the aseptic handwash.	10			
3. Place a sterile gown pack on a Mayo stand or clean, dry counter surface near the sink. Open the package containing the sterile gown and towel. Sterile gloves may be transferred or dropped onto the field in a sterile manner; otherwise, sterile gloves should be positioned nearby for easy access once the gown is applied.	10			
4. Apply cap, goggles, shoe covers (if needed), and mask.	10			
5. Open the sterile scrub pack containing the scrub brush and nail stick.	10			
6. Follow steps 4 through 16 in Procedure 10-1 for performing a surgical handwash.	10			
7. Reach down in the sterile package and lift upward on the folded gown by grasping the inside of the gown below the neckline.	10			
8. To provide a wide margin of safety, step away from the table into an area that is unobstructed.	10			
9. Keeping the inside of the gown toward your body, allow the gown to unfold. Do not touch the outside of the gown with your bare hands.	10			
10. Keeping the hands well above the waist, simultaneously slip both hands into the armholes. Do not allow the hands to extend beyond the cuffs.	10			
11. Have another medical assistant pull the gown up over your shoulders by grasping the inside shoulder and neck seams. Keep the hands within the cuffed sleeves. The gown should then be fastened at the neck and waist level in the back only. Do not allow the medical assistant to touch any part of the gown that is to remain sterile.	10			
12. Using only the outside cuff of your surgical gown from your dominant hand, pick up the glove for your nondominant hand. Lay the glove on the palm side of the outside cuff of the nondominant hand. If correctly positioned, the fingers of the glove should be pointing toward your elbow and the thumb side of the glove should be facing down.	10			
13. With both hands still tucked within the inside cuffs of the sleeves, pinch the rolled edges of the glove and stretch the glove up and over the gown cuff while working your fingers out of the cuff and into the glove.	10			
14. Gently slide your fingers into the glove.	10			
15. Pick up the second glove by placing the fingers of the gloved hand under the cuff of the second glove.	10			

Name _____ Date _____ Score _____

16. Slide the glove over the cuff of the gown on the opposite hand while working your fingers into the glove. Make certain both cuffs are folded over stockinette cuffs.	10				
17. Remember to keep the hands above the waist once gloves are applied.	10				
18. Pass the cardboard tab to the second medical assistant. Grasp the string attached to the cardboard as the medical assistant pulls the cardboard toward the outside. The cardboard will separate from the string.	10				
19. Pick up the other loose string attached to the front of the gown and tie both strings at the waist and secure	10				
20. Make sure your hands stay above the level of the waist at all times.	10				
Points Earned / Points Possible:	__ / 200				

Points possible reflect importance of step in meeting the task: Important = (5) Essential = (10). Determine score by dividing points earned by total points possible, and multiplying results by 100.

EVALUATION

Evaluator Signature: _____ Date: _____

Evaluator Comments:

Key Competencies		
ABHES	MA.A.1.9.a	Practice standard precautions and perform disinfection/sterilization techniques
CAAHEP	III.P.2	Select appropriate barrier/personal protective equipment (PPE)
	III.P.3	Perform handwashing

Name _____ Date _____ Score _____

COMPETENCY CHECKLIST
PROCEDURE 10-7   Remove an Old Dressing, Irrigate the Wound, and Apply a New Dressing

Task: To remove an old dressing, irrigate the wound, and apply a new dressing.

Condition: Given the equipment and supplies as listed in the procedure, and a student to play the part of the patient, the student will demonstrate the proper steps for removing an old dressing, irrigating a wound, and applying a new dressing, adhering to the steps listed below.

Standards: The student will have 15 minutes to complete the procedure and will need to score an 85% or above to pass the competency. Automatic failure results if any essential steps are omitted or performed incorrectly.

STEPS START TIME: END TIME:	Points Possible	First Attempt	Second Attempt	Third Attempt
1. Check the patient's chart to determine the type and strength of irrigating solution and dressing to be used, and gather the supplies.	10			
2. Identify the patient using two identifiers.	10			
3. Identify yourself.	10			
4. ***Explain the rationale for performance of the procedure, showing awareness of the patient's concerns related to the procedure being performed.***	10			
5. Ask the patient if the patient has had any problems since the surgery and make certain that the patient has been following all home care instructions.	10			
6. Have the patient expose the area.	10			
7. Place a waterproof pad under the wound area and position so that the work area is easily accessible.	10			
8. Wash hands using aseptic technique and apply appropriate PPE (nonsterile examination gloves).	10			
9. Inspect the outer covering of the bandage, ***incorporating critical thinking when performing patient care***. Make a mental note of any concerns. Was the bandage torn, dirty, or wet?	10			
10. Cut the bandage with a pair of bandage scissors along the side of the wound. Carefully remove the bandage and dressing by pulling the bandage toward the wound.	10			
11. Inspect the inner portion of the bandage for any drainage or odor. Make a mental note of your findings. Discard the bandage material into a biohazard container.	10			
12. Without touching the wound, look at the wound area and inspect it for any signs of infection, including edema, erythema, drainage, etc. Make a mental note of your findings.	10			
13. Remove gloves and wash your hands. Follow office policy regarding having the physician check the wound before redressing.	10			
14. Properly position and clean the Mayo tray with the 4 × 4s containing disinfectant. Allow the stand to air dry.	10			
15. Place one of the wrapped sterile basins on the center of the Mayo stand. Open using sterile technique.	10			
16. Open the peel-apart package containing the sterile 4 x 4s and drop the contents from the packet onto the field.	10			
17. Open sterile dressing and place it on the sterile field.	10			

Name _____ Date _____ Score _____

18. Open the sterile bandage and place it on the sterile field.	10			
19. Drop a sterile 20 mL syringe onto the sterile field.	10			
20. Pour a small amount of sterile saline into the sterile basin.	10			
21. Remove the other sterile basin from the side table and place it on the waterproof drape near the wound. Open it in a sterile manner. Instruct the patient not to touch the basin or drape.	10			
22. Thoroughly wash your hands using the alcohol-based sanitizer on the side table.	10			
23. Don a pair of sterile gloves.	10			
24. Arrange items on the tray for easy access.	5			
25. Draw up irrigating fluid from the basin with the sterile syringe. Irrigate the patient's wound so that the water runs into the basin on the sterile field	10			
26. Dry the wound with sterile gauze.	10			
27. Open the sterile dressing and place it over the wound.	10			
28. Choose a bandaging technique that best suits the patient's wound.	10			
29. Throw away all trash into proper trash receptacles and give the patient home care instructions and any prescriptions.	10			
30. Dismiss the patient and clean the room.	10			
31. Document the procedure in the patient's chart.	10			
Points Earned / Points Possible:	__ / 305			

Points possible reflect importance of step in meeting the task: Important = (5) Essential = (10). Determine score by dividing points earned by total points possible, and multiplying results by 100.

EVALUATION

Evaluator Signature: _____ Date: _____

Evaluator Comments:

DOCUMENTATION

Instructor Note: Retain work products with competency checklist.
Work Product, Procedure 10-7 (Progress Note). Procedure forms can be downloaded from the student companion website.

Key Competencies		
ABHES	MA.A.1.4.a	Follow documentation guidelines
	MA.A.1.9.a	Practice standard precautions and perform disinfection/sterilization techniques
CAAHEP	I.A.2	Incorporate critical thinking skills when performing patient care
	I.A.3	Show awareness of a patient's concerns related to the procedure being performed
	III.P.2	Select appropriate barrier/personal protective equipment (PPE)
	III.P.3	Perform handwashing
	III.P.5	Perform sterilization procedures
	III.P.8	Perform wound care
	III.P.9	Perform dressing change
	V.A.4	Explain to a patient the rationale for performance of a procedure
	X.P.3	Document patient care accurately in the medical record

Name _____ Date _____ Score _____

COMPETENCY CHECKLIST

PROCEDURE 11-1   Obtain the Height and Weight of an Adult Patient

Task: To obtain and document an adult patient's height and weight.

Condition: Given the equipment and supplies as listed in the procedure and a classmate to play the part of the patient, the student will perform and document an adult height and weight, adhering to the steps listed below.

Standards: The student will have five minutes to complete the procedure and will need to score an 85% or above to pass the competency. Automatic failure results if any essential steps are omitted or performed incorrectly.

STEPS START TIME: END TIME:	Points Possible	First Attempt	Second Attempt	Third Attempt
1. Place the scale weights at zero.	10			
2. Check that the scale is balanced and adjust, if necessary.	10			
3. Wash your hands.	10			
4. Identify the patient using at least two identifiers, identify yourself, and ***explain the rationale for performance of the procedure, showing awareness of the patient's concerns related to the procedure being performed***.	10			
5. Assess the stability of the patient.	5			
6. ***Explaining the rationale for the procedure***, have the patient remove any unnecessary clothing, such as a jacket or sweater, as well as shoes.	10			
7. Place a paper towel on the floor of the scale.	10			
8. Assist the patient onto the scale, facing the weights. ***Incorporate critical thinking skills when performing patient assessment and care***.	10			
9. Instruct the patient to stand on the center of the scale and to hold still. Move the lower weight first, then slowly move the upper weight until the scale arrow is balanced.	10			
10. Record the measurement by adding the measurement from the lower weight to the measurement from the upper weight. (When reading the measurements from the upper bar, the longer calibration markings are pound increments and the shorter line increments are in quarter- and half-pound increments.)	5			
11. Return the weights to zero.	10			
12. Assist the patient off the scale.	10			
13. Raise the calibrated height bar to a height that would be greater than the patient's height.	10			
14. Extend the bar used to measure to a horizontal position.	5			
15. Assist the patient back onto the scale platform, back toward the measurement tool. Have the patient stand as erect as possible.	10			
16. Lower the horizontal bar slowly and gently until it reaches the top of the patient's head, forming a 90° angle with the height bar.	10			
17. Assist the patient off the platform.	10			
18. Read the height measurement by reading from the top of the bar going down reading it at the junction of the stationary calibration rod and the movable calibration rod.	10			
19. Place the measurement bar back to its original position.	5			
20. Discard the paper towel.	5			

Name _____ Date _____ Score _____

21. Document the results in the patient record (if you didn't already). Convert weight into kilograms if necessary. Calculate and record BMI when using a paper chart. ***Reassure the patient of the accuracy of the test results***.	10			
Points Earned / Points Possible:	___ / 185			

Points possible reflect importance of step in meeting the task: Important = (5) Essential = (10). Determine score by dividing points earned by total points possible, and multiplying results by 100.

EVALUATION

Evaluator Signature: _____ Date: _____

Evaluator Comments:

DOCUMENTATION

Instructor Note: Retain work products with competency checklist.
Work Products, Procedure 11-1a (Progress Note) and 11-1b (Flow Sheet). Procedure forms can be downloaded from the student companion website.

Key Competencies			
ABHES	MA.A.1.9.b	Obtain vital signs, obtain patient history, and formulate chief complaint	
CAAHEP	I.P.1.e	Measure and record height	
	I.P.1.f	Measure and record weight	
	I.A.1	Incorporate critical thinking skills when performing patient assessment	
	I.A.2	Incorporate critical thinking skills when performing patient care	
	I.A.3	Show awareness of a patient's concerns related to the procedure being performed	
	II.A.1	Reassure a patient of the accuracy of the test results	
	III.P.3	Perform handwashing	
	V.P.11	Report relevant information concisely and accurately	
	V.A.4	Explain to a patient the rationale for performance of a procedure	
	X.P.3	Document patient care accurately in the medical record	

Name _____ Date _____ Score _____

COMPETENCY CHECKLIST

PROCEDURE 11-2   Obtain Oral, Aural, Axillary, and Temporal Body Temperatures

Task: To obtain and document an accurate oral, aural, axillary, and temporal body temperature reading.

Condition: Given the equipment and supplies as listed in the procedure and a classmate to play the part of the patient, the student will perform and document an oral, aural, axillary, and temporal body temperature, adhering to the steps listed below.

Standards: The student will have five minutes to complete the procedure (five minutes allowed for each type of temperature reading) and will need to score an 85% or above (on each type of temperature reading) to pass the competency. Automatic failure results if any essential steps are omitted or performed incorrectly.

STEPS START TIME: END TIME:	Points Possible	First Attempt	Second Attempt	Third Attempt
1. Wash your hands. (Gloving is optional.)	10			
2. Assemble the equipment.	10			
3. Identify the patient using two identifiers, identify yourself, and ***explain the rationale for performance of the procedure, showing awareness of the patient's concerns related to the procedure being performed***.	10			
4. *Take an oral temperature*				
a. Ask if the patient has ingested hot or cold food or beverages or smoked within the last half hour.	10			
b. Make certain that the thermometer is on the appropriate setting (oral or axillary) and cover it with a disposable probe cover. ***Incorporate critical thinking skills when performing patient assessment and care***.	10			
c. Place the thermometer in the patient's mouth under the tongue to the right or left side of the frenulum linguae.	10			
d. Instruct the patient not to clench or bite down on the thermometer and to hold the mouth closed and breathe through the nostrils, not through the mouth.	10			
e. Keep the thermometer in place until a tone or beep is heard.	10			
f. Read the digital display, remove and discard probe into the trash can and place electronic thermometer back into the base. ***Reassure the patient of the accuracy of the test results***.	10			
5. *Take an aural temperature*				
a. Place a clean probe cover over the tympanic probe and make certain the unit is turned on and in the "ready" mode.	10			
b. Straighten the aural canal to best facilitate an accurate measurement. (Pull the auricle up and back on adults and children over the age of three. Pull down and back on anyone younger than age three). ***Incorporate critical thinking skills when performing patient assessment and care***.	10			
c. Place the covered probe into the patient's ear canal, forming a tight seal and pointing the probe toward the eardrum.	10			
d. Activate the thermometer while having the patient quietly relax.	10			
e. Leave the probe in place until the unit beeps. The temperature will be displayed digitally on the thermometer. ***Reassure the patient of the accuracy of the test results***.	10			
f. Discard the probe cover in the appropriate waste container. Return the thermometer to storage.	10			

Name _____ Date _____ Score _____

6. *Take an axillary temperature*					
a. Make certain that the route setting is on axillary and place a new probe cover over the probe.	10				
b. Have the patient remove clothing that interferes with the axillary region. Offer a gown or drape for coverage. ***Incorporate critical thinking skills when performing patient assessment and care.***	10				
c. Pat the armpit with a dry paper towel if perspiration is present (or have the patient do it).	10				
d. Place the probe tight in the center of the axilla.	10				
e. Instruct or assist the patient in holding the arm tight against the body, holding the thermometer in place until the digital device emits a tone, indicating completion of the reading. ***Reassure the patient of the accuracy of the test results.***	10				
f. Remove probe and discard into trash can.	10				
7. *Take a temporal temperature*					
a. Clean the thermometer probe with an alcohol swab or place probe cover over the probe and ensure that it is working properly. ***Incorporate critical thinking skills when performing patient assessment and care.***	10				
b. Remove hats or scarves on the side of the head that is to be measured and pull hair back if applicable.	10				
c. Check the forehead for perspiration. Wipe dry if perspiration is present.	10				
d. Depress the scan button and place the probe at the midline of the forehead. Keep probe flush with the skin and slowly glide the thermometer across the forehead until the probe reaches the hairline on the side of the head over the temporal artery.	10				
e. When the reading is complete, release the scan button, lift the probe from the patient's skin, and check the display for the reading. (Take a second reading behind the ear under the mastoid process if necessary.) ***Reassure the patient of the accuracy of the test results.***	10				
f. Clean the probe with alcohol or if using a probe cover, discard in trash receptacle.	10				
For All Temperature Procedures					
8. Immediately record results on a scrap piece of paper.	10				
9. Return equipment back to its proper location.	10				
10. Wash your hands and record temperature reading in the patient record.	10				
Points Earned / Points Possible: **(For each type of temperature reading)**	___ / 120				
Points Earned / Points Possible: **(Total for all combined temperature readings)**	___ / 300				

Points possible reflect importance of step in meeting the task: Important = (5) Essential = (10). Determine score by dividing points earned by total points possible, and multiplying results by 100.

Name _____ Date _____ Score _____

EVALUATION

Evaluator Signature: _____ Date: _____

Evaluator Comments:

DOCUMENTATION

Instructor Note: Retain work products with competency checklist.

Work Products, Procedure 11-2a (Progress Note) and 11-2b (Flow Sheet). Procedure forms can be downloaded from the student companion website.

Key Competencies		
ABHES	MA.A.1.9.b	Obtain vital signs, obtain patient history, and formulate chief complaint
CAAHEP	I.P.1.b	Measure and record temperature
	I.A.1	Incorporate critical thinking skills when performing patient assessment
	I.A.2	Incorporate critical thinking skills when performing patient care
	I.A.3	Show awareness of a patient's concerns related to the procedure being performed
	II.A.1	Reassure a patient of the accuracy of the test results
	II.C.4	Convert among measurement systems
	III.P.3	Perform handwashing
	V.P.11	Report relevant information concisely and accurately
	V.A.4	Explain to a patient the rationale for performance of a procedure
	X.P.3	Document patient care accurately in the medical record

Name _____ Date _____ Score _____

COMPETENCY CHECKLIST

PROCEDURE 11-3   Obtain a Radial Pulse Rate and Respiration Rate

Task: To obtain a radial pulse rate and respiration rate.

Condition: Given the equipment and supplies as listed in the procedure and a classmate to play the part of the patient, the student will perform a radial pulse and respiration, adhering to the steps listed below.

Standards: The student will have five minutes to complete the procedure and will need to score an 85% or above to pass the competency. Automatic failure results if any essential steps are omitted or performed incorrectly.

STEPS START TIME: END TIME:	Points Possible	First Attempt	Second Attempt	Third Attempt
1. Wash your hands.	10			
2. Identify the patient using two identifiers, identify yourself, and ***explain the rationale of the procedure, showing awareness of the patient's concerns related to the procedure being performed***.	10			
3. Place the patient in a calm, quiet environment. Allow the patient to relax in a sitting position with the arm in a comfortable location. ***Incorporate critical thinking skills when performing patient assessment and care***.	10			
4. Locate the radial pulse with your second, third, and fourth fingers. The hand you use should be opposite from the hand on which you wear your watch. Never use your thumb when measuring the pulse.	10			
5. Apply slight pressure onto the radial artery. Increase pressure until the pulse is felt.	10			
6. Count the number of beats for a minimum of 30 seconds. Multiply this number by two for a full-minute rate.	10			
7. Note if there are any irregular beats that occur.	10			
8. Maintain fingers on the pulse and begin counting respirations.	10			
9. Count the number of breaths for 30 seconds. Multiply this number by two for a full-minute rate. ***Reassure the patient of the accuracy of the test results***.	10			
10. Note any irregular breath sounds.	10			
11. Wash your hands.	10			
12. Document the results of the pulse and respirations in the patient record.	10			
Points Earned / Points Possible:	___ / 120			

Points possible reflect importance of step in meeting the task: Important = (5) Essential = (10). Determine score by dividing points earned by total points possible, and multiplying results by 100.

Name _____ Date _____ Score _____

EVALUATION

Evaluator Signature: _____ Date: _____

Evaluator Comments:

DOCUMENTATION

Instructor Note: Retain work products with competency checklist.

Work Products, Procedure 11-3a (Progress Note) and 11-3b (Flow Sheet). Procedure forms can be downloaded from the student companion website.

Key Competencies		
ABHES	MA.A.1.9.b	Obtain vital signs, obtain patient history, and formulate chief complaint
CAAHEP	I.P.1.c	Measure and record pulse
	I.P.1.d	Measure and record respirations
	I.A.1	Incorporate critical thinking skills when performing patient assessment
	I.A.2	Incorporate critical thinking skills when performing patient care
	I.A.3	Show awareness of a patient's concerns related to the procedure being performed
	II.A.1	Reassure a patient of the accuracy of the test results
	III.P.3	Perform handwashing
	V.P.11	Report relevant information concisely and accurately
	V.A.4	Explain to a patient the rationale for performance of a procedure
	X.P.3	Document patient care accurately in the medical record

Name _____ Date _____ Score _____

COMPETENCY CHECKLIST
PROCEDURE 11-4   Obtain an Apical Pulse Rate

Task: To obtain an apical pulse reading.

Condition: Given the equipment and supplies as listed in the procedure and a classmate to play the part of the patient, the student will perform an apical pulse rate, adhering to the steps listed below.

Standards: The student will have five minutes to complete the procedure and will need to score an 85% or above to pass the competency. Automatic failure results if any essential steps are omitted or performed incorrectly.

STEPS START TIME: END TIME:	Points Possible	First Attempt	Second Attempt	Third Attempt
1. Wash your hands.	10			
2. Assemble the equipment. Sanitize the stethoscope.	10			
3. Identify the patient using two identifiers, identify yourself, and ***explain the rationale of the procedure, showing awareness of the patient's concerns related to the procedure being performed***.	10			
4. Instruct the patient to expose the chest area by either unbuttoning the shirt or removing clothes from the waist up. Provide a gown for privacy. ***Incorporate critical thinking skills when performing patient assessment and care***.	10			
5. Remove clothing, gown, or drape covering the left thoracic area.	10			
6. Place the stethoscope in your ears correctly.	10			
7. Locate the apical pulse.	10			
8. After warming the diaphragm of the stethoscope, place it over the apex of the heart.	10			
9. Count the beats for one full minute.	10			
10. Note any irregularities, along with the quality of sound.	10			
11. Remove the stethoscope. ***Reassure the patient of the accuracy of the test results***.	10			
12. Assist the patient in redressing or draping.	10			
13. Wash your hands.	10			
14. Record the results in the patient record.	10			
Points Earned / Points Possible:	___ / 140			

Points possible reflect importance of step in meeting the task: Important = (5) Essential = (10). Determine score by dividing points earned by total points possible, and multiplying results by 100.

Name _____ Date _____ Score _____

EVALUATION

Evaluator Signature: _____ Date: _____

Evaluator Comments:

DOCUMENTATION

Instructor Note: Retain work products with competency checklist.

Work Products, Procedure 11-4a (Progress Note) and 11-4b (Flow Sheet). Procedure forms can be downloaded from the student companion website.

Key Competencies		
ABHES	MA.A.1.9.b	Obtain vital signs, obtain patient history, and formulate chief complaint
CAAHEP	I.P.1.c	Measure and record pulse
	I.A.1	Incorporate critical thinking skills when performing patient assessment
	I.A.2	Incorporate critical thinking skills when performing patient care
	I.A.3	Show awareness of a patient's concerns related to the procedure being performed
	II.A.1	Reassure a patient of the accuracy of the test results
	III.P.3	Perform handwashing
	V.P.11	Report relevant information concisely and accurately
	V.A.4	Explain to a patient the rationale for performance of a procedure
	X.P.3	Document patient care accurately in the medical record

Name _____ Date _____ Score _____

COMPETENCY CHECKLIST

PROCEDURE 11-5   Obtain a BP Measurement Using the Palpatory Method

Task: To accurately obtain a blood pressure reading.

Condition: Given the equipment and supplies as listed in the procedure and a classmate to play the part of the patient, the student will perform a blood pressure reading, adhering to the steps listed below.

Standards: The student will have five minutes to complete the procedure and will need to score an 85% or above to pass the competency. Automatic failure results if any essential steps are omitted or performed incorrectly.

STEPS START TIME: END TIME:	Points Possible	First Attempt	Second Attempt	Third Attempt
1. Wash your hands.	10			
2. Assemble the equipment. Sanitize the stethoscope.	10			
3. Test the equipment to make sure the bulb and gauge are in working order. Tighten the bulb valve and inflate the cuff briefly.	10			
4. Remove any air from the cuff bladder.	10			
5. Identify the patient using two identifiers, identify yourself, and *explain the rationale of the procedure, showing awareness of the patient's concerns related to the procedure being performed*. Ask patient if there is any reason you can't perform blood pressure on one side or the other.	10			
6. Assess the patient's upper arm diameter to determine if the size of the cuff selected is adequate. *Incorporate critical thinking skills when performing patient assessment and care.*	10			
7. Position the patient in a quiet, comfortable position.	10			
8. Roll up the patient's sleeve or remove any clothing or garments from the arm that will be used for obtaining the BP.	10			
9. Palpate the brachial artery for a viable pulse.	10			
10. With the patient's palm facing upward, wrap the cuff around the upper arm 1 to 2 inches above the bend of the elbow. The cuff should be snug but not overly tight. The arrow on the cuff, R for right arm and L for left arm, should align with the artery. Position the arm so that it is at heart level.	10			
11. Adjust the stethoscope so that the sound is coming from the diaphragm side of the chest piece. (Lightly tapping on the bell or diaphragm with the ear pieces in place will confirm correct side.) Remove the stethoscope tips from your ears.	5			
12 Adjust the manometer so it is clipped to the cuff and is in clear view.	5			
13. Hold the bulb in the palm of your dominant hand with the valve between the thumb and first finger. Turn the valve until closed.	10			
14. With the other hand, locate the radial pulse.	10			
15. Using the bulb, squeeze and inflate the cuff while palpating the radial pulse. Continue until the pulse is no longer felt. Proceed with inflation until the cuff has been inflated 30 mmHg beyond pulse cessation.	10			
16. Slowly open the valve to release air from the cuff while palpating the radial pulse. Release at 2–3 mmHg per second. Note the pressure on the manometer when the pulse returns.	10			
17. Open the valve completely and remove all air from the cuff.	10			
18. After waiting 30 seconds, prepare to take the BP reading.	10			

Name _____ Date _____ Score _____

19. Place the stethoscope tips correctly in your ear canals. Place the chest piece over the brachial artery. Hold the stethoscope in place with the first two fingers of your hand. Do not hold with your thumb over the chest piece as you may pick up your own pulse. Avoid touching the cuff with the stethoscope. Avoid having the tubing of the stethoscope come in contact with anything.	10			
20. Tighten the valve by turning it clockwise and pump the cuff rapidly up to 20 mmHg above the palpated systolic pressure.	10			
21. Begin to release the pressure in the cuff by slowly turning the valve counterclockwise, 2–3 mmHg per second. Observe the manometer carefully. Note the measurement when the first beat is heard. This is the systolic pressure.	10			
22. Continue to deflate the cuff at this speed. Observe the manometer carefully and note the measurement when the sound ceases. This is the diastolic pressure.	10			
23. Open the valve completely to deflate the cuff quickly and remove all air from the cuff.	10			
24. Remove the stethoscope and cuff. ***Reassure the patient of the accuracy of the test results***.	10			
25. Wash your hands.	10			
26. Record the results in the patient record.	10			
Points Earned / Points Possible:	___ / 250			

Points possible reflect importance of step in meeting the task: Important = (5) Essential = (10). Determine score by dividing points earned by total points possible, and multiplying results by 100.

EVALUATION

Evaluator Signature: _____ Date: _____

Evaluator Comments:

DOCUMENTATION

Instructor Note: Retain work products with competency checklist.
Work Products, Procedure 11-5a (Progress Note) and 11-5b (Flow Sheet). Procedure forms can be downloaded from the student companion website.

Key Competencies		
ABHES	MA.A.1.9.b	Obtain vital signs, obtain patient history, and formulate chief complaint
CAAHEP	I.P.1.a	Measure and record blood pressure
	I.A.1	Incorporate critical thinking skills when performing patient assessment
	I.A.2	Incorporate critical thinking skills when performing patient care
	I.A.3	Show awareness of a patient's concerns related to the procedure being performed
	II.A.1	Reassure a patient of the accuracy of the test results
	III.P.3	Perform handwashing
	V.P.11	Report relevant information concisely and accurately
	V.A.4	Explain to a patient the rationale for performance of a procedure
	X.P.3	Document patient care accurately in the medical record

Name _____ Date _____ Score _____

COMPETENCY CHECKLIST

PROCEDURE 12-1   Prepare the Examination Room

Task: To properly prepare the examination room for a patient coming in for a complete physical exam.

Condition: Given the equipment and supplies as listed in the procedure and an exam room that has been staged for cleaning by the instructor (instructor may place artificial body fluids on exam table, simulated contaminated sponges and instruments on trays, mayo stands, sharps containers, etc.), the student will prepare an examination room, adhering to the steps listed below. The student should know what type of exam or procedures were performed prior to cleaning the exam room and the reason for the next patient's visit.

Standards: The student will have five minutes to complete the procedure and will need to score an 85% or above to pass the competency. Automatic failure results if any essential steps are omitted or performed incorrectly.

STEPS START TIME: END TIME:	Points Possible	First Attempt	Second Attempt	Third Attempt
1. Wash your hands and put on disposable gloves, practicing standard precautions.	10			
2. Remove any used exam paper and pillow coverings. Discard in an appropriate container.	10			
3. Perform disinfection/sterilization techniques, using the designated disinfectant cleaner to wipe the exam table surfaces along with any other trays or countertops that have been used during the previous exam. Always clean from an area of lesser concentration to an area of greater concentration.	10			
4. Remove gloves, discard, and wash your hands.	10			
5. Place the exam paper on the exam table. Replace the pillow cover with a clean or new cover.	10			
6. Check the function of the exam table. Is it at the correct height? If you have an electronic table, make certain that the selection controls are working properly.	5			
7. Make sure the lighting is effective.	5			
8. If the exam room contains a sink, be sure paper towels or another method for drying the hands are available and functional.	10			
9. Make sure all supplies and equipment necessary for the exam are well stocked and placed in a location easily accessible. Have gowns and drapes available. Have gloves for the provider in place. This assists the provider with the examination.	5			
10. Make one last visual sweep of the exam room to ensure that all equipment and supplies are ready and available for the next patient exam.	10			
11. If applicable, activate the room indicator to alert workers that the room is ready for the next patient.	5			
Points Earned / Points Possible:	___ / 90			

Points possible reflect importance of step in meeting the task: Important = (5) Essential = (10). Determine score by dividing points earned by total points possible, and multiplying results by 100.

Name _____ Date _____ Score _____

EVALUATION

Evaluator Signature: _____ Date: _____

Evaluator Comments:

Key Competencies		
ABHES	MA.A.1.9.a	Practice standard precautions and perform disinfection/sterilization techniques
	MA.A.1.10.c	Dispose of biohazardous materials
CAAHEP	III.P.5	Perform sterilization procedures
	III.P.10	Demonstrate proper disposal of biohazardous material

Name _____ Date _____ Score _____

COMPETENCY CHECKLIST

PROCEDURE 12-2   Position and Drape the Patient

Task: To assist patients into a variety of common positions that are used for various exams and to drape for privacy.

Condition: Given the equipment and supplies as listed in the procedure and a classmate to play the part of the patient, the student will demonstrate the proper steps for placing patients in a variety of different positions (according to exam type or procedure). The instructor may use a different order for testing from the order listed below.

Standards: The student will have 15 minutes to work through the preliminary steps and each of the listed positions and will need to score an 85% or above to pass the competency. Automatic failure results if any essential steps listed in the preliminary steps are performed incorrectly or omitted. If student misses any steps for one of the listed positions, just that position will need to be repeated.

STEPS START TIME: END TIME:	Points Possible	First Attempt	Second Attempt	Third Attempt
1. Wash your hands and use gloves if necessary, practicing standard precautions.	10			
2. Prepare the exam room, positioning the table into a low flat position, if applicable.	10			
3. Identify the patient using two identifiers, identify yourself, and ***explain the rationale for performance of the procedure, showing awareness of the patient's concerns related to the procedure being performed***.	10			
4. If a gown is to be used, provide this to the patient with instructions on opening in the front or rear. ***Demonstrate the principles of self-boundaries***, and allow the patient privacy to change into the gown. Provide assistance with gowning if requested.	10			
5. Pull out the retractable step to allow the patient to step up and be seated safely on the exam table. Once the patient is seated on the exam table, push in the retractable step and assist the patient into one of the following positions.	10			
Sitting position: a. Explain to the patient how to sit. The patient's legs should be flexed, hanging at a 90° angle over the edge of the table. The thighs should be supported on the exam table. Make certain the patient is sitting in a stable manner and be certain the patient is stable. Provide a drape for privacy and comfort. This should cover the lower extremities and lap area.	10			
Supine position: b. Ask the patient to sit at the end of the exam table. Have the patient lie back on the exam table and extend the table extension to rest the patient's legs on. Place a pillow under the patient's head and shoulders, for comfort. Place a drape over the torso and lower extremities using lengthwise draping procedure for comfort and privacy.	10			
Prone position: c. Ask the patient to sit on the end of the exam table. Have the patient lie back in the supine position and extend the table extension. Instruct the patient to roll toward you and lie on the stomach. Position the patient with the head turned to the side and the arms at the side or above the head. Place a drape on the torso and lower extremities using lengthwise draping procedure for comfort and privacy.	10			

Name _____ Date _____ Score _____

Dorsal recumbent position: d. Ask the patient to sit on the end of the exam table. Have the patient lie back in the supine position and extend the table extension. Ask the patient to bend the knees and place the feet flat on the table. Push the table extension in. Drape the patient using a diagonal draping procedure so that the corner can be easily lifted during the procedure.	10			
Sims' position: e. Ask the patient to sit on the end of the exam table. Have the patient lie back in the supine position and extend the table extension. Ask the patient to roll toward you up onto the left side. Instruct the patient to place the left arm behind the body and the right arm in front of the body. Both legs are flexed slightly with the top leg flexed at a more extreme angle. Drape using diagonal draping procedures for comfort and privacy.	10			
Fowler's position: f. Ask the patient to sit on the end of the exam table. Elevate the head of the exam table to the desired angle (Fowler's is a 90° angle and semi-Fowler's is a 45° angle). Drape the patient using a lengthwise procedure for comfort and privacy.	10			
Lithotomy position: g. Ask the patient to lie in the supine position and pull out the table extension. Extend the stirrups at the end of the exam table and instruct the patient to scoot to the end of the exam table and place the feet in the stirrups; assist the patient, as this is sometimes difficult. Drape the patient with the diamond (diagonal) drape.	10			
Knee-chest position: h. Ask the patient to lie on the exam table in the prone position. Instruct the patient to get on hands and knees and pull the knees as close to the chest as possible. Have the patient turn the head to the side and bend the arms and place them above the head. Drape the patient with the diamond (diagonal) drape.	10			
6. Instruct the patient not to tuck the drape under or around body parts.	5			
Points Earned / Points Possible:	___ / 135			

Points possible reflect importance of step in meeting the task: Important = (5) Essential = (10). Determine score by dividing points earned by total points possible, and multiplying results by 100.

Name _____ Date _____ Score _____

EVALUATION

Evaluator Signature: _____ Date: _____

Evaluator Comments:

Key Competencies			
ABHES	MA.A.1.9.c	Assist provider with general/physical examination	
	MA.A.1.9.d	Assist provider with specialty examination	
CAAHEP	I.P.8	Instruct and prepare a patient for a procedure or a treatment	
	I.P.9	Assist provider with a patient exam	
	I.A.3	Show awareness of a patient's concerns related to the procedure being performed	
	V.A.2	Demonstrate the principles of self-boundaries	
	V.A.4	Explain to a patient the rationale for performance of a procedure	

Name _____   Date _____   Score _____

COMPETENCY CHECKLIST

PROCEDURE 12-3   Assist with the General Physical Examination

Task: To assist the provider with all aspects of a complete physical examination.

Condition: Given the equipment and supplies as listed in the procedure, a classmate to play the part of the patient, and a classmate to play the part of the physician, the student will demonstrate the proper steps for assisting with a general physical exam.

Standards: The student will have 10 minutes to complete the procedure and will need to score an 85% or above to pass the competency. Automatic failure results if any essential steps are omitted or performed incorrectly.

STEPS START TIME: END TIME:	Points Possible	First Attempt	Second Attempt	Third Attempt
1. Prepare the exam room.	10			
2. Wash your hands and use gloves if necessary, practicing standard precautions.	10			
3. Prepare a tray with the equipment necessary.	10			
4. Identify the patient using two identifiers, identify yourself, and *explain the rationale for performance of the examination to the patient, showing awareness of the patient's concerns related to the examination being performed*.	10			
5. Using the patient record, begin screening the patient and obtain vital signs, height, and weight. *Incorporate critical thinking when performing patient assessment.*	10			
6. Allow the patient to use the restroom and collect a specimen if required.	10			
7. Prepare the patient for the procedure or treatment by providing a patient gown and drape. Instruct on the proper way to put on the gown. Inform the patient where personal belongings may be placed and request that cell phones and pagers be turned off.	10			
8. Place the patient in a sitting position and explain to the patient that you will be alerting the provider that the patient is ready for the exam.	10			
9. As the provider examines the patient, assist with the exam as necessary. This includes repositioning and draping the patient, active listening, handing equipment to the provider, altering lights as required, *showing awareness of a patient's concerns*, and chaperoning/reassuring the patient on delicate exams. You may also document items on the patient record as the exam proceeds.	10			
10. Following the examination, assist the patient in sitting and reorienting.	5			
11. Assist the patient from the exam table if needed. Instruct the patient to dress and inform the patient that someone will return to provide further instructions from the provider.	10			
12. Instruct the patient on any directives the provider ordered. Document instructions in the patient record.	10			
13. Accompany the patient to the checkout area and reception area.	5			
Points Earned / Points Possible:	___ / 120			

Points possible reflect importance of step in meeting the task: Important = (5) Essential = (10). Determine score by dividing points earned by total points possible, and multiplying results by 100.

Name _____ Date _____ Score _____

EVALUATION
Evaluator Signature: _____ Date: _____

Evaluator's Comments:

DOCUMENTATION
Instructor Note: Retain work products with competency checklist.
Work Products, Procedure 12-3a (Progress Note) and 12-3b (Flow Sheet). Procedure forms can be downloaded from the student companion website.

Key Competencies		
ABHES	MA.A.1.4.a	Follow documentation guidelines
	MA.A.1.9.c	Assist provider with general/physical examination
CAAHEP	I.P.8	Instruct and prepare a patient for a procedure or a treatment
	I.P.9	Assist provider with a patient exam
	I.A.1	Incorporate critical thinking skills when performing patient assessment
	I.A.3	Show awareness of a patient's concerns related to the procedure being performed
	III.P.3	Perform handwashing
	V.A.4	Explain to a patient the rationale for performance of a procedure
	X.P.3	Document patient care accuratley in the medical record

Name _____ Date _____ Score _____

COMPETENCY CHECKLIST
PROCEDURE 13-1   Snellen Chart Visual Acuity Testing

Task: To use a Snellen chart and screen for distance visual acuity.

Condition: Given the equipment and supplies as listed in the procedure and a classmate to play the part of the patient, the student will perform a visual acuity test, adhering to the steps listed below.

Standards: The student will have 10 minutes to complete the procedure and will need to score an 85% or above to pass the competency. Automatic failure results if any essential steps are omitted or performed incorrectly.

STEPS START TIME: END TIME:	Points Possible	First Attempt	Second Attempt	Third Attempt
1. Wash your hands and assemble the equipment. Clean the occluder with an alcohol wipe and allow it to air dry.	10			
2. Identify the patient using two identifiers, identify yourself, and ***explain the rationale for performance of the procedure, showing awareness of the patient's concerns related to the procedure being performed***. If the patient wears contact lenses, testing should be conducted with contacts. If the patient wears glasses, testing may be conducted both with and without glasses.	10			
3. In a well-lit area, instruct the patient to stand at the mark placed 20 feet from the eye chart. Ask the patient to cover the left eye with the occluder. Ask the patient to read the chart aloud (keeping both eyes open), beginning with the 20/200 line or with one of the several lines above the 20/20 line.	10			
4. Stand next to the chart and point to each line during testing.	10			
5. Record the results as the last line the patient can read without errors. Acuity is recorded as a fraction as follows: R. eye 20/10, L. eye 20/30, both eyes 20/20.	10			
6. ***Incorporating critical thinking skills when performing patient assessment***, observe the patient during the screening for signs of difficulty such as squinting, watering of the eyes, or repositioning of the head.	5			
7. After screening the right eye, repeat the procedure for the left eye and then with both eyes.	10			
8. Clean the occluder with alcohol, wash your hands, and document results in the patient's chart.	10			
Points Earned / Points Possible:	___ / 75			

Points possible reflect importance of step in meeting the task: Important = (5) Essential = (10). Determine score by dividing points earned by total points possible, and multiplying results by 100.

Name _____ Date _____ Score _____

EVALUATION

Evaluator Signature: _____ Date: _____

Evaluator Comments:

DOCUMENTATION

Instructor Note: Retain work products with competency checklist.
Work Product, Procedure 13-1 (Progress Note). Procedure forms can be downloaded from the student companion website.

Key Competencies		
ABHES	MA.A.1.4.a	Follow documentation guidelines
	MA.A.1.9.d	Assist provider with specialty examination
CAAHEP	I.P.9	Assist provider with a patient exam
	I.A.1	Incorporate critical thinking skills when performing patient assessment
	I.A.3	Show awareness of a patient's concerns related to the procedure being performed
	III.P.3	Perform handwashing
	V.A.4	Explain to a patient the rationale for performance of a procedure
	X.P.3	Document patient care accurately in the medical record

Name _____ Date _____ Score _____

COMPETENCY CHECKLIST
PROCEDURE 13-2   Screen Near Visual Acuity

Task: To screen near visual acuity.

Condition: Given the equipment and supplies as listed in the procedure and a classmate to play the part of the patient, the student will perform a near visual acuity test, adhering to the steps listed below.

Standards: The student will have 10 minutes to complete the procedure and will need to score an 85% or above to pass the competency. Automatic failure results if any essential steps are omitted or performed incorrectly.

STEPS START TIME: END TIME:	Points Possible	First Attempt	Second Attempt	Third Attempt
1. Wash your hands, assemble the equipment, and clean the occluder with an alcohol wipe.	10			
2. Identify the patient using two identifiers, identify yourself, and ***explain the rationale for performance of the procedure, showing awareness of the patient's concerns related to the procedure being performed.***	10			
3. With the patient in a sitting position, instruct the patient to hold the card approximately 14 inches from the eyes.	10			
4. Instruct the patient to cover the left eye with the occluder and read the chart (out loud) with the right eye.	10			
5. Record the results as the last line the patient can read without errors.	10			
6. Repeat the procedure for the left eye and both eyes together. The patient should be tested with and without corrective lenses, if worn. (Do not have the patient remove contacts.)	10			
7. Wipe the occluder with an alcohol wipe.	10			
8. Wash your hands and document results in the patient's chart.	10			
Points Earned / Points Possible:	___ / 80			

Points possible reflect importance of step in meeting the task: Important = (5) Essential = (10). Determine score by dividing points earned by total points possible, and multiplying results by 100.

Name _____ Date _____ Score _____

EVALUATION

Evaluator Signature: _____ Date: _____

Evaluator Comments:

DOCUMENTATION

Instructor Note: Retain work products with competency checklist.
Work Product, Procedure 13-2 (Progress Note). Procedure forms can be downloaded from the student companion website.

Key Competencies		
ABHES	MA.A.1.4.a	Follow documentation guidelines
	MA.A.1.9.d	Assist provider with specialty examination
CAAHEP	I.P.9	Assist provider with a patient exam
	I.A.3	Show awareness of a patient's concerns related to the procedure being performed
	III.P.3	Perform handwashing
	V.A.4	Explain to a patient the rationale for performance of a procedure
	X.P.3	Document patient care accurately in the medical record

Name _____ Date _____ Score _____

COMPETENCY CHECKLIST

PROCEDURE 13-3   Ishihara Test for Color Vision

Task: To perform a color vision screening with the Ishihara method.

Condition: Given the equipment and supplies as listed in the procedure and a classmate to play the part of the patient, the student will perform an Ishihara color vision test, adhering to the steps listed below.

Standards: The student will have 10 minutes to complete the procedure and will need to score an 85% or above to pass the competency. Automatic failure results if any essential steps are omitted or performed incorrectly.

STEPS START TIME: END TIME:	Points Possible	First Attempt	Second Attempt	Third Attempt
1. Wash your hands and assemble the equipment.	10			
2. Identify the patient using two identifiers, identify yourself, and ***explain the rationale for performance of the procedure, showing awareness of the patient's concerns related to the procedure being performed.*** The test should be conducted in a room illuminated by daylight.	10			
3. Starting with the practice plate as an example, hold the plate 30 inches from the patient and at a right angle to the patient's field of vision. Instruct the patient to identify the number formed by the colored dots. Patient should only have three seconds to read each line.	10			
4. Repeat the procedure with all plates. *Note:* Lines will have a winding line that the patient will need to trace rather than a number to read. Record the results after each plate.	10			
5. Protect the plates from light when not in use.	10			
6. Wash your hands and document results in the patient's chart.	10			
Points Earned / Points Possible:	___ / 60			

Points possible reflect importance of step in meeting the task: Important = (5) Essential = (10). Determine score by dividing points earned by total points possible, and multiplying results by 100.

Name _____ Date _____ Score _____

EVALUATION

Evaluator Signature: _____ Date: _____

Evaluator Comments:

DOCUMENTATION

Instructor Note: Retain work products with competency checklist.

Work Products, Procedure 13-3a (Progress Note) and 13-3b (Ishihara Recording Form). Procedure forms can be downloaded from the student companion website.

Key Competencies		
ABHES	MA.A.1.4.a	Follow documentation guidelines
	MA.A.1.9.d	Assist provider with specialty examination
CAAHEP	I.P.9	Assist provider with a patient exam
	I.A.3	Show awareness of a patient's concerns related to the procedure being performed
	III.P.3	Perform handwashing
	V.A.4	Explain to a patient the rationale for performance of a procedure
	X.P.3	Document patient care accurately in the medical record

Name _____ Date _____ Score _____

COMPETENCY CHECKLIST

PROCEDURE 13-4   Eye Instillation

Task: To perform an eye instillation.

Condition: Given the equipment and supplies as listed in the procedure and a classmate to play the part of the patient, the student will perform an eye instillation using sterile saline or sterile water, or will simulate performing the procedure, adhering to the steps listed below.

Standards: The student will have 10 minutes to complete the procedure and will need to score an 85% or above to pass the competency. Automatic failure results if any essential steps are omitted or performed incorrectly.

STEPS START TIME: END TIME:	Points Possible	First Attempt	Second Attempt	Third Attempt
1. Wash your hands and assemble the equipment. If the medication has been refrigerated, it must come to room temperature before instilling.	10			
2. Check medication against the provider's orders and look for the word *ophthalmic* on the label. Check the expiration date and check the label three times before administration.	10			
3. Identify the patient using two identifiers, identify yourself, and ***explain to the patient the rationale for performing this procedure, showing awareness of the patient's concerns related to the procedure being performed.***	10			
4. Wash your hands and apply gloves.	10			
5. Place the patient in a sitting or lying position and prepare the medication. For eye drops, withdraw the medication into a sterile dropper. For eye ointment, remove the cap from the tube.	10			
6. Instruct the patient to look up at the ceiling. With your fingers over a tissue, gently pull down on skin to expose the lower conjunctival sac.	10			
7. Instill the correct number of drops into the center of the lower conjunctival sac or place a thin line of ointment along the lower surface of the eyelid. *Do not touch the tip of the medication applicator to the eye.*	10			
8. Instruct the patient to close the eye and roll the eyeball around.	10			
9. Dab excess solution from the eyelid with gauze.	5			
10. *Do not return any unused medication to the bottle.* Discard the unused medication, and return the dropper to the bottle without touching the dropper to the outside of the bottle.	10			
11. Discard used equipment and supplies.	10			
12. Remove gloves and wash your hands.	10			
13. Record the procedure in the patient's chart.	10			
Points Earned / Points Possible:	___ / 125			

Points possible reflect importance of step in meeting the task: Important = (5) Essential = (10). Determine score by dividing points earned by total points possible, and multiplying results by 100.

Name _____ Date _____ Score _____

EVALUATION

Evaluator Signature: _____ Date: _____

Evaluator Comments:

DOCUMENTATION

Instructor Note: Retain work products with competency checklist.

Work Products, Procedure 13-4a (Progress Note) and 13-4b (Patient Medication Log). Procedure forms can be downloaded from the student companion website.

Key Competencies		
ABHES	MA.A.1.4.a	Follow documentation guidelines
	MA.A.1.9.d	Assist provider with specialty examination
CAAHEP	I.P.9	Assist provider with a patient exam
	I.A.3	Show awareness of a patient's concerns related to the procedure being performed
	III.P.3	Perform handwashing
	V.A.4	Explain to a patient the rationale for performance of a procedure
	X.P.3	Document patient care accurately in the medical record

Name _____ Date _____ Score _____

COMPETENCY CHECKLIST
PROCEDURE 13-5   Eye Irrigation

Task: To perform an eye irrigation using a water pick.

Condition: Given the equipment and supplies as listed in the procedure and a classmate to play the part of the patient, the student will simulate performing an eye irrigation, adhering to the steps listed below.

Standards: The student will have 15 minutes to complete the procedure and score an 85% or above to pass the competency. Automatic failure results if any essential steps are omitted or performed incorrectly.

STEPS START TIME: END TIME:	Points Possible	First Attempt	Second Attempt	Third Attempt
1. Wash your hands and assemble the equipment. *Note:* If both eyes are to be irrigated, separate supplies will be needed for each eye.	10			
2. Identify the patient using two identifiers, identify yourself, and ***explain to the patient the rationale for performing this procedure, showing awareness of the patient's concerns related to the procedure being performed***.	10			
3. Place the patient in a sitting or supine position with the head turned toward the affected eye.	10			
4. Check the expiration date of the solution and check the label three times. *Note:* Solution should be warmed to body temperature (99°F or 37.2°C).	10			
5. Place a towel on the patient's shoulder and place a basin beside the affected eye. Wash your hands again and apply gloves.	10			
6. Cleanse the eyelid from the inner to outer canthus with moistened gauze. Discard the gauze after each cleansing.	10			
7. Prepare a water pick with irrigating solution and hold the eye open with the index finger and thumb.	10			
8. Rest the bulb of the water pick on the bridge of the patient's nose. Be careful not to touch the eye or conjunctiva with the tip of the water pick.	10			
9. Instruct the patient to stare at a fixed spot and open the water pick valve, allowing the solution to flow along the lower conjunctiva from the inner to outer canthus and into the basin.	10			
10. After irrigation is complete, dry the eyelid and eyelashes from the inner to outer canthus with gauze.	10			
11. Discard supplies in an appropriate container.	10			
12. Remove gloves, wash your hands, and document the procedure in the patient's chart.	10			
Points Earned / Points Possible:	___ / 120			

Points possible reflect importance of step in meeting the task: Important = (5) Essential = (10). Determine score by dividing points earned by total points possible, and multiplying results by 100.

Name _____ Date _____ Score _____

EVALUATION

Evaluator Signature: _____ Date: _____

Evaluator Comments:

DOCUMENTATION

Instructor Note: Retain work products with competency checklist.

Work Product, Procedure 13-5 (Progress Note). Procedure forms can be downloaded from the student companion website.

Key Competencies			
ABHES	MA.A.1.4.a	Follow documentation guidelines	
	MA.A.1.9.d	Assist provider with specialty examination	
CAAHEP	I.P.9	Assist provider with a patient exam	
	I.A.3	Show awareness of a patient's concerns related to the procedure being performed	
	III.P.3	Perform handwashing	
	V.A.4	Explain to a patient the rationale for performance of a procedure	
	X.P.3	Document patient care accurately in the medical record	

Name _____ Date _____ Score _____

COMPETENCY CHECKLIST

PROCEDURE 13-6   Hearing Acuity Test

Task: To test a patient's hearing, to determine and define hearing deficits.

Condition: Given the equipment and supplies as listed in the procedure and a classmate to play the part of the patient, the student will perform a hearing acuity test, adhering to the steps listed below.

Standards: The student will have 15 minutes to complete the procedure and score an 85% or above to pass the competency. Automatic failure results if any essential steps are omitted or performed incorrectly.

STEPS START TIME: END TIME:	Points Possible	First Attempt	Second Attempt	Third Attempt
1. Review the provider's order, wash your hands, and assemble the equipment.	10			
2. Identify the patient using two identifiers, identify yourself, and **explain to the patient the rationale for performing this procedure, showing awareness of the patient's concerns related to the procedure being performed**.	10			
3. Seat the patient in a comfortable chair in a quiet, soundproof room. Provide headphones to the patient to place over the ears.	10			
4. Instruct the patient to raise the left hand if a sound is heard in the left ear, and the right hand if a sound is heard in the right ear. (Do not allow patient to see you pressing the buttons.)	10			
5. Record your findings on a special graphic form or in the patient's chart.	10			
Points Earned / Points Possible:	___ / 50			

Points possible reflect importance of step in meeting the task: Important = (5) Essential = (10). Determine score by dividing points earned by total points possible, and multiplying results by 100.

Name _____ Date _____ Score _____

EVALUATION

Evaluator Signature: _____ Date: _____

Evaluator Comments:

DOCUMENTATION

Instructor Note: Retain work products with competency checklist.

Work Product, Procedure 13-6 (Progress Note). Procedure forms can be downloaded from the student companion website.

Key Competencies		
ABHES	MA.A.1.4.a	Follow documentation guidelines
	MA.A.1.9.d	Assist provider with specialty examination
CAAHEP	I.P.9	Assist provider with a patient exam
	I.A.3	Show awareness of a patient's concerns related to the procedure being performed
	III.P.3	Perform handwashing
	V.A.4	Explain to a patient the rationale for performance of a procedure
	X.P.3	Document patient care accurately in the medical record

Name _____ Date _____ Score _____

COMPETENCY CHECKLIST
PROCEDURE 13-7   Ear Instillation

Task: To perform an ear instillation.

Condition: Given the equipment and supplies as listed in the procedure and a classmate to play the part of the patient, the student will simulate performing an ear instillation, adhering to the steps listed below.

Standards: The student will have five minutes to complete the procedure and will need to score an 85% or above to pass the competency. Automatic failure results if any essential steps are omitted or performed incorrectly.

STEPS START TIME: END TIME:	Points Possible	First Attempt	Second Attempt	Third Attempt
1. Wash your hands and assemble the equipment.	10			
2. Identify the patient using two identifiers, identify yourself, and ***explain to the patient the rationale for performing this procedure, showing awareness of the patient's concerns related to the procedure being performed.***	10			
3. Check the medication against the provider's orders and check the medication three times. Check the expiration date of the medication and verify that the medication is for otic use.	10			
4. Instruct the patient to lie with affected ear up or to sit with head slightly tilted toward the unaffected ear. Place a towel on the patient's shoulder of the affected side.	10			
5. Apply gloves.	10			
6. Grasp the top of the ear and pull up and back for adults, or grasp the earlobe and pull down and back for children under three.	10			
7. Instill the prescribed amount of medication into the ear canal by depressing the rubber bulb of the dropper. *Do not touch the tip of the dropper to the ear.*	10			
8. Instruct the patient to keep the head tilted toward the unaffected side for approximately five minutes.	10			
9. Insert a slightly moistened cotton ball into the ear canal (per the provider's orders) and instruct the patient to leave it in place for 15 minutes.	10			
10. Dispose of used equipment and supplies.	10			
11. Remove gloves and wash your hands.	10			
12. Document the procedure in the patient's chart.	10			
Points Earned / Points Possible:	___ / 120			

Points possible reflect importance of step in meeting the task: Important = (5) Essential = (10). Determine score by dividing points earned by total points possible, and multiplying results by 100.

Name _____ Date _____ Score _____

EVALUATION

Evaluator Signature: _____ Date: _____

Evaluator Comments:

DOCUMENTATION

Instructor Note: Retain work products with competency checklist.
Work Product, Procedure 13-7a (Progress Note) and 13-7b (Patient Medication Log). Procedure forms can be downloaded from the student companion website.

Key Competencies			
ABHES	MA.A.1.4.a	Follow documentation guidelines	
	MA.A.1.9.d	Assist provider with specialty examinations	
CAAHEP	I.P.9	Assist provider with a patient exam	
	I.A.3	Show awareness of a patient's concerns related to the procedure being performed	
	III.P.3	Perform handwashing	
	V.A.4	Explain to a patient the rationale for performance of a procedure	
	X.P.3	Document patient care accurately in the medical record	

Name _____ Date _____ Score _____

COMPETENCY CHECKLIST
PROCEDURE 13-8   Ear Irrigation

Task: To perform an ear irrigation.

Condition: Given the equipment and supplies as listed in the procedure and a classmate to play the part of the patient, the student will simulate performing an ear irrigation, adhering to the steps listed below.

Standards: The student will have 15 minutes to complete the procedure and will need to score an 85% or above to pass the competency. Automatic failure results if any essential steps are omitted or performed incorrectly.

STEPS START TIME: END TIME:	Points Possible	First Attempt	Second Attempt	Third Attempt
1. Wash your hands and assemble the equipment and supplies. Check the name and strength of irrigation solution as well as the expiration date. (Label should be checked 3×.)	10			
2. Identify the patient using two identifiers, identify yourself, and *explain to the patient the rationale for performing this procedure, showing awareness of the patient's concerns related to the procedure being performed*.	10			
3. Place the patient in a sitting position with the head tilted to the affected side.	10			
4. Place a towel or impervious drape over the patient's shoulder and instruct the patient to hold an ear or emesis basin under the affected ear and against the neck.	10			
5. Apply gloves and pour sterile irrigating liquid into sterile/clean basin.	10			
6. Fill irrigating syringe or device with warmed irrigating solution (around 99 degrees F [37.2 degrees C] to 100 degrees F [37.8 degrees C]). If using syringes, expel any air at the top of syringe.	10			
7. Gently pull the top of the ear up and back in adults and down and back in children three and under.	10			
8. Insert the tip of the irrigation syringe into the ear canal. Aim the irrigation solution so it flows up toward the roof of the ear canal.	10			
9. Continue the process until the desired effects are obtained.	10			
10. Dry the outer ear and if office protocol, check the inner ear with an otoscope to determine removal of foreign matter.	10			
11. Remove the towel from patient's shoulder and ear basin and have the patient lie on the affected side with towel under her head on the exam table.	10			
12. After five to ten minutes, have provider check ear for clearance of debris.	10			
13. Remove gloves and wash your hands.	10			
14. Document the procedure in the patient's chart. (Make certain you summarize what was in the return basin.)	10			
Points Earned / Points Possible:	___ / 140			

Points possible reflect importance of step in meeting the task: Important = (5) Essential = (10). Determine score by dividing points earned by total points possible, and multiplying results by 100.

Name _____ Date _____ Score _____

EVALUATION

Evaluator Signature: _____ Date: _____

Evaluator Comments:

DOCUMENTATION

Instructor Note: Retain work products with competency checklist.
Work Product, Procedure 13-8 (Progress Note). Procedure forms can be downloaded from the student companion website.

Key Competencies		
ABHES	MA.A.1.4.a	Follow documentation guidelines
	MA.A.1.9.d	Assist provider with specialty examination
CAAHEP	I.P.9	Assist provider with a patient exam
	I.A.3	Show awareness of a patient's concerns related to the procedure being performed
	III.P.3	Perform handwashing
	V.A.4	Explain to a patient the rationale for performance of a procedure
	X.P.3	Document patient care accurately in the medical record

Name _____ Date _____ Score _____

COMPETENCY CHECKLIST

PROCEDURE 14-1   Perform a Standard 12-Lead Electrocardiogram with a Multichannel Unit

Task: To perform a standard 12-lead electrocardiogram, free from artifacts and interference.

Condition: Given the equipment and supplies as listed in the procedure and a classmate to play the part of the patient, the student will perform a 12-lead ECG, adhering to the steps listed below.

Standards: The student will have 15 minutes to complete the procedure and will need to score an 85% or above to pass the competency. Automatic failure results if any essential steps are omitted or performed incorrectly.

STEPS: START TIME: END TIME:	Points Possible	First Attempt	Second Attempt	Third Attempt
1. Perform the ECG in a quiet, warm, and comfortable room away from other electrical equipment.	10			
2. Wash your hands and assemble all equipment.	10			
3. Identify the patient using at least two identifiers, identify yourself, and ***explain the rationale for the performance of the procedure*** and why it is important not to move or talk during the tracing.	10			
4. ***Show awareness of a patient's concerns related to the procedure being performed.***	5			
5. ***Intervene on behalf of the patient regarding issues/concerns that may arise.***	5			
6. Instruct the patient to remove all clothing from the waist up and to expose the lower legs. Provide drape and cape and instruct patient to put the cape on so it opens in the front.	10			
7. Prep the patient's skin by scrubbing areas where the electrodes are to be placed with alcohol and drying with a 4 × 4 gauze pad until the skin turns slightly pink. (Dry shave areas on men that are particularly hairy.)	10			
8. Place the limb electrodes on the fleshy part of the upper arm and the inner part of the calf midway between the knee and the ankle. (Electrode tabs on the arms should be facing downward, electrode tabs on the legs should be facing upward.)	10			
9. Place all six chest electrodes in the correct positions on the chest by counting down the correct intercostal spaces and locating the proper landmarks. Do not trust your eyes alone. (Electrode pad tabs should be facing downward for all chest electrodes.)	10			
10. Securely connect all lead wires to the corresponding electrodes following the body's natural contour. Be sure that lead wires are pointed downward on the legs and upward on the arms and chest. (Confirm that leads are not pulling upward once the wires are connected. If they are, make the proper adjustments.) The patient cable should lie over the patient's abdomen.	10			
11. Connect the patient cable to the machine and turn machine to the "ON" position. Enter the patient's data into the unit by using the keypad. Requested information may include the patient's name, age, gender, height, weight, and any cardiac medications currently being taken.	10			
12. Press the auto run button on the machine and allow the tracing to be recorded. Observe the standardization mark for accuracy.	10			

Name _____ Date _____ Score _____

13. Observe the tracing for problems or artifacts. ***Incorporate critical thinking skills*** when a problem is identified. Determine if any changes are needed with regard to the amplitude of the beats (gain or sensitivity control) or the heart's rhythm (paper speed).	10				
14. Allow the provider to briefly scan the tracing before disconnecting the patient from the machine.	5				
15. Disconnect the lead wires and remove the electrodes from the patient.	10				
16. Clean the equipment following manufacturer's guidelines. Replace tracing paper as needed.	5				
17. Wash your hands and document the procedure.	10				
18. Place the tracing in the patient's chart or upload into the patient's EHR.	10				
Points Earned / Points Possible:	___ / 160				

Points possible reflect importance of step in meeting the task: Important = (5) Essential = (10). Determine score by dividing points earned by total points possible, and multiplying results by 100.

EVALUATION

Evaluator Signature: _____ Date: _____

Evaluator Comments:

DOCUMENTATION

Instructor Note: Retain work products, along with completed ECG tracing, with competency checklist.
Work Product, Procedure 14-1 (Progress Note). Procedure forms can be downloaded from the student companion website.

Key Competencies		
ABHES	MA.A.1.4.a	Follow documentation guidelines
	MA.A.1.5.c	Intervene on behalf of the patient regarding issues/concerns that may arise, i.e., insurance policy information, medical bills, physician/provider orders, etc.
	MA.A.1.9.e	Perform specialty procedures including but not limited to minor surgery, cardiac, respiratory, OB-GYN, neurological, gastroenterology
CAAHEP	I.P.2.a	Perform electrocardiography
	I.A.2	Incorporate critical thinking skills when performing patient care
	I.A.3	Show awareness of a patient's concerns related to the procedure being performed
	III.P.3	Perform handwashing
	V.A.4	Explain to a patient the rationale for performance of a procedure
	X.P.3	Document patient care accurately in the medical record

Name _____ Date _____ Score _____

COMPETENCY CHECKLIST

PROCEDURE 14-2   Apply the Holter Monitor

Task: To correctly apply a Holter monitor and properly educate the patient on how to care for the monitor and electrodes, and instruct the patient on what events need to be written in the event journal or diary.

Condition: Given the equipment and supplies as listed in the procedure and a classmate to play the part of the patient, the student will apply a Holter monitor, adhering to the steps listed below.

Standards: The student will have 15 minutes to complete the procedure and will need to score an 85% or above to pass the competency. Automatic failure results if any essential steps are omitted or performed incorrectly.

STEPS START TIME: END TIME:	Points Possible	First Attempt	Second Attempt	Third Attempt
1. Wash your hands and assemble the equipment and read manufacturer's instructions. Check expiration date on electrodes. Make certain memory or flash card is in the recorder and place a new battery in the monitor following polarity diagram that came with your unit.	10			
2. Complete necessary forms and set up the patient diary by entering required information.	10			
3. Identify the patient using at least two identifiers, identify yourself, and *explain the rationale for the performance of the procedure*. Instruct the patient to disrobe from the waist up and to put a gown on so it opens in the front.	10			
4. *Show awareness of a patient's concerns related to the procedure being performed.*	5			
5. If applicable, *intervene on behalf of the patient regarding issues/ concerns* that arise when explaining the procedure.	5			
6. Prep the patient's skin: Dry shave hair, if necessary, and rub the area of skin where electrodes will be placed with an alcohol swab. Next, abrade the skin with dry gauze or prepackaged pads.	10			
7. If applicable, spread a small amount of compound benzoin tincture over the area in which each electrode will be placed.	10			
8. Remove the electrodes from the package and study the manufacturer's electrode placement diagram to see which electrode/wire will be placed on the chest first, second, third, and so on. Attach the lead wires to the electrodes in the order they will be applied to the chest.	10			
9. Peel the backing from the electrode and check to make certain the electrolyte is moist. Correctly place disposable electrodes on the proper landmarks of the chest one at a time until all electrodes have been placed on the chest.	10			
10. Be sure the electrodes adhere firmly to the skin by applying gentle pressure around the outer border of each electrode. (Avoid pressing on the center of the electrode pad as this may cause the electrolyte gel or solution to seep from the pad.)	10			
11. Make a stress loop for each electrode and wire and reinforce the electrodes to the skin with a piece of nonallergenic tape if necessary.	10			
12. Connect the patient cable to the patient input connector on the monitor and turn on the unit following manufacturer's instructions.	10			
13. Review the waveform on the LCD advancing through each channel to verify proper connection. (Follow manufacturer's instructions for this process.) *Incorporate critical thinking skills* when a problem is identified.	10			

Name _____ Date _____ Score _____

14. Make certain that the date and time are set correctly; if not, make necessary adjustments.	10			
15. Note the start time on the Holter explanation sheet and in the patient's diary. Show the patient the location of the event button and explain what should be recorded in the diary and how to care for the monitor. Refer to Health Coach (Holter Monitor Patient Pointers) for a full list of instructions that should be shared with each patient.	10			
16. Specify the exact time the patient should return to the office for removal of the monitor. (The latest models will automatically stop recording after the 24-hour period is completed). The patient should be instructed how to remove the electrodes and secure the monitor for safe keeping.	10			
17. Insert recorder in the pouch and secure the pouch to the patient's body using the belt or lanyard provided by the manufacturer.	10			
18. Dismiss the patient and wash your hands and document the procedure in the patient's chart.	10			
Points Earned / Points Possible:	___ / 170			

Points possible reflect importance of step in meeting the task: Important = (5) Essential = (10). Determine score by dividing points earned by total points possible, and multiplying results by 100.

EVALUATION

Evaluator Signature: _____ Date: _____

Evaluator Comments:

DOCUMENTATION

Instructor Note: Retain work products with competency checklist.
Work Product, Procedure 14-2 (Progress Note). Procedure forms can be downloaded from the student companion website.

Key Competencies			
ABHES	MA.A.1.4.a	Follow documentation guidelines	
	MA.A.1.5.c	Intervene on behalf of the patient regarding issues/concerns that may arise, i.e., insurance policy information, medical bills, physician/provider orders, etc.	
	MA.A.1.9.e	Perform specialty procedures including but not limited to minor surgery, cardiac, respiratory, OB-GYN, neurological, gastroenterology	
CAAHEP	I.P.2.a	Perform electrocardiography	
	I.A.2	Incorporate critical thinking skills when performing patient care	
	I.A.3	Show awareness of a patient's concerns related to the procedure being performed	
	III.P.3	Perform handwashing	
	V.A.4	Explain to a patient the rationale for performance of a procedure	
	X.P.3	Document patient care accurately in the medical record	

Name _____ Date _____ Score _____

COMPETENCY CHECKLIST

PROCEDURE 15-1 Perform a Spirometry Test

Task: To perform a spirometry test.

Condition: Given the equipment and supplies as listed in the procedure and a classmate to play the part of the patient, the student will perform a spirometry test, adhering to the steps listed below.

Standards: The student will have 15 minutes to complete the procedure and will need to score an 85% or above to pass the competency. Automatic failure results if any essential steps are omitted or performed incorrectly.

STEPS START TIME: END TIME:	Points Possible	First Attempt	Second Attempt	Third Attempt
1. Wash your hands, apply gloves, and gather the equipment.	10			
2. Calibrate the machine following the manufacturer's instructions.	10			
3. Greet and identify the patient using two identifiers.	10			
4. Introduce yourself and *explain to the patient the rationale for performance of the procedure, showing awareness of the patient's concerns related to the procedure being performed.*	10			
5. Measure the patient's height and weight if not already performed.	10			
6. Have the patient remove constricting clothing, such as belts and sports bras.	10			
7. Position the patient so that the patient is comfortable and safe.	10			
8. Program the unit with the patient's information. Information may include: the patient's name, sex, height, weight, and medication information.	10			
9. Place the nose clip on the patient's nose.	10			
10. Have the patient inhale as deeply as possible and place the mouthpiece in the mouth. (Some units have the patient take in a deep breath when the tube is in the mouth.) Seal with lips. If the patient has dentures, they are to be left in.	10			
11. Have the patient quickly and forcefully exhale following the prompts on the screen. (Press the start button according to manufacturer's instructions.)	10			
12. Repeat the test two more times. Record the results from the spirometer and attach the printout to the chart.	10			
13. If ordered, provide medication to the patient.	10			
14. Repeat the spirometry procedure, if ordered.	5			
15. Document or attach the results.	10			
16. Discard the test products and clean the equipment.	10			
Points Earned / Points Possible:	___ / 155			

Points possible reflect importance of step in meeting the task: Important = (5) Essential = (10). Determine score by dividing points earned by total points possible, and multiplying results by 100.

Name _____ Date _____ Score _____

EVALUATION

Evaluator Signature: _____ Date: _____

Evaluator Comments:

DOCUMENTATION

Instructor Note: Retain work products, along with completed PFT results, with competency checklist.
Work Product, Procedure 15-1 (Progress Note). Procedure forms can be downloaded from the student companion website.

Key Competencies		
ABHES	MA.A.1.4.a	Follow documentation guidelines
	MA.A.1.9.e	Perform specialty procedures including but not limited to minor surgery, cardiac, respiratory, OB-GYN, neurological, gastroenterology
CAAHEP	I.P.2.d	Perform pulmonary function testing
	I.A.3	Show awareness of a patient's concerns related to the procedure being performed
	III.P.3	Perform handwashing
	V.A.4	Explain to a patient the rationale for performance of a procedure
	X.P.3	Document patient care accurately in the medical record

Name _____ Date _____ Score _____

COMPETENCY CHECKLIST
PROCEDURE 15-2   Performing Peak Flow Testing

Task: To correctly perform peak flow testing, and train the patient in home testing and how to interpret results according to the individualized Asthma Action Plan.

Condition: Given the equipment and supplies as listed in the procedure and a classmate to play the part of the patient, the student will perform a spirometry test, adhering to the steps listed below.

Standards: The student will have 10 minutes to complete the procedure and will need to score an 85% or above to pass the competency. Automatic failure results if any essential steps are omitted or performed incorrectly.

STEPS START TIME: END TIME:	Points Possible	First Attempt	Second Attempt	Third Attempt
1. Assemble the equipment, including individualized Asthma Action Plan.	10			
2. Identify the patient using two identifiers, introduce yourself, and ***explain the rationale for performance of the procedure, showing awareness of the patient's concerns related to the procedure being performed***.	10			
3. Wash your hands and apply gloves.	10			
4. Have the patient remove all gum and food from mouth.	5			
5. Start pointer on flow meter at 0.	10			
6. Have the patient take in a deep breath.	10			
7. Have the patient place the mouthpiece in mouth behind the teeth, with lips tightly sealed around the tube. Move tongue out of the way.	10			
8. Direct the patient to breathe out as fast and hard as possible.	10			
9. Record the results from the gauge; move it back to 0.	10			
10. Repeat two more times.	10			
11. Record the highest reading of the three attempts.	5			
12. If providing education, give patient peak flow meter, directions, and results of personal best reading to take home.	5			
13. Reference personal best value with their Asthma Action Plan to determine if a change in treatment is indicated at the present time.	10			
Points Earned / Points Possible:	___ / 115			

Points possible reflect importance of step in meeting the task: Important = (5) Essential = (10). Determine score by dividing points earned by total points possible, and multiplying results by 100.

Name _____ Date _____ Score _____

EVALUATION

Evaluator Signature: _____ Date: _____

Evaluator Comments:

DOCUMENTATION

Instructor Note: Retain work products, along with completed PFT results, with competency checklist.
Work Product, Procedure 15-2 (Progress Note). Procedure forms can be downloaded from the student companion website.

Key Competencies			
ABHES	MA.A.1.4.a	Follow documentation guidelines	
	MA.A.1.9.e	Perform specialty procedures including but not limited to minor surgery, cardiac, respiratory, OB-GYN, neurological, gastroenterology	
CAAHEP	I.P.2.d	Perform pulmonary function testing	
	I.A.3	Show awareness of a patient's concerns related to the procedure being performed	
	III.P.3	Perform handwashing	
	V.A.4	Explain to a patient the rationale for performance of a procedure	
	X.P.3	Document patient care accurately in the medical record	

Name _____ Date _____ Score _____

COMPETENCY CHECKLIST

PROCEDURE 15-3   Perform Pulse Oximetry

Task: To correctly apply a pulse oximeter to the patient and obtain an accurate reading.

Condition: Given the equipment and supplies as listed in the procedure and a classmate to play the part of the patient, the student will perform pulse oximetry, adhering to the steps listed below.

Standards: The student will have 10 minutes to complete the procedure and will need to score an 85% or above to pass the competency. Automatic failure results if any essential steps are omitted or performed incorrectly.

STEPS START TIME: END TIME:	Points Possible	First Attempt	Second Attempt	Third Attempt
1. Identify the patient using two identifiers, and introduce yourself.	10			
2. Wash your hands and *explain to the patient the rationale for performance of the procedure, showing awareness of the patient's concerns related to the procedure being performed.*	10			
3. Have the patient remove nail polish, if necessary, and wash the hands with soap and water. Hands should be rinsed well and dried.	10			
4. Apply the pulse oximeter probe and observe the perfusion indicator. Observe both the heart rate and the SpO_2 levels.	10			
5. Leave the oximeter probe attached to the patient and give the findings to the provider. If the saturation rate is below 95%, notify the provider as soon as possible.	10			
6. Continue to monitor as long as the provider wants the patient monitored. (The patient may need to receive oxygen if oxygen is poor.)	10			
7. Remove the probe once the provider orders the probe to be removed.	5			
8. Record the results in the chart and assist the patient.	10			
Points Earned / Points Possible:	___ / 75			

Points possible reflect importance of step in meeting the task: Important = (5) Essential = (10). Determine score by dividing points earned by total points possible, and multiplying results by 100.

Name _____ Date _____ Score _____

EVALUATION

Evaluator Signature: _____ Date: _____

Evaluator Comments:

DOCUMENTATION

Instructor Note: Retain work products with competency checklist.

Work Product, Procedure 15-3 (Progress Note). Procedure forms can be downloaded from the student companion website.

Key Competencies		
ABHES	MA.A.1.4.a	Follow documentation guidelines
	MA.A.1.9.e	Perform specialty procedures including but not limited to minor surgery, cardiac, respiratory, OB-GYN, neurological, gastroenterology
CAAHEP	I.P.1.i	Measure and record pulse oximetry
	I.A.3	Show awareness of a patient's concerns related to the procedure being performed
	III.P.3	Perform handwashing
	V.A.4	Explain to a patient the rationale for performance of a procedure
	X.P.3	Document patient care accurately in the medical record

Name _____ Date _____ Score _____

COMPETENCY CHECKLIST

PROCEDURE 15-4   Obtain a Sputum Specimen and Prepare a Smear

Task: To instruct and assist the patient on obtaining a viable sputum specimen that is free of saliva and obtained from deep coughing; prepare a smear.

Condition: Given the equipment and supplies as listed in the procedure and a classmate to play the part of the patient, the student will instruct a patient how to obtain a sputum specimen and will prepare a smear, adhering to the steps listed below.

Standards: The student will have 10 minutes to complete the procedure and will need to score an 85% or above to pass the competency. Automatic failure results if any essential steps are omitted or performed incorrectly.

STEPS START TIME: END TIME:	Points Possible	First Attempt	Second Attempt	Third Attempt
Obtaining a Sputum Specimen				
1. Assemble the equipment and properly label the specimen container.	10			
2. Identify the patient using two identifiers, introduce yourself, and ***explain the rationale for performance of the procedure, showing awareness of the patient's concerns related to the procedure being performed.***	10			
3. Wash your hands and put on all of your PPE.	10			
4. Have the patient rinse out the mouth.	10			
5. Carefully remove the lid from the specimen cup and place on the counter without contaminating it.	10			
6. Instruct the patient to take in three deep breaths and to start forcefully coughing.	10			
7. Ask patient to expectorate into the center of the specimen container.	10			
8. Place the lid on the container without contaminating it and tighten it securely. Place the container in a plastic laboratory specimen bag.	10			
9. Insert the completed lab slip and send to the lab for analysis.	10			
Preparing the Smear				
1. Wash hands, apply PPE, and label the slide. Smear the sputum on a microscopic slide.	10			
2. Squeeze one drop of potassium hydroxide over the smear and place a cover slip over the smear.	10			
3. Place the slide under the microscope on low power for the provider.	10			
4. Clean the area and remove PPE. Throw PPE into appropriate trash or biohazard container.	10			
Points Earned / Points Possible:	___ / 130			

Points possible reflect importance of step in meeting the task: Important = (5) Essential = (10). Determine score by dividing points earned by total points possible, and multiplying results by 100.

Name _____   Date _____   Score _____

EVALUATION

Evaluator Signature: _____   Date: _____

Evaluator Comments:

DOCUMENTATION

Instructor Note: Retain work products with competency checklist.

Work Products, Procedure 15-4a (Progress Note) and 15-4b (Lab Requisition Form). Procedure forms can be downloaded from the student companion website.

Key Competencies		
ABHES	MA.A.1.10.c	Dispose of biohazardous materials
	MA.A.1.10.e(3)	Instruct patients in the collection of sputum specimens
CAAHEP	I.P.11.e	Obtain specimens and perform CLIA waived microbiology test
	I.A.3	Show awareness of a patient's concerns related to the procedure being performed
	III.P.2	Select appropriate barrier/personal protective equipment (PPE)
	III.P.3	Perform handwashing
	III.P.10.b	Demonstrate proper disposal of biohazardous material: regulated waste
	V.A.4	Explain to a patient the rationale for performance of a procedure

Name _____ Date _____ Score _____

COMPETENCY CHECKLIST

PROCEDURE 15-5   Administer a Nebulizer Treatment

Task: To correctly set up the nebulizer unit, select the correct medication, and administer a breathing treatment using a nebulizer.

Condition: Given the equipment and supplies as listed in the procedure and a classmate to play the part of the patient, the student will correctly simulate administering a nebulizer treatment, adhering to the steps listed below.

Standards: The student will have 15 minutes to complete the procedure and will need to score an 85% or above to pass the competency. Automatic failure results if any essential steps are omitted or performed incorrectly.

Procedure Scenario Information

Physician's Order: 2.5 mg Albuterol via Inhalation Therapy

STEPS START TIME: END TIME:	Points Possible	First Attempt	Second Attempt	Third Attempt
1. Prepare the equipment.	10			
2. Identify the patient using two identifiers, introduce yourself, and **explain to the patient the rationale for performance of the procedure, showing awareness of the patient's concerns related to the procedure being performed.**	10			
3. Wash your hands and put on gloves.	10			
4. Check order (three times) and pour the correct amount of medication and diluent into the medication dispenser. Screw the lid on the dispenser and gently mix the medication.	10			
5. Connect the medication dispenser to the mouthpiece or face mask.	10			
6. Connect the disposable tubing to the medication dispenser and nebulizer.	10			
7. Place the patient in a full Fowler's position or upright position.	10			
8. Turn the nebulizer on. When you turn the nebulizer on, you should see a mist.	10			
9. If using a face mask, place it over the patient's face so that it fits comfortably. If using a mouthpiece, instruct patient to place it in the mouth between the teeth and to purse the lips over the mouthpiece making a seal.	10			
10. Instruct the patient to take in slow deep breaths that last anywhere from two to three seconds.	10			
11. Continue treatment until the mist disappears.	5			
12. Turn off the nebulizer and remove and dispose of the mouthpiece or face mask, medicine dispenser, and tubing into the biohazard trash can.	10			
13. Instruct the patient to take in several deep breaths and to try and cough up any secretions that were loosened during the treatment.	10			
14. Wash your hands and document the procedure.	10			
15. Give the patient home care instructions.	10			
Points Earned / Points Possible:	___ / 145			

Points possible reflect importance of step in meeting the task: Important = (5) Essential = (10). Determine score by dividing points earned by total points possible, and multiplying results by 100.

Name _____ Date _____ Score _____

EVALUATION

Evaluator Signature: _____ Date: _____

Evaluator Comments:

DOCUMENTATION

Instructor Note: Retain work products with competency checklist.
Work Products, Procedure 15-5a (Progress Note) and 15-5b (Patient Medication Log). Procedure forms can be downloaded from the student companion website.

Key Competencies			
ABHES	MA.A.1.4.a	Follow documentation guidelines	
	MA.A.1.9.e	Perform specialty procedures including but not limited to minor surgery, cardiac, respiratory, OB-GYN, neurological, gastroenterology	
	MA.A.1.10.c	Dispose of biohazardous materials	
CAAHEP	I.P.7	Administer parenteral (excluding IV) medications	
	I.A.3	Show awareness of a patient's concerns related to the procedure being performed	
	III.P.3	Perform handwashing	
	III.P.10.b	Demonstrate proper disposal of biohazardous material: regulated waste	
	V.A.4	Explain to a patient the rationale for performance of a procedure	
	X.P.3	Document patient care accurately in the medical record	

Name _____ Date _____ Score _____

COMPETENCY CHECKLIST

PROCEDURE 16-1   Instruct the Patient on How to Collect a Fecal Specimen

Task: To instruct the patient on how to collect and preserve a fecal specimen.

Condition: Given the equipment and supplies as listed in the procedure and a classmate to play the part of the patient, the student will instruct the patient on the proper method for collecting a fecal specimen, adhering to the steps listed below.

Standards: The student will have 10 minutes to complete the procedure and will need to score an 85% or above to pass the competency. Automatic failure results if any essential steps are omitted or performed incorrectly.

STEPS START TIME: END TIME:	Points Possible	First Attempt	Second Attempt	Third Attempt
1. Assemble all the equipment, complete lab requisition forms, and adhere label with patient's information on specimen container.	10			
2. Identify the patient using two identifiers and identify yourself.	10			
3. Explain the provider's orders and ***rationale for ordering the procedure to the patient, showing awareness of the patient's concerns related to the procedure being performed***.	10			
4. Instruct patient to write the date and time of collection on the affixed label prior to collection.	10			
5. Instruct the patient to fully empty the bladder before the collection procedure starts. Stress the importance of not contaminating the specimen with urine, toilet tissue, or any other foreign material.	10			
6. Instruct the patient to lift the toilet seat and place the toilet hat in the bowl, following manufacturer's instructions.	10			
7. Instruct the patient to use the tongue depressors or collection spoons to collect a small portion (approximately three to four tablespoons) of the next bowel movement from different sections of the stool and to place it in the specimen container.	10			
8. Instruct the patient to place the lid tightly onto the specimen container and to return the specimen to the office or laboratory within two hours of collection. If the specimen is to be tested for O&P, it must not be refrigerated.	10			
9. Provide the patient with a copy of the printed instructions.	10			
10. Document the procedure in the patient record.	10			
Points Earned / Points Possible:	___ / 100			

Points possible reflect importance of step in meeting the task: Important = (5) Essential = (10). Determine score by dividing points earned by total points possible, and multiplying results by 100.

Name _____ Date _____ Score _____

EVALUATION

Evaluator Signature: _____ Date: _____

Evaluator Comments:

DOCUMENTATION

Instructor Note: Retain work products with competency checklist.

Work Product, Procedure 16-1 (Progress Note). Procedure forms can be downloaded from the student companion website.

Key Competencies		
ABHES	MA.A.1.4.a	Follow documentation guidelines
	MA.A.1.10.e(2)	Instruct patients in the collection of fecal specimen
CAAHEP	I.A.3	Show awareness of a patient's concerns related to the procedure being performed
	V.A.4	Explain to a patient the rationale for performance of a procedure
	X.P.3	Document patient care accurately in the medical record

Name _____ Date _____ Score _____

COMPETENCY CHECKLIST

PROCEDURE 16-2 Perform a Fecal Occult Blood Test

Task: To perform a fecal occult blood test.

Condition: Given the equipment and supplies as listed in the procedure and a classmate to play the part of the patient, the student will perform a fecal occult blood test, adhering to the steps listed below.

Standards: The student will have 10 minutes to complete the procedure and will need to score an 85% or above to pass the competency. Automatic failure results if any essential steps are omitted or performed incorrectly.

STEPS START TIME: END TIME:	Points Possible	First Attempt	Second Attempt	Third Attempt
1. Assemble the supplies.	10			
2. Identify the patient using two identifiers and identify yourself.	10			
3. ***Explain to the patient the rationale for performance of the procedure, showing awareness of the patient's concerns related to the procedure.***	10			
4. Explain special dietary instructions for the patient to follow prior to collecting the specimen, ***showing awareness of the patient's concerns regarding a dietary change.*** Start collection with the first bowel movement following three days of dietary restriction. Patients on NSAIDs or Aspirin should restrict these medications for seven days prior to testing.	10			
5. Explain how to properly collect a stool sample following the directions in Procedure 16-1.	10			
6. Explain how to properly label the cards prior to collection.	10			
7. Explain instructions for collecting the samples, and the number of samples the patient is to collect. Most guaiac test slides have two windows for each slide (A&B). The patient is to obtain a tiny section of stool using the provided spatula or spoon from one part of the stool and to spread a thin film of the stool in window A and to repeat the procedure using a different section of the stool for window B. Instruct the patient to close the front flap of the collection slide.	10			
8. Instruct the patient to repeat steps 5–7 for the second and third day of testing, using the remaining two cards.	10			
9. Review the instructions for sending the samples back to the office. These specimens are usually mailed back in a foil lined envelope and must arrive for testing within 14 days of collection.	10			
Testing Procedure				
10. When the completed test cards arrive in the office, wash your hands, gather supplies (developer), and apply gloves before testing begins. Check the expiration date on the developer.	10			
11. Correctly follow the developing instructions, including performing a control on each test following testing and interpretation of each sample. A blue color indicates a positive result for the presence of blood.	10			
12. Properly dispose of the test cards in a trash receptacle or by following institutional guidelines.	10			
13. Remove gloves and wash your hands.	10			
14. Document the procedure and the results in the patient record.	10			
Points Earned / Points Possible:	___ / 140			

Points possible reflect importance of step in meeting the task: Important = (5) Essential = (10). Determine score by dividing points earned by total points possible, and multiplying results by 100.

Name _____ Date _____ Score _____

EVALUATION

Evaluator Signature: _____ Date: _____

Evaluator Comments:

DOCUMENTATION

Instructor Note: Retain work products with competency checklist.

Work Products, Procedure 16-2a (Progress Note) and 16-2b (In-House Testing Log). Procedure forms can be downloaded from the student companion website.

Key Competencies			
ABHES	MA.A.1.4.a	Follow documentation guidelines	
	MA.A.1.10.a	Practice quality control	
	MA.A.1.10.e(2)	Instruct patients in the collection of fecal specimen	
CAAHEP	I.P.10	Perform a quality control measure	
	I.A.3	Show awareness of a patient's concerns related to the procedure being performed	
	III.P.3	Perform handwashing	
	IV.A.1	Show awareness of patient's concerns regarding a dietary change	
	V.A.4	Explain to a patient the rationale for performance of a procedure	
	X.P.3	Document patient care accurately in the medical record	

Name _____ Date _____ Score _____

COMPETENCY CHECKLIST

PROCEDURE 16-3   Assist with a Flexible Sigmoidoscopy

Task: To assist with a flexible sigmoidoscopy.

Condition: Given the equipment and supplies as listed in the procedure and classmates to play the part of the patient and provider, the student will simulate assisting the provider with a sigmoidoscopy, adhering to the steps listed below.

Standards: The student will have 15 minutes to complete the procedure and will need to score an 85% or above to pass the competency. Automatic failure results if any essential steps are omitted or performed incorrectly.

STEPS START TIME: END TIME:	Points Possible	First Attempt	Second Attempt	Third Attempt
1. Wash hands and apply gloves.	10			
2. Assemble the equipment. Ensure that all is in acceptable working condition.	10			
3. Identify the patient using two identifiers and identify yourself. ***Explain to the patient the rationale for performance of the procedure, showing awareness of the patient's concerns related to the procedure.*** Label the sterile specimen container with all pertinent patient information.	10			
4. Ask the patient to use the restroom to empty the bladder and bowel.	10			
5. Supply the patient with a gown, instructing the patient to disrobe below the waist and place the gown with the opening in the back. Provide a drape for added privacy.	10			
6. ***Demonstrating empathy***, reassure the patient that the exam should only last a few minutes.	10			
7. Assist the patient into the Sims' position and instruct the patient to breathe deeply through the mouth to relax the abdominal muscles.	10			
8. Provide the physician with suitable disposable gloves. When gloved, provide lubrication to the first digit for rectal examination.	10			
9. Lubricate the end of the flexible scope.	10			
10. ***Incorporate critical thinking skills when performing patient care***, and be prepared for any requests by the provider. Assist with suctioning during the procedure and give support to the patient.	10			
11. Hand biopsy forceps to the provider, if requested. Be certain the specimen container is maintained in a functional position. Place the biopsy specimen into the sterile container.	10			
12. Following completion of the procedure, provide tissue to the patient to remove any excess lubrication from the anal region.	5			
13. Assist the patient into a sitting position and instruct the patient to remain sitting while you assess the patient's status, ***incorporating critical thinking skills when performing patient assessment.***	10			
14. Once the patient is stable, assist with dressing, if requested, ***while demonstrating the principles of self-boundaries.***	5			
15. Prepare the specimen for transport to the laboratory. Be certain lab requests are filled out in their entirety.	10			

Name _____ Date _____ Score _____

16. Clean the equipment and examination room. Follow the manufacturer's instructions for cleaning the scope.	10			
17. Document the exam and procedure in the patient record.	10			
Points Earned / Points Possible:	___ / 160			

Points possible reflect importance of step in meeting the task: Important = (5) Essential = (10). Determine score by dividing points earned by total points possible, and multiplying results by 100.

EVALUATION

Evaluator Signature: _____ Date: _____

Evaluator Comments:

DOCUMENTATION

Instructor Note: Retain work products with competency checklist.
Work Products, Procedure 16-3a (Progress Note) and 16-3b (Outstanding Lab Results Tracking Report). Procedure forms can be downloaded from the student companion website.

Key Competencies		
ABHES	MA.A.1.4.a	Follow documentation guidelines
	MA.A.1.9.d	Assist provider with specialty examination including cardiac, respiratory, OB-GYN, neurological, gastroenterology procedures
CAAHEP	I.P.9	Assist provider with a patient exam
	I.A.1	Incorporate critical thinking skills when performing patient assessment
	I.A.2	Incorporate critical thinking skills when performing patient care
	I.A.3	Show awareness of a patient's concerns related to the procedure being performed
	III.P.3	Perform handwashing
	V.A.1.a	Demonstrate empathy
	V.A.2	Demonstrate the principles of self-boundaries
	V.A.4	Explain to a patient the rationale for performance of a procedure
	X.P.3	Document patient care accurately in the medical record

Name _____ Date _____ Score _____

COMPETENCY CHECKLIST

PROCEDURE 17-1   Instruct the Patient in Breast Self-Examination

Task: To instruct patient on how to perform a breast self-examination (BSE).

Condition: Given the equipment and supplies as listed in the procedure and a classmate to play the part of the patient, the student will correctly instruct the patient on how to perform a breast self-examination (BSE), adhering to the steps listed below.

Standards: The student will have 15 minutes to complete the education session and will need to score an 85% or above to pass the competency. Automatic failure results if any essential steps are omitted or performed incorrectly.

STEPS START TIME: END TIME:	Points Possible	First Attempt	Second Attempt	Third Attempt
1. Greet the patient, identify yourself, and ***explain the rationale for the performance*** of BSE, ***showing awareness of the patient's concerns related to the procedure being performed***.	10			
2. Give the patient a brochure and begin explaining the proper procedure for performing BSE. Explain to the patient that the breasts should be examined in the shower, in front of a mirror, and while lying down.	10			
3. Instruct the patient to examine the breasts at the same time each month, preferably a few days to a week following menstrual period.	10			
4. While the patient is in the shower, instruct her to cover the right breast with soapy lather and place the right arm over the head. Gently glide the fingers over the entire breast and axilla feeling for any lumps or thickening. Repeat the procedure with the left breast.	10			
5. When the patient is finished showering, she should stand before a mirror and look for: • Puckering or dimpling of the skin • Redness or a change in skin texture • Nipple retraction • Any change in size or shape The exam should be repeated then with the hands raised over the head and then with the hands on the hips, while pressing down.	10			
6. Instruct the patient to gently squeeze each nipple and look for any discharge.	10			
7. Instruct the patient to lie down and place a small pillow under her right shoulder and to raise her right arm over her head.	10			
8. Instruct the patient to use the pads of the first three fingers and, using firm pressure and a circular motion, examine the entire breast, including the nipple and the underarm area. Repeat the entire process with the left breast.	10			
9. Answer any questions and instruct the patient to repeat the instructions and perform an exam on the breast model. Instruct the patient to report any changes immediately.	10			
10. Document the education session in the patient's chart.	10			
Points Earned / Points Possible:	__ / 100			

Points possible reflect importance of step in meeting the task: Important = (5) Essential = (10). Determine score by dividing points earned by total points possible, and multiplying results by 100.

Name _____ Date _____ Score _____

EVALUATION

Evaluator Signature: _____ Date: _____

Evaluator Comments:

DOCUMENTATION

Instructor Note: Retain work products with competency checklist.
Work Product, Procedure 17-1 (Progress Note). Procedure forms can be downloaded from the student companion website.

Key Competencies			
ABHES	MA.A.1.4.a	Follow documentation guidelines	
	MA.A.1.9.c	Assist provider with general/physical examination	
	MA.A.1.9.d	Assist provider with specialty examination including OB-GYN procedures	
	MA.A.1.9.e	Perform specialty procedures including but not limited to OB-GYN	
	MA.A.1.9.h	Teach self-examination, disease management and health promotion	
CAAHEP	I.P.8	Instruct and prepare a patient for a procedure or a treatment	
	I.P.9	Assist provider with a patient exam	
	I.A.3	Show awareness of a patient's concerns related to the procedure being performed	
	V.A.4	Explain to a patient the rationale for performance of a procedure	
	X.P.3	Document patient care accurately in the medical record	

Name _____ Date _____ Score _____

COMPETENCY CHECKLIST
PROCEDURE 17-2   Assist with a GYN Exam and Pap Test

Task: To assist the physician with a GYN exam and Pap test.

Condition: Given the equipment and supplies as listed in the procedure, a classmate to play the part of the patient, and a classmate to play the part of the provider, the student will correctly simulate assisting the physician with a GYN exam and pap test, adhering to the steps listed below.

Standards: The student will have 15 minutes to complete the simulation and will need to score an 85% or above to pass the competency. Automatic failure results if any essential steps are omitted or performed incorrectly.

STEPS START TIME: END TIME:	Points Possible	First Attempt	Second Attempt	Third Attempt
1. Wash your hands and set up all needed equipment. Warm the speculum.	10			
2. Label the specimens. *Direct method:* Label slides with the patient's name, the date, and source (V) = vaginal, (C) = cervical, or (E) = endocervical. *ThinPrep method:* Label the specimen container with the patient's name, date, and ID number (from lab request form).	10			
3. Identify the patient using at least two identifiers, identify yourself, and instruct the patient to empty her bladder and collect the urine specimen.	10			
4. Obtain the patient's blood pressure and weight and update her medical and GYN history.	10			
5. ***Explain the rationale for performance of the procedure*** to the patient and instruct her to undress completely and to put the gown on so that it opens correctly (check provider preference), ***showing awareness of the patient's concerns related to the procedure being performed***.	10			
6. Instruct the patient to sit on the exam table until the provider enters the room.	10			
7. After the provider enters, assist the patient into the supine position and drape for the breast exam.	10			
8. Assist the patient into the lithotomy position and drape for privacy.	10			
9. Hand the warmed vaginal speculum to the provider.	10			
10. Adjust the light source for easy visualization.	10			
11. Hand the spatula and brush to the provider when using the direct method, and the broom when using the ThinPrep method.	10			
12. Apply PPE (gloves) and: *Direct method:* Hold the slides so the provider can apply the collected cells to the slides. Immediately spray the slides with fixative from a distance of six inches. Allow the slides to dry for 10 minutes before placing in a holder. *ThinPrep method (broom method):* Hold the opened vial so the provider can place the broom in the vial. Agitate the broom in the solution until all of the specimen has been suspended in the liquid. Dispose of the broom in a biohazard container.	10			
13. Squeeze lubricant on the provider's gloved fingers for the bimanual and rectal exam.	10			

Name _____ Date _____ Score _____

14. After the provider completes the exam, assist the patient into a sitting position and give her tissues for cleansing the vaginal and rectal area.	10				
15. Properly dispose of biohazardous wastes and other used supplies and soak the stainless steel speculum in a solution. Sanitize and sterilize the speculum per office protocol.	10				
16. Instruct the patient to get dressed.	10				
17. Prepare the specimen and lab requisition for transport.	10				
18. Remove gloves and wash your hands.	10				
19. Document the procedure in the patient's chart.	10				
Points Earned / Points Possible:	__/ 190				

Points possible reflect importance of step in meeting the task: Important = (5) Essential = (10). Determine score by dividing points earned by total points possible, and multiplying results by 100.

EVALUATION

Evaluator Signature: _____ Date: _____

Evaluator Comments:

DOCUMENTATION

Instructor Note: Retain work products with competency checklist.
Work Product, Procedure 17-2a (Progress Note) and 17-2b (Outstanding Lab Results Tracking Report). Procedure forms can be downloaded from the student companion website.

Key Competencies			
ABHES	MA.A.1.4.a	Follow documentation guidelines	
	MA.A.1.9.c	Assist provider with general/physical examination	
	MA.A.1.9.d	Assist provider with specialty examination including OB-GYN procedures	
	MA.A.1.9.e	Perform specialty procedures including but not limited to OB-GYN	
	MA.A.1.10.c	Dispose of biohazardous materials	
CAAHEP	I.P.8	Instruct and prepare a patient for a procedure or a treatment	
	I.P.9	Assist provider with a patient exam	
	I.A.3	Show awareness of a patient's concerns related to the procedure being performed	
	III.P.3	Perform handwashing	
	III.P.10.b	Demonstrate proper disposal of biohazardous material: regulated wastes	
	V.A.4	Explain to a patient the rationale for performance of a procedure	
	X.P.3	Document patient care accurately in the medical record	

Name _____ Date _____ Score _____

COMPETENCY CHECKLIST
PROCEDURE 17-3   Assist with the Prenatal Exam

Task: To assist with prenatal exams to monitor the progression of a pregnancy.

Condition: Given the equipment and supplies as listed in the procedure, a classmate to play the part of the patient, and a classmate to play the part of the provider, the student will correctly simulate assisting the provider with a prenatal exam, adhering to the steps listed below.

Standards: The student will have 15 minutes to complete the procedure and will need to score an 85% or above to pass the competency. Automatic failure results if any essential steps are omitted or performed incorrectly.

STEPS START TIME: END TIME:	Points Possible	First Attempt	Second Attempt	Third Attempt
1. Wash your hands and set up the equipment.	10			
2. Identify the patient using two identifiers and instruct the patient to collect a urine specimen. Dip the urine for protein and glucose.	10			
3. Obtain the patient's weight and blood pressure. Both measurements are obtained at each prenatal visit.	10			
4. *Initial visit:* **Showing awareness of the patient's concerns related to the procedure being performed**, have the patient disrobe completely and put on a gown. Assist the provider in conducting a thorough exam including a breast exam and pelvic exam. *Return visits:* The fundal height is measured and the fetal heart tones are assessed. Assist the provider by supplying a tape measure for the fundal height measurement and a fetal monitor and gel to listen to the fetal heart tones. (After the initial visit, an internal exam will not be performed again until approximately 36 weeks gestation, and thereafter.)	10			
5. After completion of the exam, assist the patient into a sitting position and have her remain there for a few minutes.	10			
6. Provide the patient with educational materials.	10			
7. Apply gloves, clean the exam room, properly dispose of used supplies, and disinfect or sterilize equipment.	10			
8. Wash hands and document the visit in patient's chart.	10			
Points Earned / Points Possible:	___ / 80			

Points possible reflect importance of step in meeting the task: Important = (5) Essential = (10) Determine score by dividing points earned by total points possible, and multiplying results by 100.

Name _____ Date _____ Score _____

EVALUATION

Evaluator Signature: _____ Date: _____

Evaluator Comments:

DOCUMENTATION

Instructor Note: Retain work products with competency checklist.

Work Product, Procedure 17-3 (Progress Note). Procedure forms can be downloaded from the student companion website.

Key Competencies		
ABHES	MA.A.1.4.a	Follow documentation guidelines
	MA.A.1.9.c	Assist provider with general/physical examination
	MA.A.1.9.d	Assist provider with specialty examination including OB-GYN procedures
	MA.A.1.9.e	Perform specialty procedures including but not limited to OB-GYN
	MA.A.1.9.h	Teach self-examination, disease management and health promotion
CAAHEP	I.P.8	Instruct and prepare a patient for a procedure or a treatment
	I.P.9	Assist provider with a patient exam
	I.A.3	Show awareness of a patient's concerns related to the procedure being performed
	III.P.3	Perform handwashing
	X.P.3	Document patient care accurately in the medical record

Name _____ Date _____ Score _____

COMPETENCY CHECKLIST

PROCEDURE 19-1   Perform Allergy Testing

Task: Perform allergy testing to identify allergens that the patient reacts toward.

Condition: Given the equipment and supplies as listed in the procedure, the student will perform the task, adhering to the standards listed below.

Standards: The student will have 45 minutes to complete the procedure and will need to score an 85% or above to pass the competency. Automatic failure results if any essential steps are omitted or performed incorrectly.

STEPS START TIME: END TIME:	Points Possible	First Attempt	Second Attempt	Third Attempt
1. Review provider's order and gather all supplies.	10			
2. Identify yourself and identify the patient using at least two identifiers.	10			
3. Ask the patient if she held her allergy medications for the prescribed amount of days before the appointment.	10			
4. ***Demonstrating professional behavior, explain to the patient the rationale for performance of the procedure, showing awareness of the patient's concerns related to the procedure being performed.*** Counsel the patient that positive reactions will likely itch, but they must not scratch.	10			
5. ***Incorporating critical thinking skills when performing patient care,*** ensure that you have all emergency medications as well as standard supplies for the procedure.	10			
6. Wash hands and apply gloves.	10			
7. Mark out a grid on the forearms or back according to your standard operating procedure (SOP). Ensure that the controls are marked appropriately.	10			
8. Clean the skin with an alcohol pad prior to skin prick or scratch.	10			
9. Dip the tip of the individual skin prick device into the purified allergen or appropriate controls based on the grid map, apply, and allow 15 minutes for full reaction.	10			
10. Identify and measure areas of induration as well as noting the erythema for each grid square.	10			
11. Remove gloves and wash hands.	10			
12. Provide patient with self-care instructions such as use of antihistamines, topical steroids, and washing site with soap and water.	10			
13. There will likely be a skin test report form that needs to be completed. This is a rather lengthy process and may be completed by the provider or medical assistant.	10			
14. Document the procedure in the patient's chart.	10			
Points Earned / Points Possible:	___ / 140			

Points possible reflect importance of step in meeting the task: Important = (5) Essential = (10). Determine score by dividing points earned by total points possible, and multiplying results by 100.

Name _____ Date _____ Score _____

EVALUATION
Evaluator Signature: _____ Date: _____

Evaluator Comments:

DOCUMENTATION
Instructor Note: Retain work products with competency checklists.
Work product, Procedure 19-1 (Progress Note). Procedure forms can be downloaded from the student companion website.

Key Competencies		
ABHES	MA.A.1.4.a	Follow documentation guidelines
	MA.A.1.11.b	Demonstrate professional behavior
CAAHEP	I.P.8	Instruct and prepare a patient for a procedure or a treatment
	I.A.2	Incorporate critical thinking skills when performing patient care
	I.A.3	Show awareness of a patient's concerns related to the procedure being performed
	III.P.3	Perform handwashing
	V.A.4	Explain to a patient the rationale for performance of a procedure
	X.A.3	Document patient care accurately in the medical record

Name _____ Date _____ Score _____

COMPETENCY CHECKLIST

PROCEDURE 20-1 Develop a 2,000-Calorie Meal Plan Utilizing Basic Principles of Nutrition

Task: To develop a 2,000-calorie daily meal plan, applying RDA information for a nutritionally balanced diet.

Condition: Given the equipment and supplies as listed in the procedure, the student will perform the task, adhering to the standards listed below.

Standards: The student will have 20 minutes to complete the procedure and will need to score an 85% or above to pass the competency. Automatic failure results if any essential steps are omitted or performed incorrectly.

Procedure Scenario Information

Mrs. Brady, an 83-year patient who lives alone, is being seen today by Dr. Parish. After taking her vital signs, you note her BMI classifies her as underweight. She tells you nothing tastes good, she doesn't feel like cooking or eating alone, and she probably doesn't get enough nutrition. After the visit, Dr. Parish asks you to develop a 2,000-calorie meal plan for Mrs. Brady to help her nutritional understanding and provide guidelines for maintaining a healthy weight.

STEPS START TIME: END TIME:	Points Possible	First Attempt	Second Attempt	Third Attempt
1. Read the patient's chart and note the patient's height and weight. Review the list of diagnoses and note those requiring dietary modifications. Review the patient's usual daily physical activity.	10			
2. Review the Daily Food Plan for 2,000 calories/day.	10			
3. Apply the food plan to the Daily Food Plan Worksheet.	10			
Points Earned / Points Possible:	___ / 30			

Points possible reflect importance of step in meeting the task: Important = (5) Essential = (10). Determine score by dividing points earned by total points possible, and multiplying results by 100.

EVALUATION

Evaluator Signature: _____ Date: _____

Evaluator Comments:

DOCUMENTATION

Instructor Note: Retain work product with competency checklist.
Work Products, Procedure 20-1 (Daily Food Plan Worksheet). Procedure forms can be downloaded from the student companion website.

Key Competencies		
ABHES	MA.A.1.2.d	Apply a system of diet and nutrition
CAAHEP	IV.P.1	Instruct a patient according to patient's special dietary needs

Name _____ Date _____ Score _____

COMPETENCY CHECKLIST

PROCEDURE 20-2   Instruct a Patient According to the Patient's Special Dietary Needs

Task: To review and develop a daily food plan with the patient, including nutrition labels and portion sizes.

Condition: Given the equipment and supplies as listed in the procedure, the student will perform the task, adhering to the standards listed below.

Standards: The student will have 15 minutes to complete the procedure and will need to score an 85% or above to pass the competency. Automatic failure results if any essential steps are omitted or performed incorrectly.

STEPS START TIME: END TIME:	Points Possible	First Attempt	Second Attempt	Third Attempt
1. Prepare for patient instruction by writing a list of talking points. Assemble teaching materials, including print copies for the patient to take home.	10			
2. Introduce yourself to the patient. Instruct the patient what educational materials she should review and ask if she has any questions.	10			
3. Ask the patient about her dietary goals and her realistic commitment to changing her diet, ***showing awareness of the patient's concerns regarding a dietary change***.	10			
4. Review and discuss the Daily Food Plan.	10			
5. Complete the Food Plan worksheet with the patient.	10			
6. Review how to read and use the nutrition facts label with the patient.	10			
7. Teach the patient how to estimate portion sizes.	10			
8. Review the amount of time the patient spends in physical activity each day.	10			
9. Provide the website address for more information on ChooseMyPlate food plans.	5			
10. Document the patient education provided in the patient's chart.	10			
Points Earned / Points Possible:	___ / 95			

Points possible reflect importance of step in meeting the task: Important = (5) Essential = (10). Determine score by dividing points earned by total points possible, and multiplying results by 100.

Name _____ Date _____ Score _____

EVALUATION

Evaluator Signature: _____ Date: _____

Evaluator Comments:

DOCUMENTATION

Instructor Note: Retain work product with competency checklist.

Work Products, 20-1a (Progress Note) and Procedure 20-1b (Daily Food Plan Worksheet). Procedure forms can be downloaded from the student companion website.

Key Competencies		
ABHES	MA.A.1.2.d(1)	Explain the importance of diet and nutrition
	MA.A.1.2.d(2)	Educate patients regarding proper diet and nutrition guidelines
	MA.A.1.4.a	Follow documentation guidelines
CAAHEP	IV.P.1	Instruct a patient according to patient's special dietary needs
	IV.A.1	Show awareness of patient's concerns regarding a dietary change
	X.P.3	Document patient care accurately in the medical record

Name _____ Date _____ Score _____

COMPETENCY CHECKLIST
PROCEDURE 21-1   Obtain the Height/Length and Weight of an Infant

Task: To obtain the height/length and weight of an infant.

Condition: Given the equipment and supplies as listed in the procedure, a classmate to play the part of the parent, and a doll or model for the role of the infant, the student will correctly simulate performing an infant height and weight measurement, adhering to the steps listed below.

Standards: The student will have 10 minutes to complete the procedure and will need to score an 85% or above to pass the competency. Automatic failure results if any essential steps are omitted or performed incorrectly.

STEPS START TIME: END TIME:	Points Possible	First Attempt	Second Attempt	Third Attempt
1. Wash your hands and assemble the equipment.	10			
2. Identify the patient using two identifiers, and identify yourself. Ask the parent to remove the child's clothing, except for the child's diaper.	10			
3. Place the infant face up on the paper on the exam table with the top of the infant's head flush with the top measuring bar of the caliper.	10			
4. Stretch the infant's legs to their full length and place the sole of the foot flush with the bottom measuring bar of the caliper. Use caution when extending the joints, ***incorporating critical thinking when performing patient assessment***. Do not pull on the neck or legs. Be gentle. Have the parent support the head and neck, if needed.	10			
5. Document your results immediately on the patient record and the growth chart.	10			
6. After completing measurement of length, place the infant on the infant scale, lined exam paper, or towel. The scale should be balanced to zero prior to the exam.	10			
7. Have the parent comfort and support the infant. Make sure that the parent does not exert additional weight.	10			
8. Obtain a reading. Remove the infant from the scale. Remove the diaper from the infant. Place the diaper on the scale and weigh.	10			
9. Calculate the infant's weight. Remember: total weight – diaper = infant weight.	10			
10. Document your results immediately on the patient record and growth chart.	10			
Points Earned / Points Possible:	__ / 100			

Points possible reflect importance of step in meeting the task: Important = (5) Essential = (10). Determine score by dividing points earned by total points possible, and multiplying results by 100.

Name _____ Date _____ Score _____

EVALUATION

Evaluator Signature: _____ Date: _____

Evaluator Comments:

DOCUMENTATION

Instructor Note: Retain work products with competency checklist.

Work Product, 21-1a (Progress Note) and 21-1b (Infant Growth Chart). Procedure forms can be downloaded from the student companion website.

Key Competencies			
ABHES	MA.A.1.4.a	Follow documentation guidelines	
	MA.A.1.9.b	Obtain vital signs	
	MA.A.1.9.c	Assist provider with general/physical examination	
CAAHEP	I.P.1.f	Measure and record weight	
	I.P.1.g	Measure and record length (infant)	
	I.A.1	Incorporate critical thinking skills when performing patient assessment	
	II.P.4	Document on a growth chart	
	III.P.3	Perform handwashing	
	X.P.3	Document patient care accurately in the medical record	

Name _____ Date _____ Score _____

COMPETENCY CHECKLIST

PROCEDURE 21-2   Obtain the Temperature of an Infant or Young Child

Task: To obtain a rectal, aural, and temporal temperature on an infant.

Condition: Given the equipment and supplies as listed in the procedure, a classmate to play the part of the parent, and a doll or model for the role of the infant, the student will correctly simulate performing a rectal, aural, and temporal temperature on an infant, adhering to the steps listed below.

Standards: The student will have 15 minutes to complete the procedure and will need to score an 85% or above to pass the competency. Automatic failure results if any essential steps are omitted or performed incorrectly.

STEPS START TIME: END TIME:	Points Possible	First Attempt	Second Attempt	Third Attempt
1. Wash your hands and assemble all the equipment. Put on gloves.	10			
2. Identify the patient using two identifiers, and identify yourself.	10			
3. ***Explain the rationale for performance of the procedure, showing awareness of the patient's and parent's concerns related to the procedure being performed.*** Have the parent remove the infant's clothing.	10			
Rectal temperature:				
4. Place the infant on the abdomen in your lap, or the infant may be placed in a supine position.	10			
5. Apply a clean probe cover and lubricant to the rectal thermometer.	10			
6. Gently insert the thermometer into the infant's rectum approximately one inch. Hold it securely. Leave the thermometer in place until the signal that indicates the reading is complete.	10			
7. Remove the thermometer. Remove the sheath and discard it in the biohazard container.	10			
8. Observe the reading, disinfect the probe with alcohol, and place the probe into its storage slot on the unit.	10			
9. Remove excess lubricant from the anal area of the infant. Discard the tissue appropriately.	5			
Aural temperature:				
10. Place the probe cover on the thermometer.	10			
11. Insert the thermometer gently into the ear canal and press the activation button. For best placement and most accurate results, pull gently down and backward on children under the age of three and up and back on children three and over.	10			
12. After the signal sounds indicating that the reading is complete, remove the thermometer and note the reading.	10			
13. Discard the probe cover in the appropriate container.	10			
Temporal temperature:				
14. Clean the thermometer with an alcohol swab and check to be sure the thermometer is in working order.	10			

Name _____ Date _____ Score _____

15. Check the forehead for any moisture and begin with the probe at the midline of the forehead. Keeping the probe flush with the skin, press and hold the scan button and slowly glide the thermometer across the forehead to the location of the temporal artery.	10				
16. Remove gloves, if worn, and accurately record the information on the patient's record indicating the method performed.	10				
Points Earned / Points Possible:	__ / 155				

Points possible reflect importance of step in meeting the task: Important = (5) Essential = (10). Determine score by dividing points earned by total points possible, and multiplying results by 100.

EVALUATION

Evaluator Signature: _____ Date: _____

Evaluator Comments:

DOCUMENTATION

Instructor Note: Retain work products with competency checklist.
Work Product, Procedure 21-2 (Progress Note). Procedure forms can be downloaded from the student companion website.

Key Competencies			
ABHES	MA.A.1.4.a	Follow documentation guidelines	
	MA.A.1.9.b	Obtain vital signs	
	MA.A.1.9.c	Assist provider with general/physical examination	
	MA.A.1.10.c	Dispose of biohazardous materials	
CAAHEP	I.P.1.b	Measure and record temperature	
	I.A.3	Show awareness of a patient's concerns related to the procedure being performed	
	III.P.3	Perform handwashing	
	III.P.10.b	Demonstrate proper disposal of biohazardous material: regulated wastes	
	V.A.4	Explain to a patient the rationale for performance of a procedure	
	X.P.3	Document patient care accurately in the medical record	

Name _____ Date _____ Score _____

COMPETENCY CHECKLIST
PROCEDURE 21-3   Perform a PKU on a Newborn

Task: To perform a PKU on a newborn.

Condition: Given the equipment and supplies as listed in the procedure, a classmate to play the part of the parent, and a doll or model for the role of the infant, the student will correctly simulate performing a heel capillary stick to obtain blood for a PKU, adhering to the steps listed below.

Standards: The student will have 15 minutes to complete the procedure and will need to score an 85% or above to pass the competency. Automatic failure results if any essential steps are omitted or performed incorrectly.

STEPS START TIME: END TIME:	Points Possible	First Attempt	Second Attempt	Third Attempt
1. Wash your hands and assemble the equipment. Complete all required information in the patient section of the test card.	10			
2. Identify the patient using two identifiers, and identify yourself.	10			
3. ***Explain the rationale for performance of the procedure to the parent or caregiver, showing awareness of the parent's concerns related to the procedure being performed.*** Put on gloves.	10			
4. Expose the infant's heel and locate the position on the heel used to obtain blood. Warm with compresses for approximately five minutes.	10			
5. Cleanse the area with the antiseptic wipe. Allow to dry.	10			
6. Securely grasp the foot to be punctured. Using the lancet, quickly puncture the heal perpendicular to the line on the sole of the foot. Discard the lancet in the sharps container.	10			
7. Gently wipe the first drop of blood away with sterile gauze and discard in the biohazards container.	10			
8. Gently squeeze the heel, expressing large drops of blood. The test card is placed, as per directions, on the puncture site.	10			
9. Fill each circle on the test card with blood, obtained directly from the puncture site. All circles must be saturated for accurate results. Place the card aside for drying.	10			
10. Cover the puncture site with gauze and apply pressure. Maintain pressure until the bleeding has stopped.	10			
11. Cover the site with a small adhesive bandage.	10			
12. Discard all materials in the appropriate container. Remove gloves and wash hands.	10			
13. Document the results of the procedure in the patient record.	10			
14. After the card is completely dry (approximately two hours), place the card in an envelope to transport to lab.	10			
Points Earned / Points Possible:	__ / 140			

Points possible reflect importance of step in meeting the task: Important = (5) Essential = (10). Determine score by dividing points earned by total points possible, and multiplying results by 100.

Name _____ Date _____ Score _____

EVALUATION

Evaluator Signature: _____ Date: _____

Evaluator Comments:

DOCUMENTATION

Instructor Note: Retain work products with competency checklist.

Work Product, Procedure 21-3a (Progress Note) and 21-3b (PKU Card). Procedure forms can be downloaded from the student companion website.

Key Competencies		
ABHES	MA.A.1.4.a	Follow documentation guidelines
	MA.A.1.10.c	Dispose of biohazardous materials
	MA.A.1.10.d(2)	Perform capillary puncture
CAAHEP	I.P.2.c	Perform capillary puncture
	I.A.3	Show awareness of a patient's concerns related to the procedure being performed
	III.P.3	Perform handwashing
	III.P.10	Demonstrate proper disposal of biohazardous material: (a) sharps, and (b) regulated wastes
	V.A.4	Explain to a patient the rationale for performance of a procedure
	X.P.3	Document patient care accurately in the medical record

Name _____ Date _____ Score _____

COMPETENCY CHECKLIST
PROCEDURE 21-4   Perform a Pediatric Injection

Task: To perform a pediatric injection.

Condition: Given the equipment and supplies as listed in the procedure, a classmate to play the part of the parent, and a doll or model to play the role of the infant, the student will correctly simulate performing a pediatric injection, adhering to the steps listed below.

Standards: The student will have 10 minutes to complete the procedure and will need to score an 85% or above to pass the competency. Automatic failure results if any essential steps are omitted or performed incorrectly.

STEPS START TIME: END TIME:	Points Possible	First Attempt	Second Attempt	Third Attempt
1. Wash your hands, assemble the equipment, and prepare the medication.	10			
2. Identify the patient using two identifiers, identify yourself, and *explain the rationale for performance of the procedure, showing awareness of the patient's and parent's concerns related to the procedure being performed.*	10			
3. Rewash your hands and put on gloves.	10			
4. Select and locate the proper site for the injection.	10			
5. Cleanse the site with an antiseptic and allow to completely air dry.	10			
6. Remove the needle cap and properly position the hand on the injection site.	10			
7. Pull the skin taut and insert the needle at a 90° angle.	10			
8. Swiftly inject the medication into the muscle.	10			
9. Remove the needle quickly at the same angle as insertion.	10			
10. Place a gauze sponge over the injection site and gently massage.	10			
11. Engage the safety device on the needle and dispose of the entire unit in the sharps container.	10			
12. Apply an adhesive bandage to the site.	10			
13. Remove the gloves and wash your hands.	10			
14. Document the procedure in the patient's chart.	10			
Points Earned / Points Possible:	__ / 140			

Points possible reflect importance of step in meeting the task: Important = (5) Essential = (10). Determine score by dividing points earned by total points possible, and multiplying results by 100.

Name _____ Date _____ Score _____

EVALUATION
Evaluator Signature: _____ Date: _____

Evaluator Comments:

DOCUMENTATION
Instructor Note: Retain work products with competency checklist.
Work Product, Procedure 21-4a (Progress Note) and 21-4b (Immunization Tracking Log). Procedure forms can be downloaded from the student companion website.

Key Competencies			
ABHES	MA.A.1.4.a	Follow documentation guidelines	
	MA.A.1.9.f	Prepare and administer oral and parenteral medications and monitor intravenous (IV) infusions	
	MA.A.1.10.c	Dispose of biohazardous materials	
CAAHEP	I.P.5	Select proper sites for administering parenteral medication	
	I.P.7	Administer parenteral (excluding IV) medications	
	I.A.3	Show awareness of a patient's concerns related to the procedure being performed	
	III.P.3	Perform handwashing	
	III.P.10.a	Demonstrate proper disposal of biohazardous material: sharps	
	V.A.4	Explain to a patient the rationale for performance of a procedure	
	X.P.3	Document patient care accurately in the medical record	

Name _____ Date _____ Score _____

COMPETENCY CHECKLIST

PROCEDURE 22-1   Splint an Arm

Task: To splint an arm.

Condition: Given the equipment and supplies as listed in the procedure, and a classmate to play the part of the patient (victim), the student will demonstrate the correct steps for applying a splint to the arm, adhering to the steps listed below.

Standards: The student will have 15 minutes to complete the procedure and will need to score an 85% or above to pass the competency. Automatic failure results if any essential steps are omitted or performed incorrectly.

STEPS START TIME: END TIME:	Points Possible	First Attempt	Second Attempt	Third Attempt
1. Wash hands.	10			
2. Assemble equipment and supplies.	10			
3. Identify the patient using two identifiers, identify yourself, and ***explain the rationale for the performance of the procedure, showing awareness of the patient's concerns. Recognize the physical and emotional effects on persons involved in an emergency situation.***	10			
4. Follow the steps on the commercial splint for preparing the splint.	10			
5. Place the arm in the position that will be used for splinting. Be sure to stabilize the injured area by stabilizing the joint above and below the injury.	10			
6. Check the pulse point distal to the injury, checking the strength of the pulse.	10			
7. Check for sensation and movement while the arm is in the splint position.	10			
8. Apply the splint following the manufacturer's instructions. If arm is to be totally immobilized, place the arm with the splint in a sling as well.	10			
9. Check distal pulse point, check fingers for sensation and movement after applying the splint.	10			
10. Apply ice to help reduce swelling.	10			
11. Wash your hands.	10			
12. Document the procedure.	10			
Points Earned / Points Possible:	__ / 120			

Points possible reflect importance of step in meeting the task: Important = (5) Essential = (10). Determine score by dividing points earned by total points possible, and multiplying results by 100.

Name _____ Date _____ Score _____

EVALUATION

Evaluator Signature: _____ Date: _____

Evaluator Comments:

DOCUMENTATION

Instructor Note: Retain work products with competency checklist.

Work Product, Procedure 22-1 (Progress Note). Procedure forms can be downloaded from the student companion website.

Key Competencies		
ABHES	MA.A.1.4.a	Follow documentation guidelines
	MA.A.1.9.g	Recognize and respond to medical office emergencies
CAAHEP	I.P.13.c	Perform first aid procedures for fractures
	I.A.3	Show awareness of a patient's concerns related to the procedure being performed
	III.P.3	Perform handwashing
	V.A.4	Explain to a patient the rationale for performance of a procedure
	X.P.3	Document patient care accurately in the medical record
	XII.A.1	Recognize the physical and emotional effects on persons involved in an emergency situation

Name _____ Date _____ Score _____

COMPETENCY CHECKLIST

PROCEDURE 22-2   Instruct a Patient to Use a Cane

Task: To instruct a patient to use a cane.

Condition: Given the equipment and supplies as listed in the procedure and a classmate to play the part of the patient, the student will demonstrate how to use a cane, adhering to the steps listed below.

Standards: The student will have 10 minutes to complete the procedure and will need to score an 85% or above to pass the competency. Automatic failure results if any essential steps are omitted or performed incorrectly.

STEPS START TIME: END TIME:	Points Possible	First Attempt	Second Attempt	Third Attempt
1. Check the provider's orders, assemble the equipment, and wash your hands.	10			
2. Identify the patient using two identifiers, identify yourself, and *explain the rationale for the performance of the procedure, showing awareness of the patient's concerns related to the procedure being performed*.	10			
3. Inspect the tip of the cane to be sure there is a rubber tip.	10			
4. Adjust the cane height so that the handle of the cane is even with the patient's hip joint and the patient's elbow is flexed at a 25º–30º angle.	10			
5. Demonstrate the correct usage of the cane:				
a. Hold the cane on the strong side.	10			
b. Move the cane and the affected leg forward at the same time.	10			
c. Move the strong leg forward, slightly in front of the cane.	10			
d. Take slow, small steps.	10			
e. Repeat b and c.	5			
6. Apply a gait belt (an added precaution) to the patient and ask the patient to practice the procedure.	10			
7. Document the patient education in the patient's chart.	10			
Points Earned / Points Possible:	___ / 105			

Points possible reflect importance of step in meeting the task: Important = (5) Essential = (10). Determine score by dividing points earned by total points possible, and multiplying results by 100.

Name _____ Date _____ Score _____

EVALUATION
Evaluator Signature: _____ Date: _____

Evaluator Comments:

DOCUMENTATION
Instructor Note: Retain work products with competency checklist.
Work Product, Procedure 22-2 (Progress Note). Procedure forms can be downloaded from the student companion website.

Key Competencies		
ABHES	MA.A.1.4.a	Follow documentation guidelines
	MA.A.1.9.j	Make adaptations with patients with special needs
CAAHEP	I.P.8	Instruct and prepare a patient for a procedure or a treatment
	I.A.3	Show awareness of a patient's concerns related to the procedure being performed
	III.P.3	Perform handwashing
	V.A.4	Explain to a patient the rationale for performance of a procedure
	X.P.3	Document patient care accurately in the medical record

Name _____ Date _____ Score _____

COMPETENCY CHECKLIST

PROCEDURE 22-3 Instruct a Patient to Use Axillary Crutches

Task: To instruct a patient on the proper use of axillary crutches.

Condition: Given the equipment and supplies as listed in the procedure and a classmate to play the part of the patient, the student will demonstrate how to use crutches, adhering to the steps listed below.

Standards: The student will have 10 minutes to complete the procedure and will need to score an 85% or above to pass the competency. Automatic failure results if any essential steps are omitted or performed incorrectly.

STEPS START TIME: END TIME:	Points Possible	First Attempt	Second Attempt	Third Attempt
1. Check the provider's orders, assemble the equipment, and wash your hands.	10			
2. Identify the patient using two identifiers, identify yourself, and *explain the rationale for the performance of the procedure, showing awareness of the patient's concerns related to the procedure being performed*.	10			
3. Inspect rubber tips at the bottom of each crutch and tighten wing nuts. Check pads on the hand grips and the axillary bars.	10			
4. Instruct the patient to stand erect and place the crutches into the axillary space. The tip of each crutch should be held about 4 to 6 inches to the side of each foot.	10			
5. Adjust the crutches so there is a two-finger width space between the axillary bar and the armpits. The elbows should be flexed at a 25°–30° angle.	10			
6. Demonstrate the proper gait and inform the patient not to move the crutches more than 6 inches in front of the body.	10			
7. Allow the patient to practice. Be sure the patient is supporting her weight on the hand grips and not the axillary bar.	10			
8. Instruct the patient to inspect the crutches regularly for damage to the rubber tips and pads and to check the tightness of the wing nuts.	10			
9. Document the patient education in the patient's chart.	10			
Points Earned / Points Possible:	___ / 90			

Points possible reflect importance of step in meeting the task: Important = (5) Essential = (10). Determine score by dividing points earned by total points possible, and multiplying results by 100.

Name _____ Date _____ Score _____

EVALUATION

Evaluator Signature: _____ Date: _____

Evaluator Comments:

DOCUMENTATION

Instructor Note: Retain work products with competency checklist.
Work Product, Procedure 22-3 (Progress Note). Procedure forms can be downloaded from the student companion website.

Key Competencies		
ABHES	MA.A.1.4.a	Follow documentation guidelines
	MA.A.1.9.j	Make adaptations with patients with special needs
CAAHEP	I.P.8	Instruct and prepare a patient for a procedure or a treatment
	I.A.3	Show awareness of a patient's concerns related to the procedure being performed
	III.P.3	Perform handwashing
	V.A.4	Explain to a patient the rationale for performance of a procedure
	X.P.3	Document patient care accurately in the medical record

Name _____   Date _____   Score _____

COMPETENCY CHECKLIST

PROCEDURE 22-4   Instruct a Patient to Use a Walker

Task: To instruct a patient to use a walker.

Condition: Given the equipment and supplies as listed in the procedure and a classmate to play the part of the patient, the student will demonstrate how to use a walker, adhering to the steps listed below.

Standards: The student will have 10 minutes to complete the procedure and will need to score an 85% or above to pass the competency. Automatic failure results if any essential steps are omitted or performed incorrectly.

STEPS START TIME: END TIME:	Points Possible	First Attempt	Second Attempt	Third Attempt
1. Assemble the equipment and wash your hands.	10			
2. Identify the patient using two identifiers, identify yourself, and *explain the rationale for the performance of the procedure, showing awareness of the patient's concerns related to the procedure being performed.*	10			
3. Inspect the walker to be sure the rubber tips and hand grips are in place.	10			
4. Adjust the height of walker, so that the hand grips of the walker are at the patient's hip level.	10			
5. After demonstrating the proper procedure, instruct the patient to stand inside the walker and grip the handles. (When gripping the handles, the patient's elbows should be flexed at a 25°–30° angle.) Ask the patient to pick the walker up (not slide it), move it forward about 6 inches, and walk into it.	10			
6. Inform the patient that all four walker legs should be on the ground before moving forward.	10			
7. Have the patient demonstrate the procedure.	10			
8. Document the patient education in the patient's chart.	10			
Points Earned / Points Possible:	___ / 80			

Points possible reflect importance of step in meeting the task: Important = (5) Essential = (10). Determine score by dividing points earned by total points possible, and multiplying results by 100.

Name _____ Date _____ Score _____

EVALUATION
Evaluator Signature: _____ Date: _____

Evaluator Comments:

DOCUMENTATION
Instructor Note: Retain work products with competency checklist.
Work Product, Procedure 22-4 (Progress Note). Procedure forms can be downloaded from the student companion website.

Key Competencies			
ABHES	MA.A.1.4.a	Follow documentation guidelines	
	MA.A.1.9.j	Make adaptations with patients with special needs	
CAAHEP	I.P.8	Instruct and prepare a patient for a procedure or a treatment	
	I.A.3	Show awareness of a patient's concerns related to the procedure being performed	
	III.P.3	Perform handwashing	
	V.A.4	Explain to a patient the rationale for performance of a procedure	
	X.P.3	Document patient care accurately in the medical record	

Name _____ Date _____ Score _____

COMPETENCY CHECKLIST

PROCEDURE 22-5 Assist a Patient from the Wheelchair to the Exam Table and Back to the Wheelchair

Task: To correctly assist a patient from a wheelchair to the exam table and from the exam table back to the chair.

Condition: Given the equipment and supplies as listed in the procedure and a classmate to play the part of the patient, the student will demonstrate how to assist a patient from the wheelchair, adhering to the steps listed below.

Standards: The student will have 10 minutes to complete the procedure and will need to score an 85% or above to pass the competency. Automatic failure results if any essential steps are omitted or performed incorrectly.

STEPS START TIME: END TIME:	Points Possible	First Attempt	Second Attempt	Third Attempt
1. Wash your hands.	10			
2. Identify the patient using two identifiers, identify yourself, and apply the gait belt around the patient's waist. Explain that you will assist them onto the exam table. ***Show awareness of the patient's concerns related to the procedure being performed***.	10			
3. Place the wheelchair close to the exam table and lock the wheels. Pull out the extension or place a step stool close to the exam table (if necessary).	10			
4. Release the footrests and move them out of the way.	10			
5. Instruct the patient to slide forward to the edge of the wheelchair and place both feet on the floor.	10			
6. Stand in front of the patient and place your feet apart with one foot slightly out front.	10			
7. Bend your knees and instruct the patient to place his hands on the armrests of the wheelchair. Place your hands around the patient's waist, grasping the gait belt. Signal the patient to stand, pushing himself upward as you lift upward on the gait belt. Pause for a few seconds after the patient is standing before proceeding.	10			
8. Assist the patient up onto the footrest one foot at a time. Pivot the patient so that the backside of the body is against the exam table. Help the patient get into a sitting position. Move the wheelchair out of the way.	10			
9. After the exam, reapply the gait belt and move the wheelchair close to the exam table. Lock the wheels.	10			
10. Pull out the extension. Grasp your hands underneath the gait belt and ask the patient to grasp you around your shoulders. Help the patient to step down onto the foot extension and then onto the floor one foot at a time. If the patient is very tall, the patient may step directly onto the floor.	10			
11. Instruct the patient to reach behind for the arms of the chair and slowly lower the patient into the chair.	10			
12. Reposition the patient's feet on the footrests and unlock the wheels.	10			
Points Earned / Points Possible:	___ / 120			

Points possible reflect importance of step in meeting the task: Important = (5) Essential = (10). Determine score by dividing points earned by total points possible, and multiplying results by 100.

Name _____ Date _____ Score _____

EVALUATION

Evaluator Signature: _____ Date: _____

Evaluator Comments:

Key Competencies		
ABHES	MA.A.1.9.j	Make adaptations with patients with special needs
CAAHEP	I.P.8	Instruct and prepare a patient for a procedure or a treatment
	I.A.3	Show awareness of a patient's concerns related to the procedure being performed
	III.P.3	Perform handwashing
	V.A.4	Explain to a patient the rationale for performance of a procedure

Name _____ Date _____ Score _____

COMPETENCY CHECKLIST

PROCEDURE 22-6   Administer Heat Therapy Treatments

Task: To administer a heat therapy treatment.

Condition: Given the equipment and supplies as listed in the procedure and a classmate to play the part of the patient, the student will simulate administering heat therapy to a patient, adhering to the steps listed below.

Standards: The student will have 15 minutes to complete the procedure and will need to score an 85% or above to pass the competency. Automatic failure results if any essential steps are omitted or performed incorrectly.

STEPS START TIME: END TIME:	Points Possible	First Attempt	Second Attempt	Third Attempt
1. Assemble the supplies and wash your hands.	10			
2. Identify the patient using two identifiers, identify yourself, and *explain the rationale for the performance of the procedure, showing awareness of the patient's concerns related to the procedure being performed*.	10			
3. Instruct the patient to remove clothing and put on a gown, if necessary, exposing the area to be treated.	10			
4. Place the patient in the proper position for the treatment.	10			
5. Administer heat therapy as ordered:				
Heating pad:				
a. Place the protective covering over the heating pad.	10			
b. Connect the cord to an electrical outlet and set the control to the setting indicated by the provider.	10			
c. Place the heating pad on the affected area (do not allow the patient to lie on the heating pad) and ask the patient how the temperature level feels.	10			
Hot water bottle:				
a. Fill the hot water bottle approximately half full with water [the water temperature should be between 105°F and 110°F (40.5°C and 43°C)].	10			
b. Compress the air out of the bottle and close the lid tightly.	10			
c. Cover the water bottle with a cloth or towel.	10			
d. Leave in place for the prescribed amount of time.	10			
Hot compress:				
a. Fill a basin with hot water [between 105°F and 110°F (40.5°C and 43°C)].	10			
b. Soak cloth or gauze in hot water and wring out excess moisture.	10			
c. Place the compress over the affected area. Cover the compress with a plastic covering.	10			
d. Re-wet the compress to maintain the correct temperature.	10			
e. Replace the compress every few minutes for the amount of time prescribed by the provider.	10			

Name _____ Date _____ Score _____

Hot pack:				
a. Hot packs are soaked in hot water, allowed to drain, and covered with a pad. They are used on larger areas of the body, such as the back or shoulder.	10			
Hot soak:				
a. Fill an appropriate-sized container with hot water [approximately 105–110°F (40.5–43°C)] and add medication to the water if ordered by the provider.	10			
b. Place the body part in the water for the prescribed amount of time.	10			
c. After the prescribed amount of time, remove the body part from the soak and dry with a towel. Inspect the area for any redness or damage.	10			
Paraffin bath:				
a. A paraffin bath, composed of melted paraffin and mineral oil, should be heated to approximately 127°F (53°C).	10			
b. Dip the affected body part in the paraffin until a thick coating of wax builds up.	10			
c. Wrap the body part in foil, plastic wrap, or a cloth for 30 minutes.	10			
d. Take the covering off and peel away the wax.	10			
6. Check with the patient periodically during any heat treatment. The patient may feel chilled during the treatment, so cover the patient with a sheet or blanket.	10			
7. Check the treatment area for signs of damage such as redness, blisters, or irritation.	10			
8. Assist the patient with dressing, if needed.	10			
9. Clean the area and wash hands.	5			
10. Document treatment in the patient's chart.	10			
Points Earned / Points Possible:	___/285			

Points possible reflect importance of step in meeting the task: Important = (5) Essential = (10). Determine score by dividing points earned by total points possible, and multiplying results by 100.

Name _____ Date _____ Score _____

EVALUATION

Evaluator Signature: _____ Date: _____

Evaluator Comments:

DOCUMENTATION

Instructor Note: Retain work products with competency checklist.

Work Product, Procedure 22-6 (Progress Note). Procedure forms can be downloaded from the student companion website.

Key Competencies		
ABHES	MA.A.1.4.a	Follow documentation guidelines
	MA.A.1.9.e	Perform specialty procedures including but not limited to minor surgery, cardiac, respiratory, OB-GYN, neurological, gastroenterology
CAAHEP	I.P.8	Instruct and prepare a patient for a procedure or a treatment
	I.A.3	Show awareness of a patient's concerns related to the procedure being performed
	III.P.3	Perform handwashing
	V.A.4	Explain to a patient the rationale for performance of a procedure
	X.P.3	Document patient care accurately in the medical record

Name _____ Date _____ Score _____

COMPETENCY CHECKLIST

PROCEDURE 22-7   Administer Cold Therapy Treatments

Task: To administer a cold therapy treatment.

Condition: Given the equipment and supplies as listed in the procedure and a classmate to play the part of the patient, the student will simulate administering cold therapy to a patient, adhering to the steps listed below.

Standards: The student will have 15 minutes to complete the procedure and will need to score an 85% or above to pass the competency. Automatic failure results if any essential steps are omitted or performed incorrectly.

STEPS START TIME: END TIME:	Points Possible	First Attempt	Second Attempt	Third Attempt
1. Assemble the supplies and wash your hands.	10			
2. Identify the patient using two identifiers, identify yourself, and *explain the rationale for the performance of the procedure, showing awareness of the patient's concerns related to the procedure being performed.*	10			
3. Instruct the patient to remove clothing and put on a gown, if necessary, exposing the area to be treated.	10			
4. Place the patient in the proper position for treatment.	10			
5. Administer the cold therapy as ordered:				
Ice bag:				
a. Check the ice bag for damage or leaks.	10			
b. Fill the bag approximately two-thirds full with small ice chips or cubes; refill as needed.	10			
c. Squeeze the bag to expel excess air and screw the top into place.	10			
d. Cover the pack with a towel for patient comfort and to help absorb any moisture.	10			
e. Keep the ice bag in place for the amount of time ordered by the provider (usually 15 to 30 minutes).	10			
Commercial ice pack:				
a. Place the gel pack in the freezer for the amount of time recommended by the manufacturer.	10			
b. If pack has a protective covering over it, place it on the affected area.	10			
c. If there is no covering on the pack, cover the pack with a cloth or towel before applying.	10			
d. Leave the pack in place for the prescribed amount of time.	10			
e. Place the bag in the freezer after use.	10			
Chemical ice pack:				
a. Inspect the bag for leaks.	10			
b. Squeeze the bag and shake.	10			
c. Cover the pack with a protective covering.	10			
d. Apply the pack to the affected area for the amount of time prescribed by the provider.	10			
e. Discard the pack after use.	10			

Name _____ Date _____ Score _____

Cold compress:				
a. Place a small volume of water in a basin, and add large ice cubes to the water.	10			
b. Soak a washcloth or gauze pad in the water and wring out any excess.	10			
c. Place an ice pack over the compress.	10			
d. Re-wet, as needed, to maintain the temperature of the compress.	10			
e. Repeat application every 2 to 3 minutes for the amount of time prescribed by the provider.	10			
Ice massage:				
a. Fill a paper cup three-fourths full of water and place in the freezer.	10			
b. Expose the area to be treated and squeeze the paper cup so the ice cube is exposed.	10			
c. Move the ice cube in a circular motion over the affected area for the prescribed amount of time, or until the patient reports numbness and burning in the area.	10			
6. Check the treatment area following the procedure for paleness, redness, blueness, or any other signs of damage.	10			
7. Assist the patient with dressing if needed.	10			
8. Clean the work area and wash hands.	5			
9. Document the treatment in the patient's chart.	10			
Points Earned / Points Possible:	___ / 305			

Points possible reflect importance of step in meeting the task: Important = (5) Essential = (10). Determine score by dividing points earned by total points possible, and multiplying results by 100.

Name _____ Date _____ Score _____

EVALUATION
Evaluator Signature: _____ Date: _____

Evaluator Comments:

DOCUMENTATION
Instructor Note: Retain work products with competency checklist.
Work Product, Procedure 22-7 (Progress Note). Procedure forms can be downloaded from the student companion website.

Key Competencies		
ABHES	MA.A.1.4.a	Follow documentation guidelines
	MA.A.1.9.e	Perform specialty procedures including but not limited to minor surgery, cardiac, respiratory, OB-GYN, neurological, gastroenterology
CAAHEP	I.P.8	Instruct and prepare a patient for a procedure or a treatment
	I.A.3	Show awareness of a patient's concerns related to the procedure being performed
	III.P.3	Perform handwashing
	V.A.4	Explain to a patient the rationale for performance of a procedure
	X.P.3	Document patient care accurately in the medical record

Name _____   Date _____   Score _____

COMPETENCY CHECKLIST

PROCEDURE 23-1   Run a Control

Task: To use quality control data to determine if it is safe to report patient results.

Condition: Given the equipment and supplies as listed in the procedure, the student will run a control to determine if it is safe to report patient results, adhering to the steps listed below.

Standards: The student will have 15 minutes to complete the procedure and will need to score an 85% or above to pass the competency. Automatic failure results if any essential steps are omitted or performed incorrectly.

STEPS START TIME: END TIME:	Points Possible	First Attempt	Second Attempt	Third Attempt
1. Wash hands and put on appropriate PPE.	10			
2. Gather all equipment and supplies needed to run control.	10			
3. Check expiration date on control and any reagents to be used.	10			
4. Read manufacturer's instructions for running the control.	10			
5. Run control according to manufacturer's instructions.	10			
6. Record results in control log, as well as the expected results.	10			
7. Dispose of testing items in the proper trash receptacle.	10			
Points Earned / Points Possible:	___ / 70			

Points possible reflect importance of step in meeting the task: Important = (5) Essential = (10). Determine score by dividing points earned by total points possible, and multiplying results by 100.

EVALUATION

Evaluator Signature: _____   Date: _____

Evaluator Comments:

DOCUMENTATION

Instructor Note: Retain work products with competency checklist.
Work Product, Procedure 23-1 (Quality Control Log). Procedure forms can be downloaded from the student companion website.

Key Competencies		
ABHES	MA.A.1.10.a	Practice quality control
CAAHEP	I.P.10	Perform a quality control measure
	III.P.2	Select appropriate barrier/personal protective equipment (PPE)
	III.P.3	Perform handwashing

Name _____ Date _____ Score _____

COMPETENCY CHECKLIST

PROCEDURE 23-2   Review and Report Laboratory Results

Task: To review and report laboratory results.

Condition: Given the equipment and supplies as listed in the procedure, and a student to play the part of the physician, the student will review a laboratory reporting form and will handle the results in an appropriate manner, adhering to the steps listed below.

Standards: The student will have 15 minutes to complete the procedure and will need to score an 85% or above to pass the competency. Automatic failure results if any essential steps are omitted or performed incorrectly.

STEPS START TIME: END TIME:	Points Possible	First Attempt	Second Attempt	Third Attempt
1. Check open orders in tasks pane of the EHR. If you notice any open orders that are past due, contact the lab to see when the results will be available. (If using paper charts, check outstanding lab log and contact lab as above.)	10			
2. Check electronic tasks pane to review results that were electronically delivered from the night before. If results need to be scanned into the EHR, do so. (If using paper charts, pull labs off of printer and attach reports to the corresponding patient charts.)	10			
3. If using paper charts, review the laboratory report form, verifying all patient and provider information. Verify that all tests ordered were performed. Follow up with lab if missing any results. (Results delivered electronically are usually initially reviewed by provider.)	10			
4. If using paper charts, check the test results with laboratory reference ranges and immediately report any panic values to the provider. Stack charts with lab reports on provider's desk, making certain that abnormal results are on top of the pile.	10			
5. After the provider has reviewed the results, check to see if there are any special instructions for the patient.	10			
6. Report the results to the patient according to office protocol. (Verify you are speaking with patient or that you can leave results with someone listed on the patient's privacy statement.) If using EHR, make tests available in patient portal. Call patients who are not electronically connected or patients who have abnormal lab results. If patient questions the validity of the results, *reassure patient of the accuracy of the results*.	10			
7. Have patient repeat back any special instructions that need to be followed.	10			
8. Document the call in the chart and any special instructions given to patient.	10			
9. Make certain that flow sheets were completed if applicable.	10			
Points Earned / Points Possible:	___ / 90			

Points possible reflect importance of step in meeting the task: Important = (5) Essential = (10). Determine score by dividing points earned by total points possible, and multiplying results by 100.

Name _____ Date _____ Score _____

EVALUATION

Evaluator Signature: _____ Date: _____

Evaluator Comments:

DOCUMENTATION

Instructor Note: Retain work products with competency checklist.

Work Products, Procedure 23-2a (Progress Note), 23-2b (Outstanding Lab Results Tracking Report), and 23-2c (Hematology Report Form). Procedure forms can be downloaded from the student companion website.

Key Competencies		
ABHES	MA.A.1.4.a	Follow documentation guidelines
	MA.A.1.7.b	Utilize Electronic Medical Records (EMR) and Practice Management Systems
CAAHEP	II.P.2	Differentiate between normal and abnormal test results
	II.P.3	Maintain lab test results using flow sheets
	II.A.1	Reassure a patient of the accuracy of the test results
	VI.P.6	Utilize an EMR
	X.P.3	Document patient care accurately in the medical record

Name _____ Date _____ Score _____

COMPETENCY CHECKLIST

PROCEDURE 23-3   Specimen Collection for Offsite Testing

Task: To collect a specimen for offsite testing.

Condition: Given the equipment and supplies as listed in the procedure and a student to play the part of the patient, the student will simulate collecting and processing a lab specimen and will complete a lab requisition form using the student's information, adhering to the steps listed below.

Standards: The student will have 15 minutes to complete the procedure and will need to score an 85% or above to pass the competency. Automatic failure results if any essential steps are omitted or performed incorrectly.

STEPS START TIME: END TIME:	Points Possible	First Attempt	Second Attempt	Third Attempt
1. Verify the provider's order in the patient's chart.	10			
2. Review the requirements of the laboratory manual for specimen collection and transport.	10			
3. If the patient is collecting the specimen at home, gather materials with any special preparation instructions, such as fasting, diet or medication restrictions, and home collection instructions.	10			
4. Create lab order in CPOE if electronic or, if using paper charts, complete lab requisition with all important information before collecting the specimen.	10			
5. Assemble the proper equipment.	10			
6. Label all specimen tubes and containers with the patient's name, the date and time of collection, your initials, and any other information required by the lab.	10			
7. Wash your hands and put on the required PPE.	10			
8. Identify the patient using two identifiers, identify yourself, and *explain the rationale for the performance of the procedure, showing awareness of the patient's concerns related to the procedure being performed*. Verify fasting compliance, and properly collect the specimen according to lab directions.	10			
9. Properly engage safety device on needle if a needle was used and dispose of in sharp's container. Care for your patient and dismiss according to institutional policies.	10			
10. Process, prepare, and store specimen according to the protocol of the lab. Be sure to include the requisition in the outside pocket of the transfer bag and place the specimen in the middle pocket of the bag.	10			
11. Properly dispose of wastes in the correct trash receptacle, clean and disinfect the area. Remove PPE and dispose of according to facility policy.	10			
12. Wash hands and document the collection in the patient's chart and lab log if applicable.	10			
Points Earned / Points Possible:	___ / 120			

Points possible reflect importance of step in meeting the task: Important = (5) Essential = (10). Determine score by dividing points earned by total points possible, and multiplying results by 100.

Name _____ Date _____ Score _____

EVALUATION
Evaluator Signature: _____ Date: _____

Evaluator Comments:

DOCUMENTATION
Instructor Note: Retain work products (progress note, lab requisition form, and lab log) with competency checklist..
Work Products, Procedure 23-3a (Progress Note), 23-3b (Outside Lab Tracking Log), and 23-3c (Lab Requisition Form).
Procedure forms can be downloaded from the student companion website.

Key Competencies		
ABHES	MA.A.1.4.a	Follow documentation guidelines
	MA.A.1.7.b	Utilize Electronic Medical Records (EMR) and Practice Management Systems
	MA.A.1.10.c	Dispose of biohazardous material
	MA.A.1.10.d	Collect, label and process specimens
	MA.A.1.10.e	Instruct patients in the collection of: (1) clean-catch mid-stream urine specimen, (2) fecal specimen, and (3) sputum specimen
CAAHEP	I.P.11	Obtain specimens
	I.A.3	Show awareness of a patient's concerns related to the procedure being performed
	III.P.2	Select appropriate barrier/personal protective equipment (PPE)
	III.P.3	Perform handwashing
	III.P.10.b	Demonstrate proper disposal of biohazardous material: regulated wastes
	V.A.4	Explain to a patient the rationale for performance of a procedure
	VI.P.6	Utilize an EMR
	X.P.3	Document patient care accurately in the medical record

Name _____ Date _____ Score _____

COMPETENCY CHECKLIST

PROCEDURE 23-4   Use the Microscope

Task: To properly use the microscope.

Condition: Given the equipment and supplies as listed in the procedure, the student will demonstrate the steps that are necessary to properly use and care for a microscope.

Standards: The student will have 15 minutes to complete the procedure and will need to score an 85% or above to pass the competency. Automatic failure results if any essential steps are omitted or performed incorrectly.

STEPS START TIME: END TIME:	Points Possible	First Attempt	Second Attempt	Third Attempt
1. Wash your hands, apply gloves, and assemble all the equipment.	10			
2. Clean the oculars and the objectives with lens paper.	10			
3. Turn on the light source and adjust the light to a low level.	10			
4. Rotate the nosepiece to the low-power (10×) objective or high-power (40×) objective according to type of specimen and provider's order and click it into place.	10			
5. Place the specimen slide on the stage and move the stage upward using the stage adjustment knobs, so the objective is in its lowest position. Observe the stage movement so that the objective does not come in contact with the slide.	10			
6. Adjust the eyepieces to a comfortable width. View the slide through the oculars, and using the coarse adjustment knob (larger knobs) to bring the specimen into focus.	10			
7. Adjust light intensity as needed.	10			
8. Using the fine adjustment knob, bring the specimen into sharp, clear focus.	10			
9. After observation of the specimen is complete, notify provider that the specimen is ready to be viewed under the scope.	10			
10. When provider is done, remove slide from the stage and clean the objective with lens paper and wipe the stage clean with tissue or gauze.	10			
11. Turn off the light source and cover the scope with a protective dust cover.	10			
Points Earned / Points Possible:	__ / 110			

Points possible reflect importance of step in meeting the task: Important = (5) Essential = (10). Determine score by dividing points earned by total points possible, and multiplying results by 100.

Name _____ Date _____ Score _____

EVALUATION

Evaluator Signature: _____ Date: _____

Evaluator Comments:

Key Competencies		
CAAHEP	III.P.3	Perform handwashing
	VI.P.8	Perform routine maintenance of administrative or clinical equipment

Name _____ Date _____ Score _____

COMPETENCY CHECKLIST
PROCEDURE 24-1   Perform Venipuncture (Syringe Method)

Task: To perform a venipuncture using the syringe method.

Condition: Given the equipment and supplies as listed in the procedure, and a student to play the part of the patient, the student will demonstrate the proper steps for performing a venipuncture using the syringe method, adhering to the steps listed below. Instructor will inform student what tests are to be drawn.

Standards: The student will have 15 minutes to complete the procedure and will need to score an 85% or above to pass the competency. Automatic failure results if any essential steps are omitted or performed incorrectly.

STEPS START TIME: END TIME:	Points Possible	First Attempt	Second Attempt	Third Attempt
1. *Incorporating critical thinking skills when performing patient care*, check the provider's order and complete the laboratory requisition form.	10			
2. Wash your hands and apply PPE.	10			
3. Assemble all the necessary equipment, and loosen the plunger by pulling it all the way back and pushing it all the way in at least one time. Label all tubes.	10			
4. Identify the patient using at least two identifiers and identify yourself.	10			
5. *Explain the rationale for the procedure, showing awareness of the patient's concerns related to the procedure being performed.*	10			
6. Verify compliance of fasting instructions and other restrictions (for instance, the need to draw blood from one side or another due to a mastectomy or the presence of a shunt).	10			
7. Visually inspect the patient's skin and veins in both arms, *incorporating critical thinking skills when performing patient assessment*. Always ask if the patient has a preference. Patients usually know which veins produce the best results.	10			
8. Select the potential site and apply the tourniquet 3 to 4 inches above the elbow. The tourniquet should not remain in place longer than one minute.	5			
9. Palpate the vein using your index finger, moving in an upward and downward direction and side to side.	10			
10. Straighten and place the arm and hand in a downward position.	10			
11. Ask the patient to make a slight fist and hold. (Do not pump the fist, as this can cause erroneous results.)	10			
12. Cleanse the site with alcohol using a circular motion.	10			
13. Allow the area to air dry, or dry wipe the area with a clean/ sterile gauze square.	10			
14. Pull the skin taut to anchor the vein.	10			
15. Insert the needle using a 15° to 30° angle and make certain that the bevel is upward.	10			
16. When blood appears in the hub of the needle, pull back on the plunger at a slow steady rate using the opposite hand.	10			

Name _____ Date _____ Score _____

17. Allow the syringe to fill completely.	10			
18. When the syringe is full, instruct the patient to open the hand.	10			
19. Release the tourniquet.	10			
20. Place a dry piece of (clean or sterile) gauze above the site, withdraw the needle, and ask the patient to apply firm pressure to the site for two to three minutes.	10			
21. Push the sheath over the needle and carefully remove it from the syringe. Discard the needle into the sharps container.	10			
22. Carefully transfer the blood from the syringe to vacuum tubes using a safety transfer device.	10			
23. Immediately mix each filled tube according to the manufacturer's instructions.	10			
24. Discard used equipment according to OSHA standards.	10			
25. Check the puncture site and apply a pressure bandage.	10			
26. Dismiss the patient.	10			
27. Clean the work area and process the specimen.	10			
28. Remove gloves and wash your hands.	10			
29. Document the procedure in the patient's chart and in the lab log.	10			
Points Earned / Points Possible:	__/ 285			

Points possible reflect importance of step in meeting the task: Important = (5) Essential = (10). Determine score by dividing points earned by total points possible, and multiplying results by 100.

Name _____ Date _____ Score _____

EVALUATION
Evaluator Signature: _____ Date: _____

Evaluator Comments:

DOCUMENTATION
Instructor Note: Retain work products with competency checklist.
Work Product, Procedure 24-1a (Progress Note), 24-1b (Outstanding Lab Results Tracking Report), and 24-1c (Lab Requisition Form). Procedure forms can be downloaded from the student companion website.

Key Competencies		
ABHES	MA.A.1.4.a	Follow documentation guidelines
	MA.A.1.9.a	Practice standard precautions and perform disinfection/sterilization techniques
	MA.A.1.10.c	Dispose of biohazardous materials
	MA.A.1.10.d(1)	Perform venipuncture
CAAHEP	I.P.2.b	Perform venipuncture
	I.A.1	Incorporate critical thinking skills when performing patient assessment
	I.A.2	Incorporate critical thinking skills when performing patient care
	I.A.3	Show awareness of a patient's concerns related to the procedure being performed
	III.P.2	Select appropriate barrier/personal protective equipment (PPE)
	III.P.3	Perform handwashing
	III.P.10	Demonstrate proper disposal of biohazardous material: (a) sharps, and (b) regulated waste
	V.A.4	Explain to a patient the rationale for performance of a procedure
	X.P.3	Document patient care accurately in the medical record

Name _____ Date _____ Score _____

COMPETENCY CHECKLIST
PROCEDURE 24-2   Perform Venipuncture (Vacuum Tube Method)

Task: To perform a venipuncture using the vacuum tube method.

Condition: Given the equipment and supplies as listed in the procedure, and a student to play the part of the patient, the student will demonstrate the proper steps for performing a venipuncture using the vacuum tube method, adhering to the steps listed below. Instructor will provide the name of the test(s) to be performed.

Standards: The student will have 10 minutes to complete the procedure and will need to score an 85% or above to pass the competency. Automatic failure results if any essential steps are omitted or performed incorrectly.

STEPS START TIME: END TIME:	Points Possible	First Attempt	Second Attempt	Third Attempt
1. *Incorporating critical thinking skills when performing patient care*, check the order and complete the laboratory requisition form.	10			
2. Wash your hands and apply PPE. Remember the amount of PPE worn may vary from one facility to the next.	10			
3. Assemble all the necessary equipment and label all tubes.	10			
4. Identify the patient using at least two identifiers. Identify yourself.	10			
5. *Explain the rationale for performance of the procedure, showing awareness of the patient's concerns related to the procedure being performed.*	10			
6. Verify compliance of fasting instructions and other restrictions (for instance, the need to draw blood from one side or another due to a mastectomy or the presence of a shunt).	10			
7. Visually inspect the patient's skin and veins in both arms, *incorporating critical thinking skills when performing patient assessment*. Always ask if the patient has a preference. Patients usually know which veins produce the best results.	5			
8. Apply a tourniquet 3 to 4 inches above the elbow. The tourniquet should not remain in place longer than one minute.	10			
9. Straighten and place the arm and hand in a downward position.	10			
10. Ask the patient to make a fist and hold. (Do not pump the fist, as this can cause erroneous results.)	10			
11. Palpate the vein and select final site. Check the direction the vein is running and the vein's depth.	10			
12. Cleanse the site with alcohol using a circular motion.	10			
13. Allow the area to air dry, or dry wipe the area with a clean/sterile piece of gauze.	10			
14. Pull the skin taut to anchor the vein.	10			
15. Using a 15° to 30° angle, insert the needle with the bevel up and tube label down.	10			
16. Using the hand that anchored the vein, grasp the flanges of the holder and push the tube until the needle punctures the stopper and blood flows into the tube.	10			

Name _____ Date _____ Score _____

17. Allow the tube to fill completely before changing the tube. Withdraw the tube and mix the additive tubes immediately.	10				
18. Change tubes until all tubes have been collected. Instruct the patient to open the hand.	10				
19. Release the tourniquet and remove the tube before removing the needle.	10				
20. Place a dry sterile or clean piece of gauze above the site, withdraw the needle, and ask the patient to apply firm pressure to the site for two to three minutes.	10				
21. Engage the safety device and discard the used equipment according to OSHA standards.	10				
22. Check the puncture site and apply a pressure bandage.	10				
23. Dismiss the patient.	10				
24. Clean the work area and process specimen.	10				
25. Remove gloves and wash your hands.	10				
26. Document the procedure in the patient's chart.	10				
Points Earned / Points Possible:	__/255				

Points possible reflect importance of step in meeting the task: Important = (5) Essential = (10). Determine score by dividing points earned by total points possible, and multiplying results by 100.

EVALUATION

Evaluator Signature: _____ Date: _____

Evaluator Comments:

DOCUMENTATION

Instructor Note: Retain work products with competency checklist.
Work Product, Procedure 24-2a (Progress Note), 24-2b (Outstanding Lab Results Tracking Report), and 24-2c (Lab Requisition Form). Procedure forms can be downloaded from the student companion website.

Key Competencies		
ABHES	MA.A.1.4.a	Follow documentation guidelines
	MA.A.1.9.a	Practice standard precautions and perform disinfection/sterilization techniques
	MA.A.1.10.c	Dispose of biohazardous materials
	MA.A.1.10.d(1)	Perform venipuncture
CAAHEP	I.P.2.b	Perform venipuncture
	I.A.1	Incorporate critical thinking skills when performing patient assessment
	I.A.2	Incorporate critical thinking skills when performing patient care
	I.A.3	Show awareness of a patient's concerns related to the procedure being performed
	III.P.2	Select appropriate barrier/personal protective equipment (PPE)
	III.P.3	Perform handwashing
	III.P.10	Demonstrate proper disposal of biohazardous material: (a) sharps, and (b) regulated wastes
	V.A.4	Explain to a patient the rationale for performance of a procedure
	X.P.3	Document patient care accurately in the medical record

Name _____ Date _____ Score _____

COMPETENCY CHECKLIST

PROCEDURE 24-3   Perform Venipuncture (Butterfly Method)

Task: To perform a venipuncture using the butterfly method.

Condition: Given the equipment and supplies as listed in the procedure, and a student to play the part of the patient, the student will demonstrate the proper steps for performing a venipuncture using the butterfly method, adhering to the steps listed below. Instructor will provide the name of the test(s) to be performed.

Standards: The student will have 10 minutes to complete the procedure and will need to score an 85% or above to pass the competency. Automatic failure results if any essential steps are omitted or performed incorrectly.

STEPS START TIME: END TIME:	Points Possible	First Attempt	Second Attempt	Third Attempt
1. *Incorporating critical thinking skills when performing patient care*, check the provider's order and complete the laboratory requisition form.	10			
2. Wash your hands and apply PPE. Remember that the types of PPE worn during a blood draw may vary from one facility to another.	10			
3. Assemble all the necessary equipment and label all tubes.	10			
4. Identify the patient using two identifiers, and identify yourself.	10			
5. *Explain the rationale for performance of the procedure, showing awareness of the patient's concerns related to the procedure being performed.*	10			
6. Verify compliance of fasting instructions and other restrictions (for instance, the need to draw blood from one side or another due to a mastectomy or the presence of a shunt).	10			
7. Visually inspect the patient's skin and veins in both arms or hands, *incorporating critical thinking skills when performing patient assessment*. Always ask if the patient has a preference. Patients usually know which veins produce the best results.	5			
8. Select the appropriate arm or hand and apply a tourniquet 3 to 4 inches above the elbow or wrist when drawing from the hand. The tourniquet should not remain in place longer than one minute.	10			
9. Ask the patient to make a fist.	10			
10. Place the fist of the patient's other hand under the elbow when drawing from the arm, or under the wrist when drawing from the hand.	10			
11. Palpate the vein and selected final site.	10			
12. Cleanse the site with alcohol using a circular motion.	10			
13. Allow the area to air dry, or dry wipe the area with a clean/ sterile gauze square.	10			
14. Pull the skin taut.	10			
15. Grasp the wings of the butterfly and insert the needle bevel up, at a 5° to 10° angle.				

Name _____ Date _____ Score _____

Vacuum tube method:				
16a. Once blood enters the tubing, push the tube onto the needle inside the tube adapter and allow it to fill completely. Remove the tube and invert additive tubes to mix before pushing in additional tubes. When the last tube is filling, release the tourniquet. When the tube is completely full, withdraw the tube and then withdraw the needle. Engage the safety device.	10			
Syringe method:				
16b. Once blood enters the hub of the needle, start pulling back on the plunger. Fill the syringe completely and ask the patient to relax the hand. Release the tourniquet, withdraw the needle, engage the safety device, and remove the needle, placing it in a sharps container. Fill the tubes using a safety transfer device, and immediately invert them to mix.	10			
For both types:				
17. Place a dry sterile or clean gauze square over the site and instruct the patient to apply firm pressure to the site for two to three minutes.	10			
18. Discard used equipment according to OSHA standards.	10			
19. Check the puncture site and apply a pressure bandage.				
20. Dismiss the patient.	10			
21. Clean the work area and process the specimen.	10			
22. Remove gloves and wash your hands.	10			
23. Document the procedure in the patient's chart.	10			
Points Earned / Points Possible:	__/ 235			

Points possible reflect importance of step in meeting the task: Important = (5) Essential = (10). Determine score by dividing points earned by total points possible, and multiplying results by 100.

Name _____ Date _____ Score _____

EVALUATION

Evaluator Signature: _____ Date: _____

Evaluator Comments:

DOCUMENTATION

Instructor Note: Retain work products with competency checklist.
Work Product, Procedure 24-3a (Progress Note), 24-3b (Outside Lab Tracking Log), and 24-3c (Lab Requisition Form).
Procedure forms can be downloaded from the student companion website.

Key Competencies			
ABHES	MA.A.1.4.a	Follow documentation guidelines	
	MA.A.1.9.a	Practice standard precautions and perform disinfection/sterilization techniques	
	MA.A.1.10.c	Dispose of biohazardous materials	
	MA.A.1.10.d(1)	Perform venipuncture	
CAAHEP	I.P.2.b	Perform venipuncture	
	I.A.1	Incorporate critical thinking skills when performing patient assessment	
	I.A.2	Incorporate critical thinking skills when performing patient care	
	I.A.3	Show awareness of a patient's concerns related to the procedure being performed	
	III.P.2	Select appropriate barrier/personal protective equipment (PPE)	
	III.P.3	Perform handwashing	
	III.P.10	Demonstrate proper disposal of biohazardous material: (a) sharps, and (b) regulated wastes	
	V.A.4	Explain to a patient the rationale for performance of a procedure	
	X.P.3	Document patient care accurately in the medical record	

Name _____ Date _____ Score _____

COMPETENCY CHECKLIST

PROCEDURE 24-4   **Perform a Capillary Puncture**

Task: To perform a capillary puncture.

Condition: Given the equipment and supplies as listed in the procedure, and a student to play the part of the patient, the student will demonstrate the proper steps for performing a capillary puncture, adhering to the steps listed below. This specimen will be sent out for testing. Instructor will provide the name of the test(s) to be performed.

Standards: The student will have 10 minutes to complete the procedure and will need to score an 85% or above to pass the competency. Automatic failure results if any essential steps are omitted or performed incorrectly.

STEPS START TIME: END TIME:	Points Possible	First Attempt	Second Attempt	Third Attempt
1. *Incorporating critical thinking skills when performing patient care*, check the provider's order and complete the laboratory requisition form.	10			
2. Wash your hands and apply PPE. The types of PPE worn during a capillary stick may vary from one facility to another.	10			
3. Assemble all the necessary equipment and label all tubes.	10			
4. Identify the patient using two identifiers and identify yourself.	10			
5. *Explain the rationale for performance of the procedure, showing awareness of the patient's concerns related to the procedure being performed.*	10			
6. Select the fleshy portion of the patient's distal middle or ring finger on the nondominant hand.	10			
7. Apply a warm compress to the area or have the patient run the hands under warm water.	10			
8. Clean the site with alcohol and allow it to air dry, or dry wipe with a gauze square.	10			
9. Grasp the finger securely and puncture the fingertip perpendicular to the whorls of the fingerprint.	10			
10. Dispose of the lancet in the sharps container according to OSHA guidelines.	10			
11. Wipe away the first drop of blood before beginning the sample collection.	10			
12. Hold the finger, applying pressure by gently squeezing and releasing the fingertip.	10			
13. Collect needed samples either in a capillary tube or microcollection tube.	10			
14. Ask the patient to apply gentle pressure with a clean or sterile gauze square to the puncture site.	10			
15. Check the puncture site and apply a bandage, if necessary.	10			
16. Dismiss the patient.	10			

Name _____ Date _____ Score _____

17. Properly dispose of all used equipment according to OSHA standards.	10				
18. Clean the work area.	10				
19. Remove gloves and wash your hands.	10				
20. Document the procedure in the patient's chart.	10				
Points Earned / Points Possible:	__ / 200				

Points possible reflect importance of step in meeting the task: Important = (5) Essential = (10). Determine score by dividing points earned by total points possible, and multiplying results by 100.

EVALUATION

Evaluator Signature: _____ Date: _____

Evaluator Comments:

DOCUMENTATION

Instructor Note: Retain work products with competency checklist.
Work Product, Procedure 24-4a (Progress Note), 24-4b (Outstanding Lab Results Tracking Report), and 24-4c (Lab Requisition Form). Procedure forms can be downloaded from the student companion website.

Key Competencies			
ABHES	MA.A.1.4.a	Follow documentation guidelines	
	MA.A.1.9.a	Practice standard precautions and perform disinfection/sterilization techniques	
	MA.A.1.10.c	Dispose of biohazardous materials	
	MA.A.1.10.d(2)	Perform capillary puncture	
CAAHEP	I.P.2.c	Perform capillary puncture	
	I.A.2	Incorporate critical thinking skills when performing patient care	
	I.A.3	Show awareness of a patient's concerns related to the procedure being performed	
	III.P.2	Select appropriate barrier/personal protective equipment (PPE)	
	III.P.3	Perform handwashing	
	III.P.10	Demonstrate proper disposal of biohazardous material: (a) sharps, and (b) regulated wastes	
	V.A.4	Explain to a patient the rationale for performance of a procedure	
	X.P.3	Document patient care accurately in the medical record	

Name _____   Date _____   Score _____

COMPETENCY CHECKLIST

PROCEDURE 25-1   Instruct a Patient on a Clean-Catch Midstream Urine Collection

Task: To instruct a patient on a clean-catch midstream urine collection.

Condition: Given the equipment and supplies as listed in the procedure, and a student to play the part of the patient, the student will demonstrate the proper steps for instructing a patient on how to obtain a clean-catch midstream urine specimen, adhering to the steps listed below.

Standards: The student will have 10 minutes to complete the procedure and will need to score an 85% or above to pass the competency. Automatic failure results if any essential steps are omitted or performed incorrectly.

STEPS START TIME: END TIME:	Points Possible	First Attempt	Second Attempt	Third Attempt
1. Wash your hands.	10			
2. Assemble the necessary equipment.	10			
3. Identify the patient using at least two identifiers, and introduce yourself by name and credentials.	10			
4. *Show awareness of a patient's concerns related to the procedure being performed. Incorporate critical thinking skills when performing patient care*.	10			
5. Label the specimen cup with the patient's name and date/time.	10			
6. Give the patient gloves (optional), towelettes, and a labeled urine specimen cup and lid.	10			
7. Assuring privacy, and using language that enables the patient's understanding, explain the clean-catch process. *Explain the rationale for performing the procedure, displaying sensitivity to the patient's rights* and feelings when explaining the process.	10			
Instruct the female patient to:				
• Open the towelettes so they are readily available. • Spread the labia apart with nondominant hand to expose the urinary meatus, use one towelette to wipe down one side of the meatus from front to back, and discard the towelette into the toilet. • With the second towelette wipe down the other side of the meatus from front to back and discard the towelette into the toilet. • Using the third towelette, wipe down the center of the meatus from front to back and discard the towelette. • Caution the patient to hold the labia apart during urination.				
Instruct the male patient to:				
• Retract the foreskin (if applicable) and cleanse the tip and the urethral opening from the tip of the penis toward the ring of the glans twice, with two separate towelettes. Discard into the toilet and keep foreskin retracted while urinating into the cup.				
For all patients:				
8. After beginning to urinate into the toilet, catch the middle portion of the urine in the specimen cup, then withdraw the cup, and finish urinating into the toilet.	10			

Name _____ Date _____ Score _____

9. Instruct the patient to place the lid tightly on the specimen container and wipe the outside of the container with a paper towel.	10			
10. Show the patient where to leave the sample, where they may wash their hands, and where to wait for further instructions.	10			
11. Document the clean-catch order.	10			
Points Earned / Points Possible:	__ / 110			

Points possible reflect importance of step in meeting the task: Important = (5) Essential = (10). Determine score by dividing points earned by total points possible, and multiplying results by 100.

EVALUATION

Evaluator Signature: _____ Date: _____

Evaluator Comments:

DOCUMENTATION

Instructor Note: Retain work products with competency checklist.
Work Product, Procedure 25-1 (Progress Note). Procedure forms can be downloaded from the student companion website.

Key Competencies			
ABHES	MA.A.1.4.a	Follow documentation guidelines	
	MA.A.1.10.d	Collect, label, and process specimens	
	MA.A.1.10.e(1)	Instruct patients in the collection of a clean-catch mid-stream urine specimen	
CAAHEP	I.A.2	Incorporate critical thinking skills when performing patient care	
	I.A.3	Show awareness of a patient's concerns related to the procedure being performed	
	III.P.3	Perform handwashing	
	V.A.4	Explain to a patient the rationale for performance of a procedure	
	X.P.3	Document patient care accurately in the medical record	

Name _____ Date _____ Score _____

COMPETENCY CHECKLIST

PROCEDURE 25-2   Perform a Physical and Chemical Urinalysis and Prepare a Microscope Slide for the Provider

Task: To perform a physical and chemical urinalysis and prepare a slide of urinary sediment for microscopic examination.

Condition: Given the equipment and supplies as listed in the procedure, and a urine specimen to test, the student will demonstrate the proper steps for performing a physical and chemical urinalysis and preparing a slide for microscopic examination, adhering to the steps listed below.

Standards: The student will have 15 minutes to complete the procedure and will need to score an 85% or above to pass the competency. Automatic failure results if any essential steps are omitted or performed incorrectly.

STEPS START TIME: END TIME:	Points Possible	First Attempt	Second Attempt	Third Attempt
1. Wash your hands and apply appropriate PPE.	10			
2. Assemble the necessary equipment.	10			
3. Gently mix the specimen.	10			
4. Pour 10 mL of the specimen into a clear, labeled centrifuge tube.	10			
5. While holding the specimen in front of a light source, assess and record the color of the urine.	10			
6. Observe the clarity of the urine by holding a printed sheet of paper behind the specimen.	10			
7. Note any unusual odor, if present.	10			
8. Measure the specific gravity using method of choice, following manufacturer's instructions.	10			
9. Cap the tube and remix the urine. Remove cap and dip the reagent strip into the tube, being certain to cover the entire strip with urine.	10			
10. After removing the strip from the cup, place the strip on its side on a paper towel to allow excess urine to be removed.	10			
11. Hold the strip next to but not against the color chart on the bottle.	10			
12. Accurately time all readings and read the results.	10			
13. Record all results. Follow office protocol for all abnormal results.	10			
14. Centrifuge the tube of urine for five minutes at 1500 rpm. Remove tube from the centrifuge.	10			
15. Invert the tube upside down without shaking to pour the supernatant off. Exactly 1 mL should remain in the tube. Add sediment stain if directed by provider. Mix the sediment well.	10			
16. Place one drop of well-mixed sediment onto a labeled glass slide and carefully place a cover slip over the drop of urine.	10			
17. Place the slide under the microscope, leaving the light off, and inform the provider that the specimen is ready to examine.	10			
18. Properly dispose of all equipment and specimens into the biohazard container, and the slide and cover slip into the sharps container.	10			

Name _____ Date _____ Score _____

19. Remove gloves and wash your hands.	10			
20. Document the procedure.	10			
Points Earned / Points Possible:	__ / 200			

Points possible reflect importance of step in meeting the task: Important = (5) Essential = (10). Determine score by dividing points earned by total points possible, and multiplying results by 100.

EVALUATION

Evaluator Signature: _____ Date: _____

Evaluator Comments:

DOCUMENTATION

Instructor Note: Retain work products with competency checklist.
Work Products, Procedure 25-2a (Progress Note), 25-2b (Urinalysis Report Form), 25-2c (In-House Urinalysis Dipstick Testing Log). Procedure forms can be downloaded from the student companion website.

Key Competencies			
ABHES	MA.A.1.4.a	Follow documentation guidelines	
	MA.A.1.10.1(b)	Perform selected CLIA waived tests that assist with diagnosis and treatment: Urinalysis	
	MA.A.1.10.c	Dispose of biohazardous materials	
	MA.A.1.10.d	Collect, label, and process specimens	
CAAHEP	I.P.10	Perform a quality control measure	
	I.P.11.c	Obtain specimens and perform: CLIA waived urinalysis	
	II.P.2	Differentiate between normal and abnormal test results	
	III.P.2	Select appropriate barrier/personal protective equipment (PPE)	
	III.P.3	Perform handwashing	
	III.P.10	Demonstrate proper disposal of biohazardous material: (a) sharps, and (b) regulated wastes	
	X.P.3	Document patient care accurately in the medical record	

Name _____ Date _____ Score _____

COMPETENCY CHECKLIST

PROCEDURE 25-3 **Utilizing a Urine Transport System for Culture and Sensitivity**

Task: To use a urine transport system to prepare a urine specimen for an outside lab for a culture and sensitivity test.

Condition: Given the equipment and supplies as listed in the procedure the student will demonstrate the proper steps for how to use a urine transport system to prepare a urine specimen for an outside lab for a culture and sensitivity test, adhering to the steps listed below.

Standards: The student will have 10 minutes to complete the procedure and will need to score an 85% or above to pass the competency. Automatic failure results if any essential steps are omitted or performed incorrectly.

STEPS START TIME: END TIME:	Points Possible	First Attempt	Second Attempt	Third Attempt
1. Wash your hands, and apply gloves and the appropriate PPE. Check the provider's order and complete the lab requisition form.	10			
2. Assemble the equipment.	10			
3. Check the expiration date on the transport system. Check that the urine specimen is properly labeled.	10			
4. Open the urine transport kit and assemble it according to the manufacturer's directions.	10			
5. Label the tubes. Insert the urine tube into the holder without piercing the stopper.	10			
6. Put the straw of the transport system into the urine specimen and push the vacuum tube onto the needle inside the tube holder.	10			
7. Allow the tube to fill completely.	10			
8. Remove the tube from the holder and properly dispose of the unit.	10			
9. Place the specimen tube into the laboratory transport bag and seal that compartment. Clean and disinfect the work area and properly dispose of contaminated supplies.	10			
10. Remove gloves and wash your hands.	10			
11. Complete the requisition and place it into its own compartment of the transport bag.	10			
12. Document the procedure in the patient's chart.	10			
Points Earned / Points Possible:	__ / 120			

Points possible reflect importance of step in meeting the task: Important = (5) Essential = (10). Determine score by dividing points earned by total points possible, and multiplying results by 100.

Name _____ Date _____ Score _____

EVALUATION

Evaluator Signature: _____ Date: _____

Evaluator Comments:

DOCUMENTATION

Instructor Note: Retain work products with competency checklist.

Work Product, Procedure 25-3 (Progress Note). Procedure forms can be downloaded from the student companion website.

Key Competencies		
ABHES	MA.A.1.4.a	Follow documentation guidelines
	MA.A.1.10.c	Dispose of biohazardous materials
	MA.A.1.10.d	Collect, label, and process specimens
CAAHEP	III.P.2	Select appropriate barrier/personal protective equipment (PPE)
	III.P.3	Perform handwashing
	III.P.10	Demonstrate proper disposal of biohazardous material: (a) sharps, and (b) regulated wastes
	X.P.3	Document patient care accurately in the medical record

Name _____ Date _____ Score _____

COMPETENCY CHECKLIST
PROCEDURE 25-4   Urinary Catheterization

Task: To obtain a sterile urine specimen by inserting a sterile catheter into the bladder while observing strict sterile technique.

Condition: Given the equipment and supplies as listed in the procedure, using a manikin simulator, the student will demonstrate the proper steps for performing a urinary catheterization, adhering to the steps listed below.

Standards: The student will have 20 minutes to complete the procedure and will need to score an 85% or above to pass the competency. Automatic failure results if any essential steps are omitted or performed incorrectly.

STEPS START TIME: END TIME:	Points Possible	First Attempt	Second Attempt	Third Attempt
1. Identify the patient using two identifiers, introduce yourself using your credentials, and *explain the rationale for performance of the procedure*.	10			
2. Wash your hands and assemble the supplies. Place the catheter kit on the Mayo stand or a nearby counter surface.	10			
3. *Showing awareness of a patient's concerns related to the procedure being performed*, instruct the patient to remove clothing from the waist down, providing privacy. Give the patient a drape, *demonstrating the principles of self-boundaries*. Assist as needed.	10			
4. Position the patient in a comfortable dorsal recumbent position, draping with only the external genitalia exposed.	10			
5. Adjust the light as needed.	10			
6. Place the catheter kit on the Mayo stand at a right angle to the patient. Open the external covering of the catheter kit. (The inside of the outer covering of the kit will now become a sterile field.)	10			
7. Carefully reach inside the kit without contaminating the field or contents of the kit and place the waterproof sterile drape from the kit underneath the penis for a male patient, or underneath the buttocks for a female patient. Touch only the corners of the drape.	10			
8. Wash hands and put on sterile gloves, using caution not to contaminate gloved hands. (From this point on, you will touch only the sterile materials inside the kit and the surface to be catheterized. If anything outside the kit is needed, ask for assistance.)	10			
9. Open the fenestrated drape and place the drape over the external genitalia.	10			
10. Prepare a cleaning solution (either sterile wipes or sterile gauze pads with an antiseptic cleanser) and apply some lubricant onto the sterile gauze pad.	10			
11. Insert the tip of the catheter into the sterile lubricant and leave the catheter on the sterile field until ready for use. Open the specimen container and place within reach.	10			
12. For a female, spread the labia with nondominant hand and cleanse the genital areas (right side, left side, and middle) from front to back with the other hand. For males, cleanse the urinary meatus in a circular motion working from the center outward. Repeat two more times.	10			

Name _____ Date _____ Score _____

13. Resting the distal end of the catheter in the urine receptacle, insert the well-lubricated tip of the catheter *slowly* into the urinary meatus. Proceed slowly and do not force the catheter in. If an obstruction is noted or pain or bleeding is present, stop the insertion.	10			
14. **Display sensitivity to the patient's rights** and feelings when collecting the specimen.	10			
15. Progress the catheter into the bladder until urine flows. Collect the initial stream in the receptacle basin, and then obtain the sample in the specimen container.	10			
16. After adequate collection, empty the remainder of the urine inside the bladder into the receptacle basin. Never leave the bladder partially full after catheterization.	10			
17. Slowly remove the catheter from the meatus and place on the table.	10			
18. Gently clean the genital region as needed and provide tissues for the patient.	10			
19. Remove gloves and wash hands. Assist the patient into a sitting position as needed.	10			
20. Discard the materials in the appropriate waste containers.	10			
21. Label the urine specimen container and attach a lab requisition form that has been filled out with all pertinent information.	10			
22. Document the procedure on the patient's record. Include any adverse reactions from the patient.	10			
Points Earned / Points Possible:	__ / 220			

Points possible reflect importance of step in meeting the task: Important = (5) Essential = (10). Determine score by dividing points earned by total points possible, and multiplying results by 100.

Name _____ Date _____ Score _____

EVALUATION

Evaluator Signature: _____ Date: _____

Evaluator Comments:

DOCUMENTATION

Instructor Note: Retain work products with competency checklist.

Work Product, Procedure 25-4 (Progress Note). Procedure forms can be downloaded from the student companion website.

Key Competencies		
ABHES	MA.A.1.4.a	Follow documentation guidelines
	MA.A.1.10.c	Dispose of biohazardous materials
	MA.A.1.10.d	Collect, label, and process specimens
CAAHEP	I.A.3	Show awareness of a patient's concerns related to the procedure being performed
	III.P.2	Select appropriate barrier/personal protective equipment (PPE)
	III.P.3	Perform handwashing
	III.P.7	Perform within a sterile field
	III.P.10	Demonstrate proper disposal of biohazardous material: (a) sharps, and (b) regulated wastes
	V.A.2	Demonstrate the principles of self-boundaries
	V.A.4	Explain to a patient the rationale for performance of a procedure
	X.P.3	Document patient care accurately in the medical record
	X.A.1	Demonstrate sensitivity to patient rights

Name _____ Date _____ Score _____

COMPETENCY CHECKLIST
PROCEDURE 26-1   Perform a Capillary Puncture and Microhematocrit Test

Task: To perform a microhematocrit.

Condition: Given the equipment and supplies as listed in the procedure, and a classmate to play the part of the patient, the student will demonstrate the proper steps for performing a microhematocrit, adhering to the steps listed below.

Standards: The student will have 15 minutes to complete the procedure and will need to score an 85% or above to pass the competency. Automatic failure results if any essential steps are omitted or performed incorrectly.

STEPS START TIME: END TIME:	Points Possible	First Attempt	Second Attempt	Third Attempt
1. Wash your hands and apply PPE.	10			
2. Assemble the equipment and supplies.	10			
3. Identify the patient using two identifiers, identify yourself with your credentials. ***Explain the rationale for the performance of the procedure, showing awareness of the patient's concerns related to the procedure being performed.***	10			
4. Perform a capillary puncture and wipe away the first drop of blood with the 2 × 2 gauze.	10			
5. Hold a heparinized capillary tube horizontal to the second drop of blood without touching the skin. • Allow the capillary tube to fill three-fourths full. • Seal the end of tube with clay or a sealing cap. • After filling the tube to the appropriate level, wipe the outside of the tube with a tissue to remove excess blood. • Repeat the procedure with a second tube. • Apply a gauze square to the puncture site.	10			
6. Place tubes in the centrifuge directly opposite each other with the sealed ends pointed outward and pushed against the gasket.	10			
7. Securely fasten both centrifuge lids.	10			
8. Set the timer for five minutes and adjust the speed if needed. (Follow manufacturer's instructions.)	10			
9. Apply a bandage on the puncture site once the bleeding has stopped.	10			
10. Allow the centrifuge to stop completely before opening both lids.	10			
11. Remove both tubes, place them on the reader, and follow directions on reader to determine the value.	10			
12. Average the results of both tubes.	10			
13. Record the results as a percentage.	10			
14. Capillary tubes should be placed in a sharps container and any contaminated gauze should be placed in the biohazard trash.	10			
15. Remove PPE and wash your hands.	10			
16. Document the procedure both in the chart and in the lab log if applicable.	10			
Points Earned / Points Possible:	__ / 160			

Points possible reflect importance of step in meeting the task: Important = (5) Essential = (10). Determine score by dividing points earned by total points possible, and multiplying results by 100.

Name _____ Date _____ Score _____

EVALUATION
Evaluator Signature: _____ Date: _____

Evaluator Comments:

DOCUMENTATION
Instructor Note: Retain work products with competency checklist.
Work Product, Procedure 26-1a (Progress Note) and 26-1b (Hematology Reporting Form). Procedure forms can be downloaded from the student companion website.

Key Competencies			
ABHES	MA.A.1.4.a	Follow documentation guidelines	
	MA.A.1.10.b(2)	Perform selected CLIA-waived tests that assist with diagnosis and treatment: Hematology testing	
	MA.A.1.10.c	Dispose of biohazardous materials	
CAAHEP	I.P.11.a	Obtain specimens and perform: CLIA waived hematology test	
	I.A.3	Show awareness of patient's concerns related to the procedure being performed	
	II.P.3	Maintain lab test results using flow sheets	
	III.P.2	Select appropriate barrier/personal protective equipment (PPE)	
	III.P.3	Perform handwashing	
	III.P.10	Demonstrate proper disposal of biohazardous material: (a) sharps, and (b) regulated wastes	
	V.A.4	Explain to a patient the rationale for performance of a procedure	
	X.P.3	Document patient care accurately in the medical record	

Name _____ Date _____ Score _____

COMPETENCY CHECKLIST
PROCEDURE 26-2   Perform a Hemoglobin Using the Hemocue System

Task: To perform a hemoglobin.

Condition: Given the equipment and supplies as listed in the procedure, and a classmate to play the part of the patient, the student will demonstrate the proper steps for performing a hemoglobin, adhering to the steps listed below.

Standards: The student will have 15 minutes to complete the procedure and will need to score an 85% or above to pass the competency. Automatic failure results if any essential steps are omitted or performed incorrectly.

STEPS START TIME: END TIME:	Points Possible	First Attempt	Second Attempt	Third Attempt
1. Verify test order, wash your hands, and apply appropriate PPE.	10			
2. Assemble the equipment, read the manufacturer's instructions, and run a control.	10			
3. Identify the patient using two identifiers, identify yourself with your credentials. ***Explain the rationale for the performance of the procedure, showing awareness of the patient's concerns related to the procedure being performed.***	10			
4. Make certain the analyzer is in the "ready" loading position. (The display will show a three flashing dashes and the Hemocue symbol.)	10			
5. Remove a cuvette from the vial or individually wrapped package. Recap vial.	10			
6. Perform capillary puncture and wipe away first drop of blood.	10			
7. Position the cuvette so that the open end is facing the drop of blood. Fill the cuvette in one continuous motion. (Do not refill a partially filled cuvette.)	10			
8. Wipe off any excess blood from the outside of the cuvette using a clean, lint-free tissue. (Do not touch the open end with the tissue.)	10			
9. Visually inspect the cuvette for any bubbles.	10			
10. Place the cuvette into the cuvette holder and gently slide the holder into the measuring position.	10			
11. Once a result displays, pull cuvette holder out of the measuring position and remove cuvette.	10			
12. Dispose of cuvette in biohazard trash or sharp's container.	10			
13. Remove PPE, wash hands, dispose of supplies, and disinfect area.	10			
14. Document result in the chart and in the lab log if applicable.	10			
Points Earned / Points Possible:	__ / 140			

Points possible reflect importance of step in meeting the task: Important = (5) Essential = (10). Determine score by dividing points earned by total points possible, and multiplying results by 100.

Name _____ Date _____ Score _____

EVALUATION

Evaluator Signature: _____ Date: _____

Evaluator Comments:

DOCUMENTATION

Instructor Note: Retain work products with competency checklist.

Work Product, Procedure 26-2a (Progress Note) and 26-2b (Hematology Reporting Form). Procedure forms can be downloaded from the student companion website.

Key Competencies			
ABHES	MA.A.1.4.a	Follow documentation guidelines	
	MA.A.1.10.a	Practice quality control	
	MA.A.1.10.b(2)	Perform selected CLIA-waived tests that assist with diagnosis and treatment: Hematology testing	
CAAHEP	I.P.10	Perform a quality control measure	
	I.P.11.a	Obtain specimens and perform: CLIA waived hematology test	
	I.A.3	Show awareness of patient's concerns related to the procedure being performed	
	II.P.3	Maintain lab test results using flow sheets	
	III.P.2	Select appropriate barrier/personal protective equipment (PPE)	
	III.P.3	Perform handwashing	
	V.A.4	Explain to a patient the rationale for performance of a procedure	
	X.P.3	Document patient care accurately in the medical record	

Name _____ Date _____ Score _____

COMPETENCY CHECKLIST
PROCEDURE 26-3   Perform an Erythrocyte Sedimentation Rate

Task: To perform an erythrocyte sedimentation rate using the Sediplast® system.

Condition: Given the equipment and supplies as listed in the procedure, the student will demonstrate the proper steps for preparing performing an ESR, adhering to the steps listed below.

Standards: The student will have 75 minutes to complete the procedure and will need to score an 85% or above to pass the competency. Automatic failure results if any essential steps are omitted or performed incorrectly.

STEPS START TIME: END TIME:	Points Possible	First Attempt	Second Attempt	Third Attempt
1. Check the provider's order, wash your hands, and apply PPE.	10			
2. Assemble the equipment.	10			
3. Mix the blood gently, but well, for two minutes.	10			
4. Remove the stopper from the sedivial and fill with 0.8 mL of blood to the indicated mark. Replace the stopper and mix the sodium citrate and blood well.	10			
5. Place the sedivial in the Sediplast rack and place the rack on a level surface free of vibrations.	10			
6. Insert the Sediplast tube through the stopper while pushing down until tube rests on the bottom of the vial and the blood reaches the zero line.	10			
7. Set the timer for one hour.	10			
8. Read the results of the ESR at exactly one hour.	10			
9. Clean the work area and properly dispose of used supplies in biohazard waste container and the tube of blood into the sharps container.	10			
10. Remove PPE and wash your hands.	10			
11. Record the results in the patient's chart and the laboratory log.	10			
Points Earned / Points Possible:	__ / 110			

Points possible reflect importance of step in meeting the task: Important = (5) Essential = (10). Determine score by dividing points earned by total points possible, and multiplying results by 100.

Name _____ Date _____ Score _____

EVALUATION

Evaluator Signature: _____ Date: _____

Evaluator Comments:

DOCUMENTATION

Instructor Note: Retain work products with competency checklist.

Work Product, Procedure 26-3a (Progress Note) and 26-3b (In-House Kit Testing Log). Procedure forms can be downloaded from the student companion website.

Key Competencies			
ABHES	MA.A.1.4.a	Follow documentation guidelines	
	MA.A.1.10.b(2)	Perform selected CLIA-waived tests that assist with diagnosis and treatment: Hematology testing	
	MA.A.1.10.c	Dispose of biohazardous materials	
CAAHEP	I.P.11.a	Obtain specimens and perform: CLIA waived hematology test	
	II.P.3	Maintain lab test results using flow sheets	
	III.P.2	Select appropriate barrier/personal protective equipment (PPE)	
	III.P.3	Perform handwashing	
	III.P.10	Demonstrate proper disposal of biohazardous material: (a) sharps, and (b) regulated wastes	
	X.P.3	Document patient care accurately in the medical record	

Name _____ Date _____ Score _____

COMPETENCY CHECKLIST

PROCEDURE 26-4   Performing a Prothrombin Time (PT) and INR

Task: To perform a Prothrombin Time and INR.

Condition: Given the equipment and supplies as listed in the procedure, the student will demonstrate the proper steps for performing a PT and INR, adhering to the steps listed below.

Standards: The student will have 15 minutes to complete the procedure and will need to score an 85% or above to pass the competency. Automatic failure results if any essential steps are omitted or performed incorrectly.

STEPS START TIME: END TIME:	Points Possible	First Attempt	Second Attempt	Third Attempt
1. Verify provider's order, gather supplies, wash hands, and apply appropriate PPE.	10			
2. Check the expiration date on the test strip label to confirm it hasn't passed its expiration date.	10			
3. Read the manufacturer's instructions to familiarize yourself with the testing procedure.	10			
4. If applicable, run a control according to manufacturer's instructions.	10			
5. Greet your patient, identify yourself and state your credentials. Identify the patient using two identifiers, and **explain the rationale for the performance of the procedure**, **showing awareness of the patient's concerns related to the procedure being performed**.	10			
6. If the unit has a code chip, insert it into the unit and turn on the coagulation unit by depressing the "On" button. (Make certain the number on the code chip corresponds with the number on the code strip label.)	10			
7. Insert the test strip into the test strip guide following manufacturer's instructions. (Make certain that the unit has detected the test strip by listening for a beep or looking for a symbol to appear on the display.)	10			
8. Perform a capillary puncture and wipe away the first drop of blood.	10			
9. Follow the manufacturer's instructions regarding when it is appropriate to apply the drop of blood to the test strip or testing apparatus.	10			
10. Apply drop of blood to the test strip following the manufacturer's instructions.	10			
11. Wait for the test result to appear and make a mental note of result or write down on a piece of scrap paper. Discard the test strip after removing from unit and place into the biohazardous waste container.	10			
12. Disinfect work area, and remove PPE.	10			
13. Document the results in the patient's chart and lab log.	10			
Points Earned / Points Possible:	__ / 130			

Points possible reflect importance of step in meeting the task: Important = (5) Essential = (10). Determine score by dividing points earned by total points possible, and multiplying results by 100.

Name _____ Date _____ Score _____

EVALUATION

Evaluator Signature: _____ Date: _____

Evaluator Comments:

DOCUMENTATION

Instructor Note: Retain work products with competency checklist.

Work Product, Procedure 26-4a (Progress Note) and 26-4b (In-House Kit Testing Log). Procedure forms can be downloaded from the student companion website.

Key Competencies			
ABHES	MA.A.1.4.a	Follow documentation guidelines	
	MA.A.1.10.b(2)	Perform selected CLIA-waived tests that assist with diagnosis and treatment: Hematology testing	
	MA.A.1.10.c	Dispose of biohazardous materials	
CAAHEP	I.P.11.a	Obtain specimens and perform: CLIA waived hematology test	
	I.A.3	Show awareness of the patient's concerns related to the procedure being performed	
	II.P.3	Maintain lab test results using flow sheets	
	III.P.2	Select appropriate barrier/personal protective equipment (PPE)	
	III.P.3	Perform handwashing	
	III.P.10	Demonstrate proper disposal of biohazardous material: (a) sharps, and (b) regulated wastes	
	V.A.4	Explain to a patient the rationale for performance of a procedure	
	X.P.3	Document patient care accurately in the medical record	

Name _____ Date _____ Score _____

COMPETENCY CHECKLIST

PROCEDURE 27-1   Collect a Throat Specimen and Perform a Rapid Strep Test

Task: To collect a throat swab and perform a rapid strep test.

Condition: Given the equipment and supplies as listed in the procedure, and a student to play the role of the patient, the student will collect a throat specimen and perform a rapid strep test, adhering to the steps listed below.

Standards: The student will have 15 minutes to complete the procedure and will need to score an 85% or above to pass the competency. Automatic failure results if any essential steps are omitted or performed incorrectly.

STEPS START TIME: END TIME:	Points Possible	First Attempt	Second Attempt	Third Attempt
1. Assemble the equipment and check the order, *incorporating critical thinking skills when performing patient care*. Check expiration date on all supplies.	10			
2. Run an external control for the rapid strep kit if necessary.	10			
3. Wash your hands and apply all PPE except mask and goggles.	10			
4. Identify the patient using at least two identifiers, identify yourself, and *explain the rationale for performance of the procedure, showing awareness of the patient's concerns related to the procedure being performed*.	10			
5. Adjust the light source so the throat is clearly visible.	10			
6. Instruct the patient to stick out the tongue and say "ahh" while depressing the tongue with the tongue depressor.	10			
7. Carefully insert the swab into the oral cavity being careful not to touch the lips, teeth, tongue, or inside cheeks. Vigorously rotate the swab in a circular motion over the back of the throat swabbing the oropharynx on both sides of the throat, and the tonsillar area, being sure to swab any reddened areas or pustules.	10			
8. While still holding the tongue down, carefully withdraw the swab from the mouth being sure not to touch the sides of the mouth, tongue, teeth, or lips.	10			
9. Place swabs in appropriate wrapper or transport media and provide patient with instructions for what they should do while waiting for the results.	10			
10. If sending the specimen to the lab for a culture, make certain it is accompanied by a lab requisition form. If performing a rapid strep test, follow the manufacturer's directions.	10			
11. Properly dispose of used equipment.	10			
12. Remove PPE and wash your hands.	10			
13. Document the procedure in the patient's chart.	10			
Points Earned / Points Possible:	__ / 130			

Points possible reflect importance of step in meeting the task: Important = (5) Essential = (10). Determine score by dividing points earned by total points possible, and multiplying results by 100.

Name _____ Date _____ Score _____

EVALUATION

Evaluator Signature: _____ Date: _____

Evaluator Comments:

DOCUMENTATION

Instructor Note: Retain work products with competency checklist.

Work Product, Procedure 27-1a (Progress Note), 27-1b (Miscellaneous Laboratory Test Report Form), 27-1c (In-House Testing Log), and 27-1d (Rapid Strep QC Log). Procedure forms can be downloaded from the student companion website.

Key Competencies			
ABHES	MA.A.1.4.a	Follow documentation guidelines	
	MA.A.1.10.a	Practice quality control	
	MA.A.1.10.b(6)(b)	Perform selected CLIA-waived tests that assist with diagnosis and treatment: Kit testing: Quick strep	
	MA.A.1.10.d(4)	Obtain throat specimens for microbiologic testing	
CAAHEP	I.P.10	Perform a quality control measure	
	I.P.11.e	Obtain specimens and perform: CLIA waived microbiology test	
	I.A.2	Incorporate critical thinking skills when performing patient care	
	I.A.3	Show awareness of a patient's concerns related to the procedure being performed	
	III.P.2	Select appropriate barrier/personal protective equipment (PPE)	
	III.P.3	Perform handwashing	
	V.A.4	Explain to a patient the rationale for performance of a procedure	
	X.P.3	Document patient care accurately in the medical record	

Name _____ Date _____ Score _____

COMPETENCY CHECKLIST
PROCEDURE 27-2 Collect a Wound Specimen

Task: To collect a wound specimen.

Condition: Given the equipment and supplies as listed in the procedure, and a student to play the role of the patient, the student will collect a wound specimen using sterile technique, adhering to the steps listed below.

Standards: The student will have 15 minutes to complete the procedure and will need to score an 85% or above to pass the competency. Automatic failure results if any essential steps are omitted or performed incorrectly.

STEPS START TIME: END TIME:	Points Possible	First Attempt	Second Attempt	Third Attempt
1. Assemble the equipment, wash your hands, and apply PPE.	10			
2. ***Incorporating critical thinking skills when performing patient care***, check the provider's order, and complete lab requisition form.	10			
3. Identify the patient using at least two identifiers, identify yourself, and ***explain the rationale for performance of the procedure, showing awareness of the patient's concerns related to the procedure being performed.***	10			
4. Wash your hands, set up a sterile tray, and drape the patient. Wash your hands again and apply sterile gloves.	10			
5. Cleanse the wound by irrigating with sterile saline prior to collection.	10			
6. If wound is dry, moisten swab with sterile saline before collection. Without touching skin or wound edges, rotate tip of swab over a 1 cm area for five seconds.	10			
7. Immediately place the swab in the appropriate transport media. Remove gloves, wash hands, and put on new gloves. Clean and dress the wound according to the provider's instructions.	10			
8. Properly dispose of contaminated equipment.	10			
9. Remove PPE and wash your hands.	10			
10. Document the collection procedure in the patient's chart.	10			
Points Earned / Points Possible:	__ / 100			

Points possible reflect importance of step in meeting the task: Important = (5) Essential = (10). Determine score by dividing points earned by total points possible, and multiplying results by 100.

Name _____ Date _____ Score _____

EVALUATION
Evaluator Signature: _____ Date: _____

Evaluator Comments:

DOCUMENTATION
Instructor Note: Retain work products with competency checklist.
Work Product, Procedure 27-2a (Progress Note) and 27-2b (Outside Lab Tracking Log). Procedure forms can be downloaded from the student companion website.

Key Competencies		
ABHES	MA.A.1.10.c	Dispose of biohazardous materials
	MA.A.1.10.d(3)	Perform wound collection procedures
CAAHEP	I.P.11.e	Obtain specimens and perform: CLIA waived microbiology test
	I.A.2	Incorporate critical thinking skills when performing patient care
	I.A.3	Show awareness of a patient's concerns related to the procedure being performed
	III.P.2	Select appropriate barrier/personal protective equipment (PPE)
	III.P.3	Perform handwashing
	III.P.10	Demonstrate proper disposal of biohazardous material: (a) sharps, and (b) regulated wastes
	V.A.4	Explain to a patient the rationale for performance of a procedure
	X.P.3	Document patient care accurately in the medical record

Name _____ Date _____ Score _____

COMPETENCY CHECKLIST
PROCEDURE 27-3   Prepare a Wet Mount

Task: To prepare a wet mount.

Condition: Given the equipment and supplies as listed in the procedure, the student will prepare a wet mount, adhering to the steps listed below.

Standards: The student will have 15 minutes to complete the procedure and will need to score an 85% or above to pass the competency. Automatic failure results if any essential steps are omitted or performed incorrectly.

STEPS START TIME: END TIME:	Points Possible	First Attempt	Second Attempt	Third Attempt
1. Assemble the equipment and supplies.	10			
2. Wash your hands and apply PPE.	10			
3. Place the swab in a test tube with 0.5 mL of saline and mix well. Deposit a drop of bacterial suspension in the middle of a clean glass slide	10			
4. Place the slide on the microscope stage and focus on high power. Alert provider the slide is ready for viewing.	10			
Points Earned / Points Possible:	___ / 40			

Points possible reflect importance of step in meeting the task: Important = (5) Essential = (10). Determine score by dividing points earned by total points possible, and multiplying results by 100.

EVALUATION

Evaluator Signature: _____ Date: _____

Evaluator Comments:

Key Competencies		
ABHES	MA.A.1.10.d	Collect, label, and process specimens
CAAHEP	I.P.11.e	Obtain specimens and perform: CLIA waived microbiology test
	III.P.2	Select appropriate barrier/personal protective equipment (PPE)
	III.P.3	Perform handwashing

Name _____ Date _____ Score _____

COMPETENCY CHECKLIST

PROCEDURE 27-4   Instruct a Patient on Fecal Specimen Collection for Ova and Parasite Testing

Task: To instruct a patient on proper specimen handling technique when collecting a fecal specimen for ova and parasite (O&P) testing.

Condition: Given the equipment and supplies as listed in the procedure, the student will demonstrate the proper steps for instructing a patient on the proper method for collecting and handling a fecal specimen for ova and parasite testing, adhering to the steps listed below.

Standards: The student will have 5 minutes to complete the procedure and will need to score an 85% or above to pass the competency. Automatic failure results if any essential steps are omitted or performed incorrectly.

STEPS START TIME: END TIME:	Points Possible	First Attempt	Second Attempt	Third Attempt
1. Wash your hands and assemble the equipment.	10			
2. Identify the patient using at least two identifiers, and identify yourself.	10			
3. Provide patient with proper instructions on medications that should be avoided prior to testing.	10			
4. Give the patient the appropriate specimen collection kits and gloves. ***Explain the rationale for performance of the procedure***. Explain that the specimens will be collected at home. Patients are given 1–3 sets of O&P collection kits. Each kit contains two to three small vials containing a preservative to hold an aliquot of the original specimen.	10			
5. Instruct the patient to:				
a. Wash hands and put on gloves. Collect the specimen in a collection hat (without contaminating the fecal specimen with urine or toilet paper).	10			
b. Start with the pink capped vial, using the collection spoon built into the vial cap, collect samples from both ends and middle of the sample. Continue adding sample into vial until you have reached the red line. Mix the contents with spoon. Recap and put the lid on the vial, making certain the lid is tight. Shake the vial until contents are fully mixed.	10			
c. Now repeat step b for the gray capped vial.	10			
d. If applicable, for empty white capped vial, fill with sample as directed. No mixing or shaking is necessary.	10			
e. Complete the requested information on each vial, remove gloves, and wash hands thoroughly.	10			
f. If doctor ordered more than one set of vials, you should wait at least 48 hours but within ten days to collect next set of specimens.	10			
g. Transfer each vial into the plastic sealable storage bag following collection. Store at room temperature.	10			
6. Encourage the patient to ask questions and give ample time for answers, ***showing awareness of the patient's concerns related to the procedure being performed***.	10			

Name _____ Date _____ Score _____

7. Supply the patient with written instructions.	10			
8. Make sure the patient understands the collection process before leaving the office and when and where to return the specimens.	10			
Points Earned / Points Possible:	__ /140			

Points possible reflect importance of step in meeting the task: Important = (5) Essential = (10). Determine score by dividing points earned by total points possible, and multiplying results by 100.

EVALUATION

Evaluator Signature: _____ Date: _____

Evaluator Comments:

DOCUMENTATION

Instructor Note: Retain work products with competency checklist.
Work Product, Procedure 27-4 (Progress Note). Procedure forms can be downloaded from the student companion website.

Key Competencies		
ABHES	MA.A.1.10.d	Collect, label, and process specimens
	MA.A.1.10.e(2)	Instruct patients in the collection of a fecal specimen
CAAHEP	I.P.11.e	Obtain specimens and perform: CLIA waived microbiology test
	I.A.3	Show awareness of a patient's concerns related to the procedure being performed
	III.P.3	Perform handwashing
	V.A.4	Explain to a patient the rationale for performance of a procedure

Name _____ Date _____ Score _____

COMPETENCY CHECKLIST
PROCEDURE 28-1   Measure Blood Glucose Using a Handheld Monitor

Task: To measure blood glucose using a hand-held monitor.

Condition: Given the equipment and supplies as listed in the procedure, and a student to play the role of the patient, the student will perform a blood glucose, adhering to the steps listed below.

Standards: The student will have 15 minutes to complete the procedure and will need to score an 85% or above to pass the competency. Automatic failure results if any essential steps are omitted or performed incorrectly.

STEPS START TIME: END TIME:	Points Possible	First Attempt	Second Attempt	Third Attempt
1. ***Incorporating critical thinking skills when performing patient care***, check the provider's order, and assemble the equipment and supplies. Check the expiration date on the reagent strip and control containers.	10			
2. Wash your hands and apply PPE.	10			
3. Calibrate the instrument and run a control sample according to the manufacturer's instructions.	10			
4. Identify the patient using two identifiers and identify yourself. ***Explain the rationale for performance of the procedure, showing awareness of the patient's concerns related to the procedure being performed***. Verify if the patient is fasting or not.	10			
5. Ask the patient to wash and dry his hands.	10			
6. Cleanse the puncture site with an antiseptic wipe, allowing the site to dry before puncturing.				
7. Turn the unit on and check to make certain that the code number on the monitor matches the code number on the reagent strip container.	10			
8. Wait until the blood drop icon appears on the monitor screen (this may vary in some units) and then puncture the site.	10			
9. Puncture the site with a safety device and dispose of it in a sharps container. Wipe away the first drop of blood.	10			
10. Advance one edge of the test strip to the drop of blood and allow the strip to absorb the drop of blood.	10			
11. Instruct the patient to apply pressure to the puncture site with a gauze pad.	10			
12. Wait for the reading to appear on the screen.	10			
13. Remove the reagent strip from the monitor and dispose of properly. Throw bloody gauze square and other waste into trash receptacle following the office policy.	10			
14. Remove gloves and wash your hands.	10			
15. Document the test results in the patient's chart and the lab log if applicable.	10			
Points Earned / Points Possible:	___ / 150			

Points possible reflect importance of step in meeting the task: Important = (5) Essential = (10). Determine score by dividing points earned by total points possible, and multiplying results by 100.

Name _____ Date _____ Score _____

EVALUATION

Evaluator Signature: _____ Date: _____

Evaluator Comments:

DOCUMENTATION

Instructor Note: Retain work products with competency checklist.

Work Product, Procedure 28-1a (Progress Note), 28-1b (Miscellaneous Laboratory Test Report Form), 28-1c (In-House Testing Log), and 28-1d (Glucose QC Log). Procedure forms can be downloaded from the student companion website.

Key Competencies		
ABHES	MA.A.1.4.a	Follow documentation guidelines
	MA.A.1.10.a	Practice quality control
	MA.A.1.10.b(3)	Perform select CLIA-waived tests that assist with diagnosis and treatment: Chemistry testing
	MA.A.1.10.c	Dispose of biohazardous materials
CAAHEP	I.P.10	Perform a quality control measure
	I.P.11.b	Obtain specimens and perform: CLIA waived chemistry test
	I.A.2	Incorporate critical thinking skills when performing patient care
	I.A.3	Show awareness of a patient's concerns related to the procedure being performed
	II.P.3	Maintain lab test results using flow sheets
	III.P.2	Select appropriate barrier/personal protective equipment (PPE)
	III.P.3	Perform handwashing
	III.P.10.b	Demonstrate proper disposal of biohazardous material: regulated wastes
	V.A.4	Explain to a patient the rationale for performance of a procedure
	X.P.3	Document patient care accurately in the medical record

Name _____   Date _____   Score _____

COMPETENCY CHECKLIST
PROCEDURE 28-2   Perform a Urine Pregnancy Test

Task: To perform a urine pregnancy test.

Condition: Given the equipment and supplies as listed in the procedure, and a urine sample on which to perform the testing, the student will perform a urine pregnancy test, adhering to the steps listed below.

Standards: The student will have 15 minutes to complete the procedure and will need to score an 85% or above to pass the competency. Automatic failure results if any essential steps are omitted or performed incorrectly.

STEPS START TIME: END TIME:	Points Possible	First Attempt	Second Attempt	Third Attempt
1. ***Incorporating critical thinking skills when performing patient care***, check the order and assemble the test kit, the patient urine sample, and all necessary supplies. Read the test kit directions.	10			
2. Wash your hands and apply gloves and other required PPE.	10			
3. Perform a control.	10			
4. Open the test unit, and using the dropper provided in the test kit, add the number of drops of urine recommended by the manufacturer to the test well.	10			
5. Allow the test to develop for precisely the recommended time. Set a timer for accurate timing of the test.	10			
6. Read the test window and determine if the results are positive or negative. Check for a line beside the control display.	10			
7. Properly dispose of used equipment, test unit, and specimen.	10			
8. Remove gloves, wash your hands, and record results in the patient's chart and the appropriate logs if applicable.	10			
Points Earned / Points Possible:	___ / 80			

Points possible reflect importance of step in meeting the task: Important = (5) Essential = (10). Determine score by dividing points earned by total points possible, and multiplying results by 100.

Name _____ Date _____ Score _____

EVALUATION
Evaluator Signature: _____ Date: _____

Evaluator Comments:

DOCUMENTATION
Instructor Note: Retain work products with competency checklist.
Work Product, Procedure 28-2a (Progress Note), 28-2b (Miscellaneous Laboratory Test Report Form), 28-2c (In-House Testing Log), and 28-2d (Pregnancy QC Log). Procedure forms can be downloaded from the student companion website.

Key Competencies		
ABHES	MA.A.1.4.a	Follow documentation guidelines
	MA.A.1.10.a	Practice quality control
	MA.A.1.10.b(6)(a)	Perform select CLIA-waived tests that assist with diagnosis and treatment: Kit testing: Pregnancy
	MA.A.1.10.b(6)(c)	Perform select CLIA-waived tests that assist with diagnosis and treatment: Kit testing: Dip Sticks
	MA.A.1.10.c	Dispose of biohazardous materials
	MA.A.1.10.d	Collect, label, and process specimens
CAAHEP	I.P.10	Perform a quality control measure
	I.P.11.d	Obtain specimens and perform: CLIA waived immunology test
	I.A.2	Incorporate critical thinking skills when performing patient care
	II.P.3	Maintain lab test results using flow sheets
	III.P.2	Select appropriate barrier/personal protective equipment (PPE)
	III.P.3	Perform handwashing
	III.P.10.b	Demonstrate proper disposal of biohazardous material: regulated wastes
	X.P.3	Document patient care accurately in the medical record

Name _____ Date _____ Score _____

COMPETENCY CHECKLIST
PROCEDURE 28-3 Perform a CLIA-Waived Mono Test

Task: To perform a CLIA-waived mono test.

Condition: Given the equipment and supplies as listed in the procedure, and a capillary specimen on which to perform the testing, the student will perform a CLIA-waived mono test, adhering to the steps listed below.

Standards: The student will have 15 minutes to complete the procedure and will need to score an 85% or above to pass the competency. Automatic failure results if any essential steps are omitted or performed incorrectly.

STEPS START TIME: END TIME:	Points Possible	First Attempt	Second Attempt	Third Attempt
1. ***Incorporating critical thinking skills when performing patient care***, check the order and assemble the test kit, the patient sample, and all necessary supplies.	10			
2. Wash your hands and apply gloves and other required PPE.	10			
3. Perform a finger puncture and then perform the test following the manufacturer's directions. Be sure to run a control along with the test.	10			
4. Properly dispose of all equipment.	10			
5. Remove gloves and wash your hands.	10			
6. Record the results in the laboratory log and also document the results in the patient's chart.	10			
Points Earned / Points Possible:	___ / 60			

Points possible reflect importance of step in meeting the task: Important = (5) Essential = (10). Determine score by dividing points earned by total points possible, and multiplying results by 100.

Name _____ Date _____ Score _____

EVALUATION

Evaluator Signature: _____ Date: _____

Evaluator Comments:

DOCUMENTATION

Instructor Note: Retain work products with competency checklist.

Work Product, Procedure 28-3a (Progress Note), 28-3b (Miscellaneous Laboratory Test Report Form), 28-3c (In-House Testing Log), and 28-3d (Mono QC Log). Procedure forms can be downloaded from the student companion website.

Key Competencies		
ABHES	MA.A.1.4.a	Follow documentation guidelines
	MA.A.1.10.a	Practice quality control
	MA.A.1.10.b(4)	Perform select CLIA-waived tests that assist with diagnosis and treatment: Immunology testing
	MA.A.1.10.c	Dispose of biohazardous materials
CAAHEP	I.P.10	Perform a quality control measure
	I.P.11.d	Obtain specimens and perform: CLIA waived immunology test
	I.A.2	Incorporate critical thinking skills when performing patient care
	II.P.3	Maintain lab test results using flow sheets
	III.P.2	Select appropriate barrier/personal protective equipment (PPE)
	III.P.3	Perform handwashing
	III.P.10	Demonstrate proper disposal of biohazardous material: (a) sharps, and (b) regulated wastes
	X.P.3	Document patient care accurately in the medical record

Name _____ Date _____ Score _____

COMPETENCY CHECKLIST
PROCEDURE 30-1   Write a Prescription

Task: To create a prescription.

Condition: Given the equipment and supplies as listed in the procedure and a student to play the part of the physician, the student will demonstrate the correct procedure for creating a prescription, adhering to the steps listed below.

Standards: The student will have 10 minutes to complete the procedure and will need to score an 85% or above to pass the competency. Automatic failure results if any essential steps are omitted or performed incorrectly.

Sample Procedure Scenario

Create a prescription for patient Sydney Heller, 1234 Hickory Hills, Polaris, NY 01298, DOB 02/04/20XX. Dr. Trent Valentine prescribed her Amoxicillin Capsules, 250 mg, one capsule by mouth twice per day for 10 days, no refills.

STEPS START TIME: END TIME:	Points Possible	First Attempt	Second Attempt	Third Attempt
1. Assemble the chart, order for medication, and prescription pad.	10			
2. Read the order and ask any questions if you do not understand the order.	10			
3. Write in the patient's name, address, and age or date of birth.	10			
4. If not already on the form, write the superscription, or Rx symbol.	10			
5. Fill in the information included in the inscription (name of the drug, form of the drug, and strength of the medication).	10			
6. Fill in the information that should be included in the subscription. This usually refers to the dispense amount. (The dispense amount should include the number itself followed by the written amount in parentheses.)	10			
7. Fill in the information included in the signature (instructions for taking).	10			
8. If applicable, check the box that states: Do Not Substitute or Dispense As Written.	10			
9. Circle or write the amount of refills.	10			
10. Insert the DEA number if applicable.	10			
11. Give the prescription to the physician to read and sign.	10			
12. Document the order in the patient's record.	10			
Points Earned / Points Possible:	__ / 120			

Points possible reflect importance of step in meeting the task: Important = (5) Essential = (10). Determine score by dividing points earned by total points possible, and multiplying results by 100.

Name _____ Date _____ Score _____

EVALUATION

Evaluator Signature: _____ Date: _____

Evaluator Comments:

DOCUMENTATION

Instructor Note: Retain work products with competency checklist.
Work Product, Procedure 30-1 (Prescription). Procedure forms can be downloaded from the student companion website.

Key Competencies		
ABHES	MA.A.1.4.a	Follow documentation guidelines
	MA.A.1.6.c	Prescriptions: (1) Identify parts of prescriptions, (2) Identify appropriate abbreviations that are accepted in prescription writing, (3) Comply with legal aspects of creating prescriptions, including federal and state laws
	MA.A.1.6.e	Comply with federal, state, and local health laws and regulations
CAAHEP	X.P.3	Document patient care accurately in the medical record

Name _____ Date _____ Score _____

COMPETENCY CHECKLIST

PROCEDURE 30-2   Administer an Oral Medication

Task: To administer oral medication.

Condition: Given the equipment and supplies as listed in the procedure and a classmate to play the part of the patient, the student will demonstrate the correct procedure for administering an oral medication, adhering to the steps listed below.

Standards: The student will have 10 minutes to complete the procedure and will need to score an 85% or above to pass the competency. Automatic failure results if any essential steps are omitted or performed incorrectly.

STEPS START TIME: END TIME:	Points Possible	First Attempt	Second Attempt	Third Attempt
1. Working in a well-lit area, verify the physician's order. Be certain to follow the Seven Rights of Drug Administration.	10			
2. Wash your hands and apply gloves (gloves are optional). Assemble the medication and supplies. Check the label on the medication bottle as you retrieve it from the cabinet (**Medication check #1**).	10			
3. Compare the written drug order with the drug label before preparing the drug. Make certain that you have the right drug and the right dose (**Medication check #2**). Perform dosage calculation if necessary.	10			
4. Check the expiration date of the drug.	10			
5. Loosen the lid and remove it from the bottle. Place the lid on the counter so that the inside of the lid is pointing upward. Pour the correct amount of pills into the cap of the medication vial without contaminating the inside of the cap, and then into the medicine cup. (When measuring a liquid form of medication, palm the label before pouring and hold the medication cup at eye level. Read the volume at the lowest point of the curve in the liquid, or at the meniscus.)	10			
6. Replace the medication in its proper storage area. Read the label once again before returning it to verify that it is the correct drug and dosage (**Medication check #3**).	10			
7. Properly transport the medication to the patient. Be careful not to touch the medication or the inside of the container.	10			
8. Identify the patient, using a minimum of two identifiers.	10			
9. Identify yourself, and *explain the rationale for the performance of the procedure to the patient, showing awareness of the patient's concerns related to the procedure being performed*.	10			
10. Give the patient the medication to swallow and observe the patient to make sure there is no difficulty in taking the medication. With a pill, allow the patient to have plenty of water to ensure the medication has passed from the esophagus into the stomach. Do not give the patient water when giving a liquid medication unless you have confirmed with the package insert and the physician that it is okay to do so.	10			
11. Properly dispose of the medication cup and other disposable equipment into the garbage and remove gloves and wash hands.	10			

Name _____ Date _____ Score _____

12. Provide the patient with any relevant educational materials and ask the patient to repeat back any instructions to confirm that the patient comprehends the information.	10			
13. Document the procedure in the patient's record.	10			
Points Earned / Points Possible:	__ / 130			

Points possible reflect importance of step in meeting the task: Important = (5) Essential = (10). Determine score by dividing points earned by total points possible, and multiplying results by 100.

EVALUATION

Evaluator Signature: _____ Date: _____

Evaluator Comments:

DOCUMENTATION

Instructor Note: Retain work products with competency checklist.

Work Product, Procedure 30-2a (Progress Note) and 30-2b (Medication Log). Procedure forms can be downloaded from the student companion website.

Key Competencies		
ABHES	MA.A.1.4.a	Follow documentation guidelines
	MA.A.1.9.f	Prepare and administer oral and parenteral medications and monitor intravenous (IV) infusions
CAAHEP	I.P.4	Verify the rules of medication administration: (a) right patient, (b) right medication, (c) right dose, (d) right route, (e) right time, and (f) right documentation
	I.P.6	Administer oral medications
	I.A.3	Show awareness of a patient's concerns related to the procedure being performed
	II.P.1	Calculate proper dosages of medication for administration
	III.P.3	Perform handwashing
	V.A.4	Explain to a patient the rationale for performance of a procedure
	X.P.3	Document patient care accurately in the medical record

Name _____ Date _____ Score _____

COMPETENCY CHECKLIST

PROCEDURE 31-1   Calculate a Medication Dosage for Administration

Task: To calculate a medication dosage for administration.

Condition: Given the equipment and supplies as listed in the procedure, the student will demonstrate the correct procedure for calculating a medication dosage for administration, adhering to the steps listed below.

Standards: The student will have 10 minutes to complete the procedure and will need to score an 85% or above to pass the competency. Automatic failure results if any essential steps are omitted or performed incorrectly.

Sample Procedure Scenario

Order: 0.5 g of Duricef p.o.r
Supply: Duricef 500 mg tablets

STEPS START TIME: END TIME:	Points Possible	First Attempt	Second Attempt	Third Attempt
1. Obtain medication order, medication vial or bottle, pencil, a piece of scrap paper, and calculator.	10			
2. Compare the order with the medication label a minimum of three times to make certain you have the correct medication. (Check the name of the medication, the strength, and the expiration date.)	10			
3. Compare the order with the medication label to make certain the prescribed units match the available units. (If not, do a metric conversion to get both into like units.)	10			
4. Calculate the correct dosage by applying the appropriate formula. ***Incorporate critical thinking skills when performing patient care.***	10			
5. Write down the amount of medication to administer on the piece of scrap paper.	10			
Points Earned / Points Possible:	__ / 50			

Points possible reflect importance of step in meeting the task: Important = (5) Essential = (10). Determine score by dividing points earned by total points possible, and multiplying results by 100.

EVALUATION

Evaluator Signature: _____ Date: _____

Evaluator Comments:

Key Competencies		
ABHES	MA.A.1.6.b	Demonstrate accurate occupational math and metric conversions for proper medication administration
CAAHEP	I.A.2	Incorporate critical thinking skills when performing patient care
	II.P.1	Calculate proper dosages of medication for administration

Name _____ Date _____ Score _____

COMPETENCY CHECKLIST
PROCEDURE 32-1   Withdraw Medication from a Vial

Task: To withdraw medication from a vial.

Condition: Given the equipment and supplies as listed in the procedure, the student will demonstrate the correct procedure for withdrawing medication from a vial, adhering to the steps listed below.

Standards: The student will have 7 minutes to complete the procedure and will need to score an 85% or above to pass the competency. Automatic failure results if any essential steps are omitted or performed incorrectly.

STEPS START TIME: END TIME:	Points Possible	First Attempt	Second Attempt	Third Attempt
1. Wash your hands and apply gloves.	10			
2. Assemble the equipment.	10			
3. Work in a quiet and well-lit area.	10			
4. Select the correct medication from the storage area and check the drug label (**Medication Check #1**).	10			
5. Check the expiration date.	10			
6. Compare the medication with the physician's order (**Medication Check #2**).	10			
7. Calculate the correct dose to be given, if needed. ***Incorporate critical thinking skills when performing patient care***. Verify the correct calculations with the physician if necessary.	10			
8. Open the syringe and attach the needle to the syringe.	10			
9. Open the antiseptic wipe and clean the vial stopper.	10			
10. Holding the syringe at eye level, pull back on the plunger of syringe to draw an amount of air into the syringe equal to the amount of medication to be withdrawn from the vial.	10			
11. Check to make sure the needle is firmly attached to the syringe and remove the cap from the needle.	10			
12. Insert the needle through the rubber stopper until it reaches the empty space between the stopper and the fluid level.	10			
13. Push forward on the plunger to inject air into the vial. Keep the needle above the fluid level.	10			
14. Invert the vial while holding onto the syringe and plunger. Hold the vial and syringe without contaminating the needle or hub of the syringe. These parts of the syringe must remain sterile.	10			
15. Hold the syringe at eye level and withdraw the proper amount of medication.	10			
16. Keep the tip of needle below the fluid level.	10			
17. Remove any air bubbles in the syringe by tapping or flicking the side of the syringe where the bubbles are located.	10			
18. Remove any air remaining in the tip of the syringe. Check to make certain that you still have the correct amount of medication. If you do not, make the appropriate adjustments to confirm you have the correct amount before removing the needle from the vial.	10			
19. Remove the needle from the rubber stopper of the vial.	10			
20. Replace the needle cap on the syringe or replace with a new needle and cap setup.	10			

Name _____ Date _____ Score _____

21. Read the medication label, record the date the vial was opened, and place your initials on the vial. Replace the medication vial in the correct storage cabinet (**Medication Check #3**).	10			
22. Place the syringe on to a clean tray with other items necessary for the injection, including an alcohol wipe, a gauze pad, and an adhesive bandage.	10			
Points Earned / Points Possible:	__ / 220			

Points possible reflect importance of step in meeting the task: Important = (5) Essential = (10). Determine score by dividing points earned by total points possible, and multiplying results by 100.

EVALUATION

Evaluator Signature: _____ Date: _____

Evaluator Comments:

Key Competencies		
ABHES	MA.A.1.9.f	Prepare and administer oral and parenteral medications and monitor intravenous (IV) infusions
	MA.A.1.10.c	Dispose of biohazardous materials
CAAHEP	I.P.4	Verify the rules of medication administration: (a) right patient, (b) right medication, (c) right does, (d) right route, (e) right time, and (f) right documentation
	I.A.2	Incorporate critical thinking skills when performing patient care
	III.P.3	Perform handwashing
	III.P.10	Demonstrate proper disposal of biohazardous material: (a) sharps, and (b) regulated waste

Name _____ Date _____ Score _____

COMPETENCY CHECKLIST
PROCEDURE 32-2   Withdraw Medication from an Ampule

Task: To withdraw medication from an ampule.

Condition: Given the equipment and supplies as listed in the procedure, the student will demonstrate the correct procedure for withdrawing medication from an ampule, adhering to the steps listed below.

Standards: The student will have 7 minutes to complete the procedure and will need to score an 85% or above to pass the competency. Automatic failure results if any essential steps are omitted or performed incorrectly.

STEPS START TIME: END TIME:	Points Possible	First Attempt	Second Attempt	Third Attempt
1. Wash your hands and apply gloves.	10			
2. Assemble the equipment.	10			
3. Work in a quiet and well-lit area.	10			
4. Select the correct medication from the storage area and check the drug label (**Medication Check #1**).	10			
5. Check the expiration date.	10			
6. Compare the medication with the physician's order (**Medication Check #2**).	10			
7. Calculate the correct dose to be given, if needed. ***Incorporate critical thinking skills when performing patient care.***	10			
8. Open the syringe and filter needle and assemble, if necessary.	10			
9. Tap the stem of the ampule lightly, or snap the wrist of the arm holding the ampule, to remove any medication in the neck of the ampule.	10			
10. Open the antiseptic wipe and clean the ampule container. Allow the ampule to dry completely.	10			
11. Place a piece of gauze around the neck of the ampule. Hold the ampule firmly between the fingers and the thumbs of both hands.	10			
12. Break off the stem by snapping it quickly and firmly away from the body. Discard the top in a sharps container and carefully set the ampule down on a flat, firm surface.	10			
13. Check to make sure the filter needle is firmly attached to the syringe and remove the cap from the needle.	10			
14. Insert the needle into the ampule below the fluid level. Hold the ampule at a slight angle while advancing the needle within the glass body. Completely draw up all the medication into the syringe.	10			
15. Remove the needle from the ampule without allowing the needle to touch the edges of the ampule.	10			
16. Dispose of the ampule into the sharps container. Check the medication label before discarding the ampule (**Medication Check #3**).	10			
17. Remove any bubbles in the syringe.	10			
18. Pull back slightly on the plunger to draw the medication from the needle into the syringe, engage the safety device, and remove the filter needle.	10			
19. Open a new needle for administering medication to the patient and attach it correctly to the syringe.	10			

Name _____ Date _____ Score _____

20. Remove the cap from the needle and push slightly forward on the plunger to remove air that is within the tip of the syringe and shaft of the needle.	10			
21. Replace the needle cap on the syringe following institutional policy.	10			
22. Prepare the medication tray. Place a bandage, a gauze pad, an antiseptic wipe, and the syringe on a medication tray for transporting to the exam room to administer the injection to the patient.	10			
Points Earned / Points Possible:	__ / 220			

Points possible reflect importance of step in meeting the task: Important = (5) Essential = (10). Determine score by dividing points earned by total points possible, and multiplying results by 100.

EVALUATION

Evaluator Signature: _____ Date: _____

Evaluator Comments:

Key Competencies		
ABHES	MA.A.1.9.f	Prepare and administer oral and parenteral medications and monitor intravenous (IV) infusions
	MA.A.1.10.c	Dispose of biohazardous materials
CAAHEP	I.P.4	Verify the rules of medication administration: (a) right patient, (b) right medication, (c) right does, (d) right route, (e) right time, and (f) right documentation
	I.A.2	Incorporate critical thinking skills when performing patient care
	III.P.3	Perform handwashing
	III.P.10	Demonstrate proper disposal of biohazardous material: (a) sharps, and (b) regulated waste

Name _____   Date _____   Score _____

COMPETENCY CHECKLIST

PROCEDURE 32-3   Reconstitute a Powdered-Base Medication with a Diluent

Task: To reconstitute a powdered-base medication.

Condition: Given the equipment and supplies as listed in the procedure, the student will demonstrate the correct procedure for reconstituting a powdered-base medication, adhering to the steps listed below.

Standards: The student will have 7 minutes to complete the procedure and will need to score an 85% or above to pass the competency. Automatic failure results if any essential steps are omitted or performed incorrectly

STEPS START TIME: END TIME:	Points Possible	First Attempt	Second Attempt	Third Attempt
1. Wash your hands and apply gloves.	10			
2. Assemble the equipment.	10			
3. Work in a quiet and well-lit area.	10			
4. Select the correct medication and diluent from the storage area, and check both drug labels (**Medication Check #1**).	10			
5. Check the expiration date on both labels.	10			
6. Compare the medication with the physician's order (**Medication Check #2**).	10			
7. Calculate the correct dose to be given, if needed. ***Incorporate critical thinking skills when performing patient care***. Verify the correct calculations with the provider if necessary.	10			
8. Open the syringe and needle and assemble, if necessary.	10			
9. Clean both the powder vial and the reconstituting fluid vial stopper with alcohol before use.	10			
10. Pull back on the plunger to fill the syringe with the amount of air equal to the amount of diluting liquid required for reconstitution from the vial containing the diluent.	10			
11. Check to make sure the needle is firmly attached to the syringe and remove the needle cap.	10			
12. Insert the needle into the diluent vial.	10			
13. Push in the plunger, forcing the air from the syringe into the vial of diluent.	10			
14. Invert the vial in the dominant hand, holding between the thumb and index finger.	10			
15. Keep the needle immersed in the solution while drawing the solution into the barrel of the syringe.	10			
16. Check for air bubbles and determine that the exact amount of diluent is withdrawn from the vial before removing the needle from the vial.	10			
17. Carefully remove the needle from the vial.	10			
18. Insert the needle into the vial containing the powdered medication.	10			
19. Add the appropriate amount of reconstituting liquid to the powdered drug, slowly rotating vial while injecting fluid into it.	10			
20. Replace the needle cap on the syringe following institutional policy.	10			

Name _____ Date _____ Score _____

21. Roll the vial between the hands to thoroughly mix the medication.	10			
22. Record the new date of expiration on the label of the medication vial.	10			
23. Recheck the medication label before returning the vial to the proper storage area (**Medication Check #3**).	10			
24. Prepare to administer the medication to the patient. Place a bandage, a gauze pad, an antiseptic wipe, and the syringe on a medication tray for transporting to the exam room to administer the injection to the patient.	10			
Points Earned / Points Possible:	__ / 240			

Points possible reflect importance of step in meeting the task: Important = (5) Essential = (10). Determine score by dividing points earned by total points possible, and multiplying results by 100.

EVALUATION

Evaluator Signature: _____ Date: _____

Evaluator Comments:

Key Competencies		
ABHES	MA.A.1.9.f	Prepare and administer oral and parenteral medications and monitor intravenous (IV) infusions
	MA.A.1.10.c	Dispose of biohazardous materials
CAAHEP	I.P.4	Verify the rules of medication administration: (a) right patient, (b) right medication, (c) right does, (d) right route, (e) right time, and (f) right documentation
	I.A.2	Incorporate critical thinking skills when performing patient care
	III.P.3	Perform handwashing
	III.P.10	Demonstrate proper disposal of biohazardous material: (a) sharps, and (b) regulated waste

Name _____ Date _____ Score _____

COMPETENCY CHECKLIST

PROCEDURE 32-4   Mix Two Medications into One Syringe

Task: To mix two medications into one syringe.

Condition: Given the equipment and supplies as listed in the procedure, the student will demonstrate the correct procedure for mixing two medications into one syringe, adhering to the steps listed below.

Standards: The student will have 7 minutes to complete the procedure and will need to score an 85% or above to pass the competency. Automatic failure results if any essential steps are omitted or performed incorrectly.

STEPS START TIME: END TIME:	Points Possible	First Attempt	Second Attempt	Third Attempt
1. Wash your hands and apply gloves.	10			
2. Assemble the equipment.	10			
3. Work in a quiet and well-lit area.	10			
4. Select the correct medications from the storage area and check their drug labels (**Medication Check #1**).	10			
5. Check the expiration dates on both vials.	10			
6. Compare the medications with the physician's order (**Medication Check #2**).	10			
7. Calculate the correct doses to be given, if needed. *Incorporate critical thinking skills when performing patient care*. Verify the correct calculations with the provider if necessary.	10			
8. Open the syringe and needle and remove them from their packaging. Attach the needle to the syringe.	10			
9. Clean the rubber stopper of both vials with an alcohol wipe.	10			
10. Determine which medication is the primary medication vial. Do not do anything with the primary medicine at this point.	10			
11. Draw up an amount of air into the syringe that is equal to the amount of medication required from the second vial.	10			
12. Check to make sure the needle is firmly attached to the syringe and remove the needle cap.	10			
13. Insert the needle into the second vial and push the air from the syringe into the vial to replace the medication that will be taken out later. Do not allow the needle to touch the liquid.	10			
14. Carefully remove the needle from the vial.	10			
15. Draw up an amount of air into the syringe that is equal to the amount of medication required to be taken from the primary vial.	10			
16. Insert the needle into the primary vial. Push forward on the plunger, forcing air from the syringe into the primary vial without contacting the medication.	10			
17. Invert the vial in the dominant hand, holding it between the thumb and index finger.	10			
18. Keep the needle immersed in the solution while drawing the solution into the barrel of the syringe.	10			

Name _____ Date _____ Score _____

19. Remove any air remaining in the tip of the syringe. If there is medication lacking in the syringe, pull back on the plunger so that the correct amount of medication is drawn into the syringe.	10				
20. Remove the needle from the stopper of the first vial, engage the safety device, and discard into a sharps container. Replace the needle with a new needle.	10				
21. Smoothly insert the needle into the secondary vial.	10				
22. Invert the vial and slowly withdraw the medication required from the vial. Do not allow any medication from the first vial to be inadvertently injected into the second vial. Pulling slowly to avoid creating air bubbles, pull the plunger back to the correct calibration mark on the syringe.	10				
23. Remove the needle from the second vial.	10				
24. Check for air bubbles and remove them from the syringe.	10				
25. Check again that the total amount of medication in the syringe is the correct total to be administered.	10				
26. Replace the needle cap on the syringe following institutional policy.	10				
27. Recheck the medication labels of both vials before returning the vials to the proper storage area (**Medication Check #3**).	10				
28. Prepare to administer the medication to the patient. Place a bandage, a gauze pad, an antiseptic wipe, and the syringe on a medication tray for transporting to the exam room to administer the injection to the patient.	10				
Points Earned / Points Possible:	__ / 280				

Points possible reflect importance of step in meeting the task: Important = (5) Essential = (10). Determine score by dividing points earned by total points possible, and multiplying results by 100.

EVALUATION

Evaluator Signature: _____ Date: _____

Evaluator Comments:

Key Competencies		
ABHES	MA.A.1.9.f	Prepare and administer oral and parenteral medications and monitor intravenous (IV) infusions
	MA.A.1.10.c	Dispose of biohazardous materials
CAAHEP	I.P.4	Verify the rules of medication administration: (a) right patient, (b) right medication, (c) right does, (d) right route, (e) right time, and (f) right documentation
	I.A.2	Incorporate critical thinking skills when performing patient care
	III.P.3	Perform handwashing
	III.P.10	Demonstrate proper disposal of biohazardous material: (a) sharps, and (b) regulated waste

Name _____ Date _____ Score _____

COMPETENCY CHECKLIST
PROCEDURE 32-5   Load a Cartridge into an Injector Device

Task: To load a cartridge into an injector device.

Condition: Given the equipment and supplies as listed in the procedure, the student will demonstrate the correct procedure for loading a cartridge or injector device, adhering to the steps listed below.

Standards: The student will have 7 minutes to perform the procedure and will need to score an 85% or above to pass the competency. Automatic failure results if any essential steps are omitted or performed incorrectly.

STEPS START TIME: END TIME:	Points Possible	First Attempt	Second Attempt	Third Attempt
1. Wash your hands and apply gloves.	10			
2. Assemble the equipment.	10			
3. Work in a quiet and well-lit area.	10			
4. Select the correct medication from the storage area and check the drug label (**Medication Check #1**).	10			
5. Check the expiration date.	10			
6. Compare the medication with the physician's instructions (**Medication Check #2**).	10			
7. Calculate the correct dose to be given, if needed. *Incorporate critical thinking skills when performing patient care*.	10			
8. Pick up the cartridge unit holder (the injector).	10			
9. Turn the ribbed collar toward the open position until it stops.	10			
10. Hold the injector with the open end up and fully insert the sterile cartridge-needle unit.	10			
11. Firmly tighten the ribbed collar of the unit at the syringe base by turning the ribbed collar toward the "close" arrow. (Hold the cartridge to prevent it from swiveling inside the holder while tightening.)	10			
12. Thread the rod of the plunger into the cartridge unit until a slight resistance is felt.	10			
13. Prepare the medication for injection into the patient at this time. Place a bandage, a gauze pad, an antiseptic wipe, and the syringe on a medication tray for transporting to the exam room. Check the medication label one last time (**Medication Check #3**).	10			
14. After use, do not recap the needle.	10			
15. Disengage the plunger rod from the cartridge unit holder while holding the needle down and away from the fingers or hands over a sharps unit.	10			
16. Unscrew the ribbed collar of the cartridge unit holder.	10			
17. Allow the needle cartridge unit to drop into the sharps container.	10			
18. Cleanse the cartridge holder with an antiseptic cleanser and allow to dry.	10			
19. Cleanse the work area and remove gloves and wash your hands.	10			
Points Earned / Points Possible:	__ / 190			

Points possible reflect importance of step in meeting the task: Important = (5) Essential = (10). Determine score by dividing points earned by total points possible, and multiplying results by 100.

Name _____ Date _____ Score _____

EVALUATION
Evaluator Signature: _____ Date: _____

Evaluator Comments:

Key Competencies			
ABHES	MA.A.1.9.f	Prepare and administer oral and parenteral medications and monitor intravenous (IV) infusions	
	MA.A.1.10.c	Dispose of biohazardous materials	
CAAHEP	I.P.4	Verify the rules of medication administration: (a) right patient, (b) right medication, (c) right does, (d) right route, (e) right time, and (f) right documentation	
	I.A.2	Incorporate critical thinking skills when performing patient care	
	III.P.3	Perform handwashing	
	III.P.10	Demonstrate proper disposal of biohazardous material: (a) sharps, and (b) regulated waste	

Name _____ Date _____ Score _____

COMPETENCY CHECKLIST
PROCEDURE 32-6   Administer an Intradermal Injection

Task: To administer an intradermal injection.

Condition: Given the equipment and supplies as listed in the procedure, and a classmate or injection pad to perform the injection on, the student will demonstrate the correct procedure for administering an intradermal injection, adhering to the steps listed below.

Standards: The student will have 10 minutes to complete the procedure (not including the post-injection observation) and will need to score an 85% or above to pass the competency. Automatic failure results if any essential steps are omitted or performed incorrectly.

STEPS START TIME: END TIME:	Points Possible	First Attempt	Second Attempt	Third Attempt
1. Wash your hands.	10			
2. Assemble the equipment. Follow the Seven Rights of Drug Administration.	10			
3. Identify the patient using two identifiers, identify yourself, and *explain the rationale for performance of the procedure, showing awareness of the patient's concerns related to the procedure being performed*.	10			
4. Ask patient about drug allergies or latex allergies.	10			
5. Select the proper injection site (anterior forearm or middle of back).	10			
6. Cleanse the site with antiseptic and allow to air dry completely. (Cleanse in a circular motion working outward to an area of 2 to 3 inches.)	10			
7. Prepare the equipment and apply gloves.	10			
8. Remove the needle cap. Pull the cap straight off, never twist.	10			
9. Stretch the skin taut at the site of administration.	10			
10. Insert the needle at a 10° to 15° angle with the bevel upward just under the skin.	10			
11. Inject the medication slowly and steadily. A wheal should form.	10			
12. Remove the needle quickly at the same angle of insertion.	10			
13. Do not press on or massage the injection site. Do not apply a bandage to the site.	10			
14. Properly engage the safety device on the needle and dispose of the needle-syringe unit in the sharps container.	10			
15. Remove gloves and wash your hands.	10			
16. Give proper patient education for caring for the site and inform the patient to wait 20 to 30 minutes.	10			
17. Perform postinjection observation and document the procedure in the patient's chart and the appropriate logs.	10			
Points Earned / Points Possible:	__ / 170			

Points possible reflect importance of step in meeting the task: Important = (5) Essential = (10). Determine score by dividing points earned by total points possible, and multiplying results by 100.

Name _____ Date _____ Score _____

EVALUATION
Evaluator Signature: _____ Date: _____

Evaluator Comments:

DOCUMENTATION
Instructor Note: Retain work products with competency checklist.
Work Product, Procedure 32-6a (Progress Note) and 32-6b (Medication Log). Procedure forms can be downloaded from the student companion website.

Key Competencies		
ABHES	MA.A.1.4.a	Follow documentation guidelines
	MA.A.1.9.a	Practice standard precautions and perform disinfection/sterilization techniques
	MA.A.1.9.f	Prepare and administer oral and parenteral medications and monitor intravenous (IV) infusions
	MA.A.1.10.c	Dispose of biohazardous materials
CAAHEP	I.P.4	Verify the rules of medication administration: (a) right patient, (b) right medication, (c) right does, (d) right route, (e) right time, and (f) right documentation
	I.P.5	Select proper sites for administering parenteral medication
	I.P.7	Administer parenteral (excluding IV) medications
	I.A.3	Show awareness of a patient's concerns related to the procedure being performed
	III.P.2	Select appropriate barrier/personal protective equipment (PPE)
	III.P.3	Perform handwashing
	III.P.10	Demonstrate proper disposal of biohazardous material: (a) sharps, and (b) regulated waste
	V.A.4	Explain to a patient the rationale for performance of a procedure
	X.P.3	Document patient care accurately in the medical record

Name _____ Date _____ Score _____

COMPETENCY CHECKLIST
PROCEDURE 32-7   Administer a Subcutaneous Injection

Task: To administer a subcutaneous injection.

Condition: Given the equipment and supplies as listed in the procedure, and a classmate or injection pad to perform the injection on, the student will demonstrate the correct procedure for administering a subcutaneous injection, adhering to the steps listed below.

Standards: The student will have 10 minutes to complete the procedure (not including the post-injection observation) and will need to score an 85% or above to pass the competency. Automatic failure results if any essential steps are omitted or performed incorrectly.

STEPS START TIME: END TIME:	Points Possible	First Attempt	Second Attempt	Third Attempt
1. Wash your hands.	10			
2. Assemble the equipment. Follow the Seven Rights of Drug Administration.	10			
3. Identify the patient using two identifiers, identify yourself, and **explain the rationale for performance of the procedure, showing awareness of the patient's concerns related to the procedure being performed**.	10			
4. Ask the patient about drug allergies, latex allergies, or adhesive allergies.	10			
5. Select the proper injection site (fatty tissue of the arms, thighs, or stomach).	10			
6. Cleanse the site with antiseptic and allow to air dry completely. (Cleanse in a circular motion working outward to an area of 2 to 3 inches.)	10			
7. Prepare the equipment and apply gloves.	10			
8. Remove the needle cap. Pull the cap straight off, never twist.	10			
9. Grasp or pinch the tissue lightly with one hand.	10			
10. Insert the needle at a 45° angle with the other hand, using a quick and smooth motion.	10			
11. Stabilize the needle within the tissue. Check the guidelines of your office in regard to aspiration.	10			
12. Inject the medication slowly and steadily.	10			
13. Remove the needle quickly at the same angle of insertion.	10			
14. Place a gauze sponge over the injection site and gently massage the area, if applicable.	10			
15. Properly engage the needle's safety device and dispose of the needle and syringe into the sharps container. Apply a bandage to the site to prevent the patient's clothes from becoming contaminated with blood.	10			
16. Remove gloves and wash your hands.	10			
17. Give proper patient educational materials and waiting instructions.	10			
18. Perform post-check of the patient and site 20 to 30 minutes following the procedure.	10			
19. Chart the procedure correctly on the progress note and appropriate logs.	10			
Points Earned / Points Possible:	__ / 190			

Points possible reflect importance of step in meeting the task: Important = (5) Essential = (10). Determine score by dividing points earned by total points possible, and multiplying results by 100.

Name _____ Date _____ Score _____

EVALUATION

Evaluator Signature: _____ Date: _____

Evaluator Comments:

DOCUMENTATION

Instructor Note: Retain work products with competency checklist.

Work Product, Procedure 32-7a (Progress Note) and 32-7b (Medication Log). Procedure forms can be downloaded from the student companion website.

Key Competencies		
ABHES	MA.A.1.4.a	Follow documentation guidelines
	MA.A.1.9.a	Practice standard precautions and perform disinfection/sterilization techniques
	MA.A.1.9.f	Prepare and administer oral and parenteral medications and monitor intravenous (IV) infusions
	MA.A.1.10.c	Dispose of biohazardous materials
CAAHEP	I.P.4	Verify the rules of medication administration: (a) right patient, (b) right medication, (c) right does, (d) right route, (e) right time, and (f) right documentation
	I.P.5	Select proper sites for administering parenteral medication
	I.P.7	Administer parenteral (excluding IV) medications
	I.A.3	Show awareness of a patient's concerns related to the procedure being performed
	III.P.2	Select appropriate barrier/personal protective equipment (PPE)
	III.P.3	Perform handwashing
	III.P.10	Demonstrate proper disposal of biohazardous material: (a) sharps, and (b) regulated waste
	V.A.4	Explain to a patient the rationale for performance of a procedure
	X.P.3	Document patient care accurately in the medical record

Name _____ Date _____ Score _____

COMPETENCY CHECKLIST
PROCEDURE 32-8   Administer an Intramuscular Injection

Task: To administer an intramuscular injection.

Condition: Given the equipment and supplies as listed in the procedure, and a classmate or injection pad to perform the injection on, the student will demonstrate the correct procedure for administering an intramuscular injection, adhering to the steps listed below.

Standards: The student will have 10 minutes to complete the procedure (not including the post-injection observation) and will need to score an 85% or above to pass the competency. Automatic failure results if any essential steps are omitted or performed incorrectly.

STEPS START TIME: END TIME:	Points Possible	First Attempt	Second Attempt	Third Attempt
1. Wash your hands.	10			
2. Assemble the equipment. Follow the Seven Rights of Drug Administration.	10			
3. Identify the patient using two identifiers, identify yourself, and *explain the rationale for performance of the procedure, showing awareness of the patient's concerns related to the procedure being performed.*	10			
4. Ask the patient about drug allergies, latex allergies, or adhesive allergies.	10			
5. Locate the proper injection site (deltoid, ventrogluteal, or vastus lateralis).	10			
6. Cleanse the site with antiseptic and allow to air dry completely. (Cleanse in a circular motion working outward to an area of 2 to 3 inches.)	10			
7. Prepare the equipment and apply gloves.	10			
8. Remove the needle cap. Pull the cap straight off, never twist.	10			
9. Stretch the tissue to hold the skin taut with your nondominant hand.	10			
10. Using your dominant hand, insert the needle at a 90° angle using a quick and smooth motion.	10			
11. Stabilize the needle within the tissue.	10			
12. Aspirate if instructed to do so to ensure the needle is not in a blood vessel. If blood enters the syringe, do not inject, but remove the needle immediately. If there is no bloody return into the needle, proceed with the injection process.	10			
13. Inject the medication slowly and steadily.	10			
14. Remove the needle quickly at the same angle of insertion.	10			
15. Place a gauze sponge over the injection site and gently massage the area, if applicable.	10			
16. Engage the safety device on the needle, and dispose of the needle-syringe unit in the sharps container.	10			
17. Place an adhesive bandage over the site and remove gloves and wash your hands.	10			
18. Give related patient educational materials and proper waiting instructions.	10			
19. Perform post-check of the patient and site 20 to 30 minutes following the procedure.	10			
20. Chart the procedure correctly on the progress note and appropriate logs.	10			
Points Earned / Points Possible:	__ / 200			

Points possible reflect importance of step in meeting the task: Important = (5) Essential = (10). Determine score by dividing points earned by total points possible, and multiplying results by 100.

Name _____ Date _____ Score _____

EVALUATION
Evaluator Signature: _____ Date: _____

Evaluator Comments:

DOCUMENTATION
Instructor Note: Retain work products with competency checklist.
Work Product, Procedure 32-8a (Progress Note) and 32-8b (Medication Log). Procedure forms can be downloaded from the student companion website.

Key Competencies		
ABHES	MA.A.1.4.a	Follow documentation guidelines
	MA.A.1.9.a	Practice standard precautions and perform disinfection/sterilization techniques
	MA.A.1.9.f	Prepare and administer oral and parenteral medications and monitor intravenous (IV) infusions
	MA.A.1.10.c	Dispose of biohazardous materials
CAAHEP	I.P.4	Verify the rules of medication administration: (a) right patient, (b) right medication, (c) right does, (d) right route, (e) right time, and (f) right documentation
	I.P.5	Select proper sites for administering parenteral medication
	I.P.7	Administer parenteral (excluding IV) medications
	I.A.3	Show awareness of a patient's concerns related to the procedure being performed
	III.P.2	Select appropriate barrier/personal protective equipment (PPE)
	III.P.3	Perform handwashing
	III.P.10	Demonstrate proper disposal of biohazardous material: (a) sharps, and (b) regulated waste
	V.A.4	Explain to a patient the rationale for performance of a procedure
	X.P.3	Document patient care accurately in the medical record

Name _____ Date _____ Score _____

COMPETENCY CHECKLIST
PROCEDURE 33-1   Performing Basic First Aid in the Medical Office Setting

Task: To properly apply basic first aid steps in the medical office setting.

Condition: Given the equipment and supplies as listed in the procedure, and a few classmates to play the parts of the victim and provider, the student will demonstrate the correct steps for performing basic first aid in the medical office setting, adhering to the steps listed below.

Standards: The student will have 15 minutes to complete each basic first aid procedure and will need to score an 85% or above to pass the competency. Automatic failure results if any essential steps are omitted or performed incorrectly.

STEPS START TIME: END TIME:	Points Possible	First Attempt	Second Attempt	Third Attempt
1. *Demonstrate self-awareness in responding to an emergency situation.* Identify the patient using two identifiers, identify yourself, and observe the area *recognizing the physical and emotional effects on persons involved in an emergency situation.*	10			
2. Wash hands and apply PPE. Assemble equipment and supplies. *Show awareness of a patient's concerns related to the procedure being performed.*	10			
3. *Incorporate critical thinking skills when performing patient assessment and care. Explain to a patient the rationale for performance of a procedure.*	10			
4. *For Bleeding Emergencies:*				
a. If the area is already bandaged and blood is seeping through the bandage, apply 4 × 4s over the top of the existing bandage. If no bandage is present, apply sterile/clean 4 × 4s over the bleeding wound and apply pressure	10			
b. While still applying direct pressure to the site, elevate the arm above the level of the heart.	10			
c. Apply direct pressure to the artery between the point of attachment and the site of the injury. Compress the artery against the bony surface of the limb. (Use the brachial artery for the upper limbs and the femoral artery for the lower limbs.) Continue to apply direct pressure and elevate the extremity.	10			
d. If bleeding is still uncontrolled, a tourniquet should be applied. The provider should apply the tourniquet just above the affected area. Once applied, the tourniquet should not be loosened. Attach a note to the patient's clothes, close to the tourniquet, stating when the tourniquet was applied.	10			
e. Treat the patient for shock and help the patient to remain calm while waiting for the EMS.	10			
f. Continue to monitor the patient for breathing and heart function.	10			
g. Document the incident.	10			
h. Dispose of soiled bandages in the biohazardous trash and clean and disinfect the area.	10			
5. *To Treat Shock:*				
a. Recognize that the patient may be going into shock and take the patient's vital signs. The symptoms of shock include an increase in pulse and respiration; pale, cool, clammy skin; and restlessness.	10			

Name _____ Date _____ Score _____

b. Alert the provider or activate the EMS.	10			
c. Elevate the patient's legs. You may use pillows or blankets if the exam table does not have a mechanism to elevate the legs	10			
d. Place a sheet or blanket over the patient to keep the patient warm.	10			
e. Monitor the patient's airway, breathing, and circulation, ***demonstrating critical thinking when performing patient assessment***.	10			
f. Keep the patient calm and reassure the patient that help is on the way.	10			
6. *For Possible Fractures:*				
a. Recognize possible fracture. If open fracture, control bleeding and treat for shock. If closed, elevate limb and apply ice.	10			
b. Notify provider and get ready to send patient for radiographs (X-rays).	10			
c. Obtain casting supplies and assist provider with casting if applicable.	10			
7. *For Syncope Episodes:*				
a. Recognize symptoms of syncope and immediately have patient lay down elevating feet above the head. (If possible, place patient in Trendelenburg position.)	10			
b. Apply cold compresses to patient's forehead and neck.	10			
c. Place a blanket or sheet over patient if the patient is cold.	10			
d. Monitor patient's vital signs and have them evaluated by provider before releasing.	10			
e. If patient actually faints, break fall if possible. Check for injuries and place patient in Trendelenburg position. Notify provider as soon as possible. Monitor vital signs.	10			
8. *For Seizures or Convulsions:*				
a. Recognize that patient is having a seizure. (Wash hands and apply gloves when possible.)	10			
b. Notify provider as soon as possible.	10			
c. Clear area of items that may cause injury to patient.	10			
d. Try to keep patient on side, if possible.	10			
e. Once seizing subsides, place pillow underneath patient's head and a blanket over patient.	10			
f. Allow patient time to rest. Have provider assess patient for release.	10			
9. *For a Diabetic Emergency:*				
a. Recognize signs of a diabetic emergency. Ask assessment questions as described in this chapter. Signs of insulin shock include bounding pulse; shallow respiration; pale, cool, and clammy skin; shaking; headache; possibly anger. Signs of diabetic ketoacidosis or coma include thread pulse; deep and rapid respirations; red, hot, and dry skin; possible fruity odor coming from mouth; drowsiness; and intense thirst.	10			
b. Notify provider right away and obtain order for blood glucose testing.	10			
c. Test patient's blood glucose and obtain vital signs.	10			
d. If patient's blood glucose is low, offer sugary liquid or sugary snack. If patient's blood glucose is high, prepare insulin and wait for order to administer.	10			
e. Have provider assess patient for release.	10			
f. Be prepared to call EMS if applicable.	10			

Name _____ Date _____ Score _____

10. Provide patient education.	10			
11. Clean exam table, floor, and so on with disinfectant and dispose of trash in proper receptacles.	10			
12. Document procedure in the patient's chart.	10			
Points Earned / Points Possible:	__ /400			

Points possible reflect importance of step in meeting the task: Important = (5) Essential = (10). Determine score by dividing points earned by total points possible, and multiplying results by 100.

EVALUATION

Evaluator Signature: _____ Date: _____

Evaluator Comments:

DOCUMENTATION

Instructor Note: Retain work products with competency checklist.
Work Product, Procedure 33-1 (Progress Note). Procedure forms can be downloaded from the student companion website.

Key Competencies		
ABHES	MA.A.1.4.a	Follow documentation guidelines
	MA.A.1.9.g	Recognize and respond to medical office emergencies
	MA.A.10.c	Dispose of biohazardous materials
CAAHEP	I.P.13	Perform first aid procedures for: (a) bleeding, (b) diabetic coma or insulin shock, (c) fractures, (d) seizures, (e) shock, and (f) syncope
	I.A.1	Incorporate critical thinking skills when performing patient assessment
	I.A.2	Incorporate critical thinking skills when performing patient care
	I.A.3	Show awareness of patient's concerns related to the procedure being performed
	III.P.2	Select appropriate barrier/personal protective equipment (PPE)
	III.P.3	Perform handwashing
	III.P.10	Demonstrate proper disposal of biohazardous material: (a) sharps, and (b) regulated waste
	V.A.4	Explain to a patient the rationale for performance of a procedure
	X.P.3	Document patient care accurately in the medical record
	XII.C.2	Identify safety techniques that can be used in responding to accidental exposure to: (a) blood, (b) other body fluids, (c) needle sticks, and (d) chemicals
	XII.A.1	Recognize the physical and emotional effects on persons involved in an emergency situation
	XII.A.2	Demonstrate self-awareness in responding to an emergency situation